I0093384

Ensnared by AIDS

Cultural Contexts of HIV and AIDS in Nepal

Second Edition

SIL International
Publications in Ethnography 42

Series Editor

Mike Cahill

Volume Editor
Lynn Frank

Managing Editor
Bonnie Brown

Compositor
Judy Benjamin

Graphic Artist
Barbara Alber

Cover Photo
Courtesy of Ram Sarraf, *The Himalayan Times*

Ensnared by AIDS

Cultural Contexts of HIV and AIDS in Nepal

Second Edition

David K. Beine

SIL International®
Dallas, Texas

© 2014 by SIL International®
Library of Congress Catalog No: 2014952110
ISBN13: 978-1-55671-350-7
ISSN: 0-0895-9897

Printed in the United States of America

All rights reserved. No part of this publication may be reproduced, stored in a retrieval system, or transmitted in any form or by any means—electronic, mechanical, photocopy, recording, or otherwise—without the express permission of the SIL International. However, short passages generally understood to be within the limits of fair use, may be quoted without permission.

Copies of this and other publications of the SIL International® may be obtained from

SIL International Publications
7500 W. Camp Wisdom Road
Dallas, TX 75236-5629 USA

Voice: +1-972-708-7404
Fax: +1-972-708-7363
publications_intl@sil.org
www.sil.org/resources/publications

Contents

List of Figures

List of Tables

Preface to the Second Edition

Much has changed in the world of HIV and AIDS over the past ten years. From the medical side, treatments and preventative measures have emerged that have changed the face of the disease. And these changes have not been without effect upon Nepal. Having said that, history and culture, which were impacting the trajectory and form of the epidemic in Nepal ten years ago, continue to do so. In this second edition I update the medical changes worldwide and in Nepal; address the demographic, historical, cultural and political changes (or lack thereof) which continue to impact prevention and treatment programs; and present an update on the current epidemiological situation. And it will be obvious that culture, at least in the context of Nepal, still matters.

The astute reader will notice that the subtext of the book has changed slightly in this second edition. In the earlier edition the title combined the acronyms HIV and AIDS into a single unit (HIV/AIDS). This was convention at that time. Today these two terms are more often separated into two terms, HIV and AIDS, in order to purposively distinguish HIV, the virus that causes AIDS—from AIDS, the dreaded deadly disease caused by untreated HIV. This is often done to disassociate HIV (which is now treatable) from AIDS, which often carries a strong stigma, in part because of is fatal nature. This change in terminology is reflective of the changing cultural model of HIV and AIDS in the West where we have gone from "dying of AIDS" (the old cultural model) to "living with HIV" (the new cultural model). The title of this book, therefore, reflects this wider understanding of HIV and AIDS, even though this is still far from being a reality for many HIV sufferers in Nepal, as we will see later in this book. Likewise, I have attempted to change this convention wherever possible throughout the second edition, retaining the earlier convention only in the case of quotations or where using the latter convention might cause confusion.

Along with great changes in the world over the past ten years, cultural models of HIV and AIDS have begun to shift slightly in Nepal, while at the same time many elements of the earlier model are perpetuated and reinforced. The danger of books is that they can lock our understanding of any phenomenon into the "ethnographic present." In this second edition I will not only elucidate the earlier model of HIV and AIDS in Nepal, but I will also cursorily comment on the changes I have noticed, both in the national narratives (via media, INGOs, NGOs and doctors) and personal narratives of those living with HIV. It would require a whole volume based on careful research (another forthcoming book I am working on) to fully elucidate the changing cultural model and its constituent components. And finally, in this second edition, I reflect on the remaining problems in the "fight" (to employ a western illness schema) against HIV and AIDS in Nepal.

Preface to the First Edition

He deceived me. He persuaded me, promising to take me to a glittering town. He deceived me, promising to take me on a running motor car. He promised to employ me in the carpet industry and then told me to be happy with an income of one or two hundred rupees. I am a girl of the village and was easily deceived. I got entangled in the threads of the carpet looms. He told me he would take me into another profession. He said "Raxaul," as it sounded but took me to Bombay. I learned that he had sold me for 12,000 rupees. He pushed me down into living hell.

That *didi* [sinful woman] uttered sweet words. With smiles she said that my stars would now shine bright, but when I refused, I was beat. Don't ask me then through what hell I've been up till now! I spent nine years in that hell and my life was totally shattered. One day a cold caught me. I found myself with diarrhea and chest pains. One day a doctor came to give me a check-up, the didi gestured and I agreed.

She gave me 2,000 rupees and a train ticket and they sent me home with many incurable diseases. I was not cured and my ailments made me desperate. The blood exam revealed that I have the fatal AIDS.

Alas, my life is reaching an end, and it ends in nothing then. O straight-forward girls of the village, please look at me! Don't get coaxed in the sweet words of those sinful souls. (Ramesh 1993)

I was once told, "If you want to know the depth of a Nepali's emotion about a certain experience, ask them to write a song about it."[1] The quote above is a translated stanza from a song written by a Nepali woman about

---

[1] In the 2003 edition, this section was titled, "Chapter One, Introduction."

the depth of her experience with life, and ultimately with the disease called AIDS.[2] I often found people matter-of-factly telling me their heart-wrenching life stories that broke my heart and left me in a state of emotional disarray and emptiness. It seems that personal emotions are not publicly displayed in Nepali society.

Perhaps, as I assert in the latter part of this book, the responses (mostly unemotional) to their tragic situation is due, at least in part, to their deeply held Vedic worldview of their own anticipated reincarnation. Or perhaps it is due to their underlying attitude of fatalism. Or perhaps, as has been suggested above, it is just their style. Whatever it is, it often perplexed me.

This book is about HIV and AIDS. More specifically, it is about cultural models, particularly the cultural models of HIV and AIDS currently being negotiated in Nepal. It is also about the cognitive illness schemata that underlie and inform these cultural models.[3] The way that people make sense of illness is, in part, culturally determined. Existing beliefs and presuppositions shared by a community (cultural knowledge) regarding illness play a significant role in shaping an understanding of newly emerging illnesses in any given culture. This cultural knowledge is organized as cultural models, which are utilized to "make meaning" of new situations such as the HIV and AIDS epidemic. These cultural constructions (cultural models) of illness can also contribute to the spread of the epidemic. HIV and AIDS is a relatively new and rapidly growing problem in Nepal. Little is known about how the populace of Nepal understands the illness, locally known only as *AIDS rog*,[4] or about the process taking place to develop a cultural model of HIV and AIDS.

This research, utilizing a cognitive anthropological approach in tandem with a discourse analysis approach, focuses on the meaning of HIV and AIDS in Nepal. The results may have practical application for HIV and AIDS prevention programs in Nepal as well as theoretical implications by testing

---

[2]Although HIV/AIDS is a conventional notation these days, I use both "HIV" and "AIDS" throughout this book. I tend to use the notation "HIV" when referring to the infection and disease biomedically and "AIDS" when referring to the disease in the Nepali context. I do this because "AIDS" is the most common notation used in Nepal. Thus far, there has been little association made among the general public in Nepal between HIV and AIDS.

[3]Ronald Casson (1983) suggests that "schemata" is the plural form of "schema." Many authors use "schema" in a plural sense. I will use "schemata" myself as the plural for "schema" but will retain the use of "schemas" when used this way by other authors.

[4]*Rog* is a generic word used for a disease but usually used only in this type of grammatical structure with a certain class of diseases such as sexual diseases *(yon rog)*, tuberculosis *(chhe rog)*, and leprosy *(kusta rog)*. We will see later that AIDS has been cognitively categorized as a member of the same class with these other diseases.

the cross-linguistic validity of the narrative analysis model. It may also be theoretically important for providing a better understanding of how people incorporate new ideas into their established cognitive systems.

The title for this book, *Ensnared by AIDS,* comes from the mouths of many of the informants. The Nepali word *phasnu,* used by many to describe their condition, carries with it the meaning of being ensnared like a bird in a hunting net. For instance, Prabita, lamenting the discovery of her HIV status, told me, "Now I, a free and innocent girl, am ensnared." Rajina, regretting how she was tricked into marriage and sold into prostitution by a deceitful man, claimed, "He ensnared me, showing me many hollow things." And Hari, saddened by his fatal condition, said, "I just know that I am ensnared and will probably die."

Because the research was conducted using the Nepali language, I use Nepali words extensively throughout this book. Since these words may be new to many readers, I provide a glossary of the Nepali terms used. I also include the English meanings in single quotes next to the Nepali word the first time the word is used in each new chapter, as a reminder.

The conclusions of chapter six (a narrative discourse analysis) are drawn from thousands of pages of translated materials. My original notes include (1) a transcription of each of the thirty stories (in the Nepali Devanagri script), (2) a word-for-word English translation below each Nepali sentence, and (3) a free translation rendering it more understandable to mother tongue English speakers. Because the database for this project was so extensive, I have included only the English free translations for each text. Although including these texts in this book necessitates many extra pages, I feel that it is important to hear the voices of those struggling with AIDS in Nepal. After all, this book is ultimately about them and for them.

This book is about AIDS in Nepal. In the end, however, it is really about people. There are many faces of the AIDS epidemic in Nepal, but behind these faces are real people. Many of the storytellers in this book will be dead by the time these words are finally read. Many of them are men and women like you and me, who over the course of this research became good friends. It is my hope that this book will honor them and that it will, in some way, contribute to a lessening of the future personal tragedies of others in the tiny Himalayan nation of Nepal.

Background

Although the current reported number of HIV cases in Nepal is relatively small (just under 21,000) it is widely accepted that a much larger problem lies hidden under these official statistics. Traditionally researchers have focused upon the structural epidemiology of the illness (Mann 1992; Sabatier 1988; Sabatier 1989; Shannon et al. 1991) tracing the spread of AIDS worldwide along trucking routes and through high-risk communities such as commercial sex workers. Researchers once predicted that many of these same structural factors would become major determinants in the development of AIDS in Nepal (Seddon 1995; Suvedi et al. 1994). And in fact, structural factors have played a significant role in the spread of HIV, particularly among high-risk communities in Nepal.

Recently, scholars have begun to focus more attention on the social epidemiology of AIDS (Farmer 1992, Feldman and Johnson 1990; Fleming et al. 1988; Herdt and Lindenbaum 1992; Muir 1991; Schoepf 1990). Several authors (Brown 1993; Green 1992; Taylor 1990) have pushed us beyond the structural epidemiological explanations by adequately demonstrating that cultural beliefs can also be a critical factor in the spread of AIDS. People's perceptions about AIDS have been found to be crucial factors associated with its spread (Caprara 1993; Shah 1991). These perceptions of the illness, or the "meaning" of AIDS, are socially constructed (Herzlich 1989; Sontag 1988; Treichler 1992) by members of a society and are then developed into a cultural model (Farmer 1994), which is subsequently reinforced by society.

Although some work has been done on HIV and AIDS in Nepal, no one has examined the cultural models and underlying illness schemata that are being used to make sense of HIV and AIDS. This book brings together the results of two major studies designed to identify shared perceptions regarding HIV and AIDS as well as underlying illness schemata that inform these cultural models.

The studies, utilizing traditional ethnoscience methods in tandem with discourse analysis methods, were conducted over a sixteen-month period between January 1998 and May 1999. The primary research sites were the small rural village of Saano Dumre in Gorkha District, and various non-governmental organizations (NGOs) in and around the capital city of Kathmandu. More specific details about the sites, the people interviewed, and the research contexts will be discussed in the following chapters. The use of multiple methods provides a more complete picture of the cultural model of AIDS in Nepal, accurately reflecting the cognitive categories arrived at through cognitive anthropological methods, while better reflecting the multivocalic diversity present in any culturally constructed meaning.

The studies will reveal that there are, indeed, cultural models of HIV and AIDS in Nepal. We will see several cultural models being expressed by various communities in Nepal, but we will also see the emergence of a dominant cultural model of AIDS formed through the weaving together of Western models and schemata with traditional Nepali cultural models of illness and traditional illness schemata. An understanding of these models is crucial as it is these cultural models that people are employing to make sense of AIDS and it is these same cultural models that people use to determine appropriate behavior to exhibit toward those who have HIV and AIDS. And a cursory re-examination of some of these same factors ten years after the first edition of this book was published will reveal that some elements of the cultural model are slowly shifting while others remain the same.

The purpose of this book is to examine the HIV and AIDS situation in Nepal in depth. Although a thorough coverage of the subject necessitates an investigation of the structural factors contributing to the spread of the disease, I will focus primarily on the social side of AIDS in Nepal—in particular, upon the newly emerging cultural models of AIDS and their underlying illness schemata.

Format of the book

This book is divided into four main parts: (1) "Background and theoretical underpinnings," (2) "The projects," (3) "The findings," and (4) "In their own words." These parts are described below.

Background and theoretical underpinnings

The purpose of part one is to (1) introduce the reader to Nepal (the context in which this study takes place), (2) explore in general the concept of AIDS as both fact and social construction, (3) examine in particular the current AIDS situation in Nepal, (4) introduce the theoretical concepts of cultural models and illness schemata, and (5) introduce the cognitive methodology on which the findings of this book are based.

In chapter one, I briefly introduce the country of Nepal. Many of the facts about her history, economy, educational system and religion have played an important part in fostering the current AIDS situation. Many of these same cultural features have also been influential in the production of cultural models that I will discuss at length in subsequent chapters.

In chapter two, I look at AIDS in particular. AIDS is a biomedical fact. It is also a socially constructed disease. In addition, other factors are making it a socioeconomic disease. The result of the mixing of biomedical fact and social construction is that different meanings are attributed to AIDS from culture to culture. The resultant cultural models are also malleable as the nature of the disease (the biomedical facts) itself changes, or as our socially determined understanding of the disease changes.

In chapter three, I discuss the current AIDS "crisis" in Nepal in particular, including the statistics and prognosis for impact upon the tiny country, and examine the various types of research that have been conducted in Nepal in respect to AIDS. I also introduce the major discourses on AIDS that have been presented by NGOs, the media and others, as well as discuss the various approaches being taken by international aid agencies and local authorities to help with the growing problem. Finally, I introduce the major components of a newly emerging cultural model of HIV and AIDS.

In chapter four, I examine the theoretical frameworks upon which this research is based. I introduce the "cultural model" concept and examine cultural models as both product of and producer of culture. I also introduce the idea of schema theory, examining the various kinds of schemata, discussing what they are and how they are proposed to work, and I introduce recent modifications to the schema concept that inform this research. I also examine the cognitive methodologies employed in two different studies, focusing attention on the value of combining multiple methods in this type of social research.

The background information provided in part one will facilitate a better understanding of the findings (and the implications) of the projects presented in part two.

The projects

In part two, I present the findings of two different studies, which were conducted in tandem, in order to discover the different meanings attributed to HIV and AIDS by various groups in Nepal. The goal of these studies was to discover if there are any widely shared meanings (dominant cultural model) associated with HIV and AIDS as well as to discover underlying illness schemata associated with HIV and AIDS.

The use of multiple methods of analysis in ethnomedical research has been suggested as a way to increase the validity of such research (Browner et al.1988; Stone and Campbell 1984; Viney 1991; Van Gelder 1996). Hence, the methodology followed during this research, approaching the meaning of AIDS in Nepal, included both a cognitive ethnomedical approach as well as a discourse analysis approach. Two major studies, using the two different approaches, were conducted in order to study the emergence of various cultural models of AIDS in Nepal and their constituent elements.

In chapter five, I present the findings of an ethnosemantic study designed to elicit the conceptions regarding HIV and AIDS among a rural Nepali community. The investigation of rural conceptions of AIDS took place within the larger context of a study on conceptions of illness in a Nepali village. I present the full study here as elements of wider illness schemata are identified, which transfer to HIV and AIDS as well. Through this study we can see how traditional concepts have influenced understanding of the new illness known as *"AIDS rog."* This study, using primarily an ethnomedical cognitive approach, ultimately sought to determine whether a salient cultural model of HIV and AIDS still exists among the people of a rural Nepali village. The village of Saano Dumre in Gorkha District was selected as the study site. Besides illuminating cultural models of HIV and AIDS, this study also examines the apparent changes that have taken place in regard to health beliefs over the past twenty-five years. Using the methods of cognitive anthropology, I explore several health-related topics including categories of illness, treatment-seeking order, factors influencing health, perceived causes of illness (including factors which facilitate a greater susceptibility to illness), ideas about transmission of illness, villagers' perceptions about what has changed over the past twenty-five years, and ideas regarding the efficacy of traditional and Western medicines.

Chapter six presents the findings of a narrative discourse analysis project conducted among HIV-positive persons in Nepal. Thirty texts were collected from HIV-positive persons in both urban and rural settings. Besides illuminating elements of the dominant cultural model that have emerged as a result of the various governmental prevention campaigns, these narratives also express common themes of shared meanings of HIV and AIDS not held by members of the wider culture. Furthermore, the texts demonstrate that a slightly different understanding of HIV and AIDS is held between rural and urban dwellers regarding the disease and between urban males and females. These common themes, as well as the illness schemata that underlie these narratives, are the focus of the chapter.

In chapter seven, I examine the emerging cultural models intimated by the two studies. We will see several sub-group cultural models being expressed by various communities in Nepal, but we will also see the emergence of a dominant cultural model of HIV and AIDS. I will also further examine the underlying illness schemata that are made evident through the findings of both studies. An understanding of the various cultural models (and their constituent schemata) is essential because it is these cultural models that people employ to make sense of AIDS and it is these same cultural models that people use to determine appropriate behavior to exhibit toward those who have HIV and AIDS.

The findings

In chapter eight, I examine the making of the dominant cultural model of HIV and AIDS in Nepal. I will focus mainly on the creation of this model, since it is being disseminated widely and seems to be having the greatest impact in shaping people's understandings of HIV and AIDS, and I expect this cultural model will continue to do so in the coming years. We will see the strong influence of Western cultural models (and schemata) upon the dominant cultural model. However, we will discover that cultural models are also influenced by biology. I will examine the role of NGOs, doctors, policy makers and the media, as well as underlying biologically based schemata in the making of a dominant cognitive model of HIV and AIDS in Nepal. We will see that the resultant dominant cultural model of HIV and AIDS in Nepal is a type of hybrid based on the combination of the traditional and the new (especially when traditional ideas reinforce the new ideas) as well as a product of universal biology.

Chapter nine will conclude the analytical portion of this book by sum-marizing the findings, examining the implications of the findings, and intro-ducing a few remaining issues that intrigue me. In particular, I will address the issue of the negative impact of current foreign aid projects, make some recommendations for future prevention efforts and discuss why I encoun-tered less depression than expected among AIDS sufferers.

In their own words

I reserve the last chapter of this book, chapter ten, for those struggling with AIDS in Nepal to tell their own stories. Quite often in this type of social research the voices of the research participants are never heard. Their stories are real. And they are tragic. These people's stories often left me empty and saddened at the hard circumstances of their lives. It is my hope that these stories from their own mouths will compel readers to consider what part they can play in helping to curb the growing HIV and AIDS pandemic. These stories represent only thirty struggling voices. There are thousands more like them in Nepal alone. And millions more like them around the world.

Acknowledgements

I would be remiss if I did not thank the many that helped me bring this book to completion. First of all I would like to thank Mr. Dwarika Shrestha for his friendship and hard work on this project. Without his able assistance during the research phase, this project would not have been remotely possible. Next, I would like to thank Dr. Ganesh Gurung and the Department of Anthropology at Tribhuvan University for their sponsorship of this project. I would also like to thank Dr. Nirmal Man Tuladhar and the Center for Nepali and Asian Studies for their most gracious help in many areas. I would also like to thank the entire membership at Prerana for their most gracious cooperation. Further, I would like to thank Rajendra Shrestha at Freedom Center; Mrs. Amina Lama at Maiti Nepal; Mrs. Shanta Sapkota at Peace Rehabilitation Center [the entire staff at ABC Nepal; Dr. Bhadra at B. P. Memorial; Dr. Bal K. Suvedi and Dr. Bhoj Raj Joshi of the Nepal Medical Council; Shiba Hari Maharjan of LALS; Dr. Vijaya Lal Gurubacharya and Dr. B. B. Karki of the National Center; Sally Smith of the United Mission to Nepal; Ms. Prakriti K. C. and Dr. Mark Zimmerman at Patan Hospital; all the staff at Amp Pipal Hospital, Gorkha District and all of the residents of Saano Dumre, Gorkha District. I am indebted to the above individuals for their assistance. Without their help many of the goals of this project could never have been realized.

I would also like to thank the members of my doctoral committee, Dr. Linda Stone, Dr. Barry Hewlett, and Dr. John Bodley for their help in improving this manuscript. I would also like to thank my wife and children for supporting me through the long grueling process.

Finally, I wish to thank those men and women who shared with me their stories. May the details of their lives that make up this book bring about a solution to the looming problem of HIV and AIDS in Nepal.

Abbreviations

AIDS	Acquired Immunodeficiency Syndrome
ART	Antiretroviral Therapy
CDC	Center for Disease Control
CMA	Critical Medical Anthropology
FHI	Family Health International
FSW	Female Sex Worker
HIV	Human Immunodeficiency Viruses
HSCB	HIV and AIDS and STI Control Board
IDU	Injecting Drug User
INGO	International Non-governmental Organization
IOM	Institute of Medicine
IS	Idiosyncratic Schemata
KAB	Knowledge And Behavior
KAP	Knowledge And Practices
MARP	Most At Risk Population
MCP	Multiple Concurrent Partners
MDP	Millenium Development Goal
NAC	National AIDS Council
NACC	National AIDS Coordination Committee
NAP	National Action Plan
NCASC	National Center for AIDS and STD Control
NSP	National Strategic Plan
PEMA	Political Economy Medical Anthropology
PEPFAR	President's Emergency Plan for AIDS Relief
PIMS	Primitive Innate Mental Schemas, or universal schemata
PLHIV	People Living with HIV
PWA	Person with AIDS
PLWHA	People living with HIV and AIDS
SAE	Semi-autonomous Entity

STD	Sexualy Transmitted Disease
STI	Sexually Transmitted Infection
USAID	United States Agency for International Development
VDRL	Venereal Disease Research Lab

Part One

Background and Theoretical Underpinnings

1

Nepal

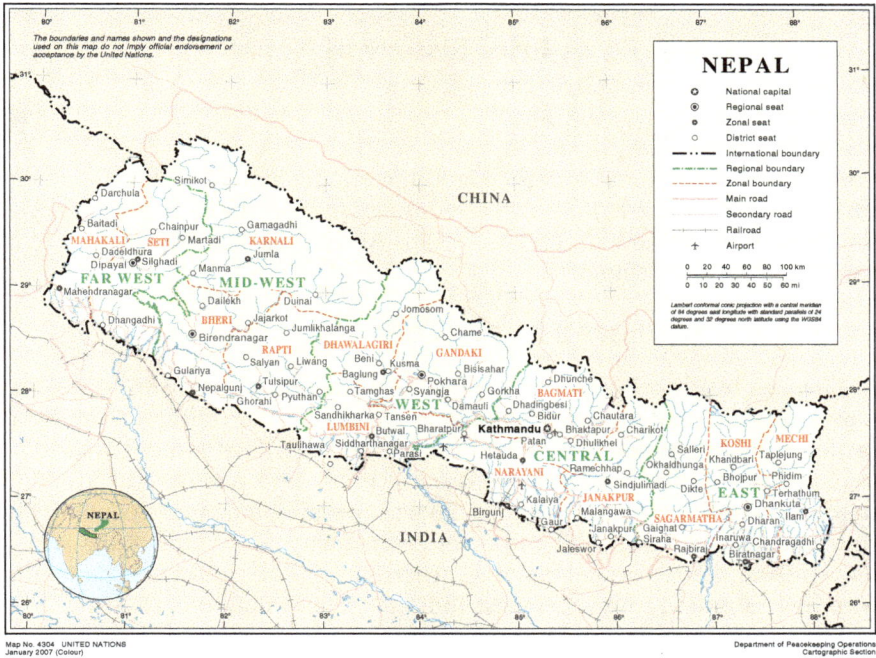

Figure 1.1 Map of Nepal, map no. 4304, January 2007
(United Nations, used by permission)

Many aspects of history have played a part in formulating and fostering the current AIDS situation in Nepal, including population demographics, economy, geography, the educational system, medical systems, and overriding religious philosophy, as well as the current political structure. Because of the relationship of these factors to the current AIDS situation, they are introduced in this chapter.[1] Nepal is a small, landlocked nation sandwiched between Chinese-controlled Tibet and India (fig. 1.1). With a population of 26.6 million (Central Bureau of Statistics 2012), the country of Nepal is best known for its legendary Himalayan mountain range. It boasts nine of only fourteen mountains in the world over eight thousand meters (26,247 feet), including the tallest, *Sagarmatha* (the Nepali term for Mt. Everest). The country also claims tropical jungles (currently being lost at an alarming rate) which are home to Bengal tigers, elephants, and rhinoceroses. The diversity of landscape mirrors the collage of cultures. The country is home to more than a dozen cultures—each with its own language, with multiple dialects, from three major ethnic groups,[2] which have settled over thousands of years, through sequential historical migrations (Savada 1991; Anderson 1987).

1.1 A brief history of Nepal

1.1.1 Pre-history: ?–500 B.C.

Archaeological finds from the Neolithic era demonstrate that this region was occupied, but little is known about these early settlers. Legends suggest that they were the cow-herding Gopals or Ahir tribes, but this remains to be confirmed by archaeologists.

1.1.2 Ancient Nepal: 500 B.C.– 700 A.D.

The first historical inhabitants of the Kathmandu Valley were the Kirati, a people of Mongolian origin following a proto-Hindu religion.[3] The Kirati settled the Kathmandu Valley and established small settlements with limited central authority. These eventually grew into a powerful kingdom that saw the reign of twenty-nine kings. The kingdom was economically strengthened by trade with countries as far away as Sri Lanka and was at its zenith in the fourth century B.C. Then the Khasa, pastoral Aryan tribes who had migrated into northwest India between 2000 and 1500 B.C., began to slowly inhabit the Terai region, which today is part of Nepal. These

---

[1]This history is culled from Burbank (1992), Savada (1991), and Anderson (1987).

[2]Savada (1991:xxxiv) refers to these three groups as (1) Indo-Nepalese (others refer to this group as "Rajputs," an Indo-Aryan group originating in Rajasthan, India); (2) Tibeto-Nepalese (this would be refugee Tibetans); and (3) indigenous Nepalese (others refer to these peoples as Tibeto-Burman).

[3]Both Burbank (1992) and Anderson (1987) use the spelling *Kirati,* while Savada (1991) uses *Kiratas.*

tribes (following a Vedic Hindu religion) grew into confederations of tribes or small kingdoms that were often at war with one another. From one of these small kingdoms of the Terai came Prince Siddhartha Gautama (the Buddha), whose followers and missionaries carried the new Buddhist religion as far as Mongolia to the north (crossing Nepal and Tibet en route) and Sri Lanka to the south. Buddhism was established in the Kathmandu Valley and throughout most of Nepal. It added unique features to the Kirati and Khasa cultures of modern-day Nepal such as a belief in the divinity of the monarchy.

About 300 A.D. the Licchavis (a Khasa tribe from northern India) invaded Kathmandu, driving out her Kirati population. The Kirati were pushed to the east where they settled in the hills as simple farmers. Today's Rais and Limbus (two of Nepal's indigenous groups) trace their ancestry to them. The Licchavis invasion brought with it one of the most significant and lasting changes to Nepali culture, namely the Hindu caste system. The Licchavis dynasty was centered in Kathmandu but its widespread roaming armies managed to produce the first true Nepali state. It is also certain that the Licchavis looked back to their Indian homeland, which exerted a powerful cultural influence upon the people of Nepal, especially in terms of their Hindu religion (which was syncretized with the established Buddhism and leftover animism) and art. By the end of their dynasty in 750 A.D., the political system mirrored that of the Rajas of India: they were absolute monarchs in theory but actually interfered minimally in their subjects' lives due to the mountainous geography. The economy during the Licchavis dynasty was based mainly on agriculture. The king established a system of hierarchical political leaders that descended to the local level while it allowed the dynasty to maintain control of the wider area. This political system would later (i.e., in the late twentieth century) serve as a model for the political development of modern Nepal. The Licchavis also continued the tradition of trade with Tibet and India (including the export of Buddhism with the marriage of one of her Licchavis princesses to the king of Tibet, whom she converted).

1.1.3 Medieval Nepal: 750–1750

Around 750 A.D. Nepal began to enter what some have called its "Dark Ages," about which little is known. It seems there were constant struggles among prominent families and royal lineages (still all Rajputs) for the throne, and leadership changed several times during this period of instability. Kathmandu was also invaded twice by growing foreign powers during the early years of this period (Tibet in 705 A.D. and Kashmir in 782 A.D.), but both attempts proved futile. The most profound change upon Nepali culture that can be traced to this time period is the move away from Buddhism on the part of the kings toward a stronger Vedic-Hindu devotion.

In 1200 the Mallas (Khasa groups who had ruled kingdoms in Rajasthan from the early 600s) began to inhabit Nepal and (perhaps through marriage or political struggle) assumed the throne. The rule of the early Mallas was far from peaceful. North-Indian Malla kingdoms plundered Kathmandu five times between 1244 and 1311. Worse, an earthquake devastated the valley in 1245, killing a third of its populace. Meantime, Hindu kingdoms of northern India were being broken up by the invading Muslims, sending waves of Hindu migrants into Nepal who established dozens of tiny hilltop kingdoms (forty-six in west and central Nepal). A rival Malla kingdom from western Nepal also attacked Kathmandu six times in an attempt to gain control and the city was invaded in 1345 by Muslim sultans from Bengal who plundered and destroyed the city. The result of the medieval period was the dissolution of the Nepali state that the Licchavis had founded, to a collection of feudal hilltop kingdoms scattered throughout the region that were constantly at war with one another.

1.1.4 The re-unification of Nepal: The Shah dynasty 1750–1846

It was from one of these tiny hilltop kingdoms (Gorkha) that Prithvi Narayan Shah arose as king to conquer the surrounding kingdoms, finally conquering the three kingdoms of the Kathmandu Valley twenty-three years later. Thus, Shah emerged as the king of a newly unified Nepal in 1768 and implementing a policy of protectionism, expelled all foreigners, a policy that remained in force until 1951. The Gorkha dynasty expanded, annexing parts of Kashmir (under British control) and Tibet (under Chinese control) to the new state of Nepal. Nepal's excursions into Tibet bothered China, who sent troops to surround the Kathmandu Valley. The Nepali king appealed for help to the British, who were then given their first chance to visit the country, but the dispute with China was inadvertently solved without British intervention. Then in 1810, the British, bothered by further expansion of Nepal into British territory, itself went to war with Nepal. The war lasted six years and was devastating to Nepal, whose borders shrank dramatically as territory was given up to the British. As a condition of the Treaty of Friendship, which ended the war, a single British official was allowed residence in Nepal, although he was forbidden from traveling outside the valley.

1.1.5 The Ranas: 1846–1951

In 1846 the shrewd army general Jung Bahadur Rana accomplished a military coup, establishing himself as prime minister and reducing the king to a prisoner in his own palace in a puppet monarchy. He later declared himself king and turned his interests solely to the opulent development of his own family's estate. The hereditary prime ministership established by the Rana regime lasted until 1951. It was a period of time when, to quote one historian, "the rest of the country stayed frozen in the middle ages" (Burbank 1992:24).

1.1.6 The return of the Shahs: 1951–1990

In 1947, Nepal witnessed the first open political protest against the Ranas. In 1951, the puppet king Tribhuvan (of the Shah line) left the palace ostensibly for a picnic but instead sought asylum in the Indian embassy and escaped to India. Meantime, the Nepali National Congress (NCC), an outlawed opposition party, took control of the Terai (the southern region of Nepal). The Ranas, knowing their days were numbered, formed an interim government with the NCC and King Tribhuvan was returned to Nepal, promising democracy. Although he died shortly thereafter, Tribhuvan's son Mahendra oversaw the first democratic elections in 1959. A year later, frustrated with the corruption and chaos of the newly elected officials, Mahendra again took direct control and the newly elected politicians were exiled to India. Mahendra established the Panchayat, a system where the prime minister, the cabinet, and local government officials were chosen by the king, and in which criticism of the monarchy was a criminal offense. This system mirrored the earlier Licchavis system of government.

Mahendra's son Birendra ascended the throne in 1972, carrying on the direct-rule policy of his father. He also continued the Panchayat system of government. Strong opposition to the Panchayat government throughout the 1970s led King Birendra to call for a national referendum in 1980. The referendum gave voters the opportunity to support or reject the Panchayat system of government. A very small majority (55%) voted to retain the Panchayat form of government. The narrow margin of victory suggested that many were still unhappy with the current political system and the country witnessed growing protests to Birendra's reign throughout the 1980s.

1.1.7 Democracy, civil war, and Federal Democratic Republic: 1990–present

In 1990, the people of Nepal, inspired by the fall of communism throughout Eastern Europe and the Soviet Union and motivated by the worsening economic conditions at home (caused largely by a trade dispute with India), began violent pro-democracy demonstrations. The political unrest grew and the violence increased until May 1990, when the king agreed to end the Panchayat system and establish a representative democracy (although it retained a constitutional monarchy). The first free elections were held a year later in 1991.

The years since the nation's first democratic elections can be understatedly characterized as politically unstable. The centrist Nepali Congress party won the first multi-party elections in 1991 and the Communists became the leading opposition party. Then in 1994, mid-term elections were called after the ruling Congress government lost a parliamentary confidence vote, resulting in a hung parliament, and the Communists, who emerged as the single largest party, formed a minority government. Then the minority Communist government soon fell and was followed by several successive weak coalition governments. All of these governments recognized a constitutional monarchy, retaining earlier ties to the crown within the political system.[4]

In 1996, spurred on by their frustration with the inability to affect change through the political process, one group of the Communist party splintered off to create the Communist Party of Nepal (Maoists) and subsequently declared a "Peoples War," which decimated Nepal's infrastructure and economy and paralyzed the country over the next decade. The civil war, which cost the country over fifteen thousand lives with countless others missing, tortured or displaced, lasted for ten years until the signing of a UN-led peace accord between the government of Nepal and the Maoists in 2006.[5] The country has yet to fully recover.

The years between 1996 and 2006 saw two parallel governments in operation: the unstable government of Nepal (which mainly operated in a vacuum from within the Kathmandu Valley) and a parallel Maoist government that clandestinely operated throughout most of the rest of the country. Regarding the former, the Nepali Congress won an absolute majority of seats in parliament in 1999 and formed a majority government, with Krishna Prasad Bhattarai as the prime minister. An internal power struggle soon ensued within the Nepali Congress party, however, and led to the ouster of Bhattarai and his replacement by his long-time rival within the party, Girija Prasad Koirala, in March 2000. This government lasted little over a year when Koirala resigned in July 2001 and was replaced by his rival Sher Bahadur Deuba.

In June 2001 a national tragedy threw the already fragile central government (which still held loyalties to the crown) into further nebulousness. King Birendra (who still held much political currency), Queen Aiswarya, and seven other members of the royal family were killed by Crown Prince

---

[4]In a constitutional monarchy the king remains head of state (including controlling the army) while the prime minister functions as head of the government.

[5]The Nepal constitution forbade the use of the army against its own citizenry. For this reason the army (under control of the king and then later the parliament) could not be used to fight the Maoists. Therefore, a highly-trained para-military force known as the Armed Police Force was established to fight the Maoists. Beyond the blue khaki uniforms worn by these soldiers (instead of green khakis worn by the army), it was relatively difficult to distinguish this force from the regular army (as opposed to the regular police who were relatively undisciplined, undertrained and poorly resourced).

Dipendra, who was reportedly angered over his parents' choice of his arranged marriage. The crown prince then allegedly shot himself as well and within days Birendra's brother Gyanendra assumed the throne as king of Nepal.[6]

In May 2002 the country was thrown into further political uncertainty. The king dissolved parliament upon the recommendation of Prime Minister Deuba, who had been threatened with censure by his own party for supporting the extension of an official state of emergency. After a short one-week direct rule by King Gyanendra, Lokendra Bahadur Chand became prime minister in October 2002, followed by Surya Bahadur Thapa (2003–2004) and Sher Bahadur Deuba again (2004–2005). Then, on February 1, 2005, citing incompetence by the central government to properly manage the ongoing Maoist insurgency, King Gyanendra suspended the constitution and once again assumed direct authority. The king's action sparked massive public protests, now referred to as *Loktantra Āndolan* 'Democracy Movement'.[7] Just over a year later he buckled under pressure, restoring the previous parliament on April 24, 2006. Girija Prasad Koirala was elected as prime minister. One of the first orders of business taken up by the newly reinstated parliament was a promise to hold elections within a year for a new parliament that would take up the task of writing a new constitution and usher in a new political era for Nepal. Three days later, on April 27, the Maoists announced a unilateral truce. And on May 1, Maoist leader Dr. Baburam Bhattarai acknowledged that if the Constituent Assembly (CA) elections were found to be free and fair, they would abide by the results. The Maoists were again ready to re-enter the political process of Nepal.

After two postponements in 2007, the long awaited Constituent Assembly election was finally held on April 8, 2008. The Communist Party of Nepal (Maoists) won 220 out of 575 elected seats and became the largest party in the CA. On May 28, 2008, the newly elected Constituent Assembly approved a temporary constitution abolishing the Hindu monarchy, declaring Nepal a secular state, placing the army under the command of the parliament rather than the king and stripping the king and his family of all royal privileges. The royal family would now live as equal citizens of the land, paying taxes and being subject to its laws. Nepal, the last remaining Hindu kingdom in the world, was now officially declared the Federal Democratic Republic of Nepal.

Over the next four years the elected Constituent Assembly would itself be caught in a constant quagmire of political in-fighting, positioning and

[6]Many Nepali people do not believe this official account, suggesting instead it was likely an internal palace coup.

[7]This is the name that has been given to the political protests that ensued in 2006. The movement is also commonly referred to as *Jana Andolan-II* (the Second People's Movement), harkening back to the *Jana Andolan* of 1990, which ushered in the democracy of the current era of Nepal.

bickering, and more prime ministers would come and go. Girija Prasad Koirala continued in the role as prime minister of the new Federal Democratic Republic of Nepal from May to August 2008 before being forced to resign. Then Maoist strong-man Prachanda was elected as prime minister by the Constituent Assembly in August of that same year and was expected to oversee the transition from monarchy to republic but he was forced to resign in May 2009 after his controversial sacking of a Nepali army general. He was followed by Madhav Kumar Nepal of the Communist Party of Nepal (Unified Marxist-Leninist), who resigned in 2011 amidst further serious political deadlock.[8] He was followed by Jhala Nath Kanal (February 2011–August 2011), and finally Maoist second-in-command Baburam Bhattarai (August 2011–March 2013). After its failure to draft a new constitution (having been given two years and two more one-year extensions to do so), the Constituent Assembly was finally dissolved on May 28, 2012. New elections were called for, and the date of November 2012 was set, in hopes of electing new members to a new Constituent Assembly that all hoped could get the job done.[9] In the interim, Baburam Bhattarai stayed on as head of a "caretaker government," the elections were again postponed, and on March 14, 2013, Chief Justice Khil Raj Regmi was sworn in as the head of a new "interim election government" tasked with carrying out the election process. This is where the process sits as of the publication of this book.

One of the most devastating effects of all of this political turmoil is a loss of hope for the future of Nepal. The general public is very frustrated with the gamesmanship being played at a time when the politicians should be engaged in nation building. One commentator accuses the Constituent Assembly of "procedural maneuvers instead of being honestly involved in drafting a proper constitution of the country and building the nation for which they were elected" and Nepal's political process of "'forever recycling leaders' [the same old politicians] that haunts the house of Nepal from the fifties" (NACSS 2009). Reflecting on the implications to healthcare, another commentator concludes that "the superficial changes in political structure have not brought about any changes in the life of ordinary people" and that "the state of health service development is no way different now than it was during the active [civil war] conflict period" (Ghimire 2011). What happens next will ultimately be the domain of the historians. One thing is universally accepted, however, namely that further political instability will only further detour the prevention and treatment of HIV and AIDS in Nepal.

---

[8]Much of the political deadlock of this period stemmed from two key disputed issues: (1) integration of former People's Liberation Army (Maoist) fighters into the National Nepal Army and (2) the creation of ethnic-based states in Nepal.

[9]The *Kathmandu Post* (2013) reported that in its first year extension, the Constituent Assembly managed to meet only seven times for a total of only ninety-five minutes before dissolving in disagreement. The estimated cost for the CA to this point was 110 billion Nepalese Rupees (or $1.25 billion US).

1.2 General cultural features

Many aspects of Nepal's current-day cultural features have been shaped by elements of her past history. And many of these same general features play a role in shaping and promoting the HIV and AIDS epidemic in Nepal. In the remainder of this chapter I will discuss many contemporary aspects of Nepal's culture, focusing cursorily on the resultant impact on the spread of HIV and AIDS in the former Himalayan kingdom. Some of these factors will be taken up again more at length in subsequent chapters.

1.3 Population demographics

David Seddon (1995:4) has commented that many of the demographic characteristics of Nepal play an important role in determining the pattern of development of the HIV and AIDS epidemic in the country. According to the latest figures available, Nepal's population is now 26.6 million, of which 33 percent are under the age of fourteen, 62 percent are between age fifteen and sixty-four, and only 5 percent are over age sixty-five. The population growth rate is 1.35 percent and the sex ratio for the total population is 0.94 male/1 female (NPHC 2011). The latest estimated birth rate is 21.85 births/1,000 population and the death rate is 6.75 deaths/1,000 population. Infant mortality is listed at 43.13 deaths/1,000 live births and life expectancy is 66.51 years for the total population. The total fertility rate is 2.41 children born per woman (CIA 2013). Later in this book we will see how these population demographics combine with other key characteristics (such as the amount of arable land), to "push" people to migrate, which increases their risk factor for contracting HIV and AIDS, further facilitating the spread of HIV and AIDS in Nepal.

1.4 Economy

Although Nepal has seen some statistical improvement in its economic condition since the first edition of this book was published a decade ago, the country remains one of the world's least developed nations. Nepal is listed as 157/187 (30th poorest) in the Human Development Index Rankings (UNDP 2013), with a Gross Domestic Product (GDP) per capita income of $1,300 and approximately one quarter of its population still living below the poverty line (CIA 2013). Nepal is mainly an agrarian society where nearly 75 percent of the population is economically dependent upon agriculture, which makes up over one-third of Nepal's GDP (CIA 2013). Given the declining ability for Nepalese to meet their own basic agricultural needs due to the growing population and land degradation, future economic prospects are poor. Nepal is an underdeveloped nation with strong economic ties to India as a result of Nepal's geographic proximity, historical relationships, and landlocked status. Also, Nepal has historically relied heavily upon foreign aid to meet her needs. Foreign aid (as a percentage of the GNP) had grown from 8 percent in 1984 to nearly 13 percent in 1987 (latest figures available, Savada 1991). Likewise, foreign aid accounted for 64 percent of the development expenditures between 1956 and 1990 (latest figures available, Savada 1991). And latest figures estimate foreign aid to make up 5–6 percent of the GDP, 55 percent of Nepal's capital expenditure and 25 percent of its total expenditure (Dahal 2008).

To understand Nepal's present economic condition it is necessary to understand its economic past. Nepal, under the despotic leadership of the rogue prime minister's hereditary line (the Ranas), practiced a protectionist policy of isolationism and was cut off from the rest of the world for over a hundred years (1846–1950). Karan and Ishii (1994) observe:

> Nepal's chaotic political development in the first half of the nine-teenth century precluded any real attention to the economic needs of its people. When autocratic stability was imposed by the prime ministers of the Rana regime after 1846, the administrative struc-ture was reinforced to provide economic aggrandizement for the extensive Rana family, to the extent that Nepal's revenues, land ownership, and economic opportunities were almost totally the prerogatives of the ruling family. (Karan and Ishii 1994:1)

Prior to this period Nepal had also suffered under the consequences of a two-year war (1814–1816) with the British (Anderson 1987:20–23), which had been preceded by the consolidation (through warfare) in 1769 of sev-eral tiny hilltop kingdoms into the Kingdom of Nepal under the leader-ship of Prithvi Narayan Shah (EIU 1996:71). It was King Prithvi Narayan Shah who first established the modern nation-state known today as Nepal (Savada 1991:15–19). Nepal, therefore, had suffered the consequences of underdevelopment (as a result of political instability and despotic rule) for nearly two hundred years. Blaikie, Cameron, and Seddon (1979:25) observe that "Nepal had no economic planning of any kind prior to 1951."

The year 1951 saw the overthrow of the Rana government and the re-turn of the rightful royal monarch to the throne. King Mahendra Shah took control of Nepal in 1951, ending its "virtual economic seclusion" (Johnson 1983:155) and marking Nepal's emergence into the modern world. Shah threw Nepal's doors open to the outside world and attempted to lift Nepal from its poverty by guiding the revitalization of the country through its introduction into the global community as a fully functioning economic member (Bista 1991:1). Nepal's economy, however, was still "rooted in the medieval past" (Karan and Ishii 1994:1).

Since 1951, Nepal has pursued various economic strategies with lim-ited success (Bista 1991:1; Savada 1991:107). In 1955 the government announced the first of several five-year economic development plans (Uppal 1977:17; Lohani 1984:181; Karan and Ishii 1994:1) designed to facilitate economic and social development. However, by the mid 1990s "the development strategies introduced in the 1950s and 1960s had not had the results predicted by their advocates" (Schloss 1983) and Nepal "had not advanced economically in the last 45 years" (EICU 1996:79). Although the last decade has certainly seen some statistical economic improvement, many would contend that the civil war actually set Nepal's economic development back a decade and that any statistical improvement noted has mostly been limited to the capital city of Kathmandu.

Bikaas is the Nepali word meaning 'development'. *Bikaas* has been a major theme for Nepal ever since it opened its doors to the world in the 1950s. At that time Nepal quickly adopted an attitude toward economic development that was intended to raise it out of its poverty and bring it into the world economy. Despite the attempts, Nepal remains one of the least developed countries (LDC) in the world.

Economic development has taken various forms in Nepal in the last half-century, which have received reproach from multiple critics. Several authors stress the negative effects of economic development models upon Nepali culture (Pandy 1992; Pigg 1993; Pigg 1995b; Shrestha 1993; Zurick 1993) and upon the environment (Bell 1994; Ecologist 1993; Economist 1993; Hausler 1993; Nicholson-Lord 1994; Sill 1991; Singh 1993). To be fair, however, Schloss (1983:1) points out that in evaluating the economic and political consequences of the development paradigms pursued by Nepal over the last fifty years, we must realize that although the results of economic development methods followed throughout the eight five-year plans have had only a minimal impact upon most Nepalis, "it is also evident that *no* [emphasis his] development strategy would have done any better without the development of these basic infrastructure [those pursued under the first five plans] programs. Kathmandu made the right choice in the 1950s."

Schloss also tells us "it is only now that alternative options on growth models are feasible" (1983:1). Recently international planners have begun to examine the problems created by the development strategies pursued and have begun to look at sustainable solutions to the issues raised (Gevers 1991; Zimmerer 1991; Zurick 1992). The government of Nepal has been slow to respond to these concerns but some headway is now beginning to be forged. It is clear, however, that Nepal still has a long way to go. As discussed further in chapter three, many aspects of Nepal's economy have created various push/pull factors that have, in turn, created greater exposure to the wider world. Unfortunately, this has also created a greater exposure to HIV and AIDS.

1.5 Geography

Although much of Nepal's underdevelopment is owed to history, much also
is owed to her topography. The area of Nepal is 147,181 square kilometers
(56,136 square miles), approximately the size of Tennessee (Guido-O'Grady
1995). In just over one hundred miles (as the crow flies), Nepal's altitude
climbs from about two hundred meters (685 feet) in the south to over 8,800
meters (29,035 feet) on the peak of Mt. Everest in the north (Burbank
1992:8). According to recent figures (CIA 2013), only sixteen percent of
Nepal's land is arable. Lohani (1984) divides Nepal into three topographical
and ecological zones: (1) the mountains (the northern third of the country),
which are sparsely populated (10% of Nepal's population) and difficult to
farm (5% of the total cultivated land), (2) the mid-hills (the middle area
of the country), which exhibit a higher population density (53% of Nepal's
population live here) and low agricultural yields on terraced farms, and
(3) the Terai (the lower third, bordering India), where population density
is lower (37% of Nepal's population) and agricultural productivity higher
(65% of cultivated land).[10] As can be noted from these figures, cultivation
in the mid-hills is less productive per capita than in the Terai, where
the land is more suitable for farming and the population less dense. One
publication suggests that "the difficult topography of the country has posed
a serious problem in transporting and marketing agricultural products" (EIU
1996:78). Steep terrain also exacerbates deforestation and erosion.

Perhaps more significant than topography is Nepal's status as a landlocked country. According to Blaikie, Cameron, and Seddon (1979:12),
sixteen of the twenty-five least developed countries in the world are landlocked. There seems to be a link between a nation's being landlocked and its
status as a least developed country. According to several authors (Blaikie et
al. 1979; Karan and Ishii 1994; UN 1993), Nepal's landlocked situation has
also added significantly to its economic woes. Karan and Ishii (1994) make
the following observation:

> As a direct result of its disadvantageous geographical situation
> [landlocked], Nepal has experienced difficulties and restrictions
> in its trade and development. Its foreign trade is largely dependent
> on transit facilities provided by India. The ever-increasing costs of
> transit and transportation have led to higher-priced imports and
> exports. The consequences of the landlocked situation is difficult
> to quantify, but Nepal's lack of access to the sea is compounded
> by its remoteness and its isolation from world markets, which are
> among the reasons for its relative poverty. Overall growth, export

---

[10]Lohani suggests that agriculture is intensive near water sources in the hill-
region and that output per acre is, therefore, higher, but labor productivity remains
low due to a high person-land ratio.

expansion, and the utilization of foreign capital resources generate demands for international transport services. Greater difficulties and the cost of these services constitute an extra hurdle for Nepal's development. (Karan and Ishii 1994:5–6)

Many aspects of Nepal's geography make growing enough to feed one's family and earning a sufficient living difficult. Insufficient food supply, in turn, pushes people out of the villages to seek supplemental employment in larger cities or other countries where they are more vulnerable to lifestyles that subject them to HIV and AIDS.

1.6 Education

Although primary education is compulsory and has been provided free since 1975, only 52 percent of primary school age children were enrolled by 1984 (Savada 1991:94). This figure represented 70 percent of the primary school age boys and only 30 percent of the primary school age girls at that time. At the secondary level, only 18 percent of school age children were enrolled by 1984. Recent reporting of the UNDP's Millennial Development Goal Indicators regarding school enrollment demonstrates a massive improvement on these figures to a current net enrollment rate of 94 percent in primary education and a literacy rate of 86 percent among persons of ages fifteen to twenty-four (UNDP 2013). Despite the dramatic improvement from the 1970s, overall literacy rates countrywide remain lagging. Current statistics (CIA 2013) estimate the literacy rate for the total population to be 60 percent. And low literacy levels countrywide have led to a problem for educators (since many prevention strategies rely on literacy). Gender, geography, and caste also continue to play a part in who gets educated in Nepal. Countrywide, the literacy rate is 48 percent for females while it is 73 percent for males, indicating a continuing gender divide (CIA 2013). Beyond gender, urban literacy rates are 77 percent while rural rates are 57 percent (Bureau of Statistics 2011). And Dahal (2008) has demonstrated a remaining significant differentiation in literacy rates according to caste affiliation as well. Savada considers social class (mainly defined in Nepal by caste) historically as a limiting factor to education in Nepal and writes:

> Despite general accessibility, education still nonetheless primarily served children of landlords, businessmen, government leaders, or other elite members of the society, for they were the only ones who could easily afford to continue beyond primary school... Higher caste families could afford to send their children overseas to obtain necessary degrees... Higher caste families also had the necessary connections to receive government scholarships to study abroad. (Savada 1991:97–98)

According to the People's Awareness Campaign Nepal, there are now over forty-nine thousand schools (including higher secondary), 415 colleges, five universities, and two academies of higher studies served by over 222,000 teachers across the country (PACN 2011). During the 1980s it was reported, however, that only 60 percent of the primary teachers and only 35 percent of the secondary teachers have had formal training (Savada 1991). These are the most current figures available.

The curriculum in Nepal's schools has been greatly influenced by models used in the United States. A national curriculum was developed with the assistance of the United Nations Educational, Scientific and Cultural Organization (UNESCO). Savada (1991:96) states:

> The goal of primary education was to teach reading, writing and arithmetic, and to instill discipline and hygiene. Lower secondary education emphasized character formation, a positive attitude toward manual labor, and perseverance. Higher secondary education stressed manpower requirements and preparation for higher education. National development goals were stressed through the curriculum.

Regarding the promotion of "a positive attitude toward manual labor" as an early goal of the primary education model as noted by Savada above, Bista (1991) identifies a much stronger resident Nepali cultural feature that works to counter this value toward manual labor among the educated. He writes,

> Scholarship in the Sanskritic tradition is associated with privilege and never with labor. Education is traditionally the prerogative of the upper classes; to be educated is a powerful symbol of status. Education is not seen as a means of acquiring skills that can be used productively to secure economic prosperity but is seen as an end in itself which once achieved signifies higher status... To become educated is to be effectively removed from the workforce. (Bista 1991:5–6)

Or to put it bluntly, once hands have taken up the book they should never again touch the plow. Bista concludes that such cultural features of Nepali society "are retarding and diminishing its efforts to develop" (Bista 1991:1). David Watters (2011), observing the impact of this cultural belief on the rural youths sent off for education from far-western Nepal, writes, "Many students returned home and became thugs, perfecting the criminal practices they had witnessed in the towns" and "most honest, hardworking villagers [and here he is referring to the Tibeto-Burman Kham people who are not willing to give up manual labor for the sake of an education as the Indo-Aryans are] were thus understandably wary of Nepali education and

wanted no part of it." This is a remaining cultural feature that is inhibiting Nepal's progress and yet few have ventured to address it as it relates to
education paradigms.[11]

Another little-discussed (and possibly related) problem regarding education is the impact that the form of educational curriculum had upon the
Maoist insurgency in Nepal. The curriculum in Nepal as noted above focuses
heavily upon the three Rs (reading, writing and arithmetic) at the expense
of a focus upon a more village-appropriate education (perhaps more techni-
cal or vocational in nature). Thus, rural youths were educationally trained
for types of jobs that simply were not available in the rural areas of Nepal.
And fewer and fewer of these types of jobs were available in the city either,
as unemployment and oversupply skyrocketed. As a result, frustration rose
among the well-educated rural youth toward the existing conditions. This
frustration, in turn, led to sympathy for the Maoist message. And many
well-educated rural youths joined the Maoist movement in response.

The "Maoist problem" had a major impact on the spread of HIV and
AIDS in Nepal in many direct and indirect ways.[12] The most obvious impact
was that during the conflict, many of the rural schools were forcibly closed
by the Maoists as they were considered agents of imperialistic, capitalis-
tic Nepali hegemony. These schools had been the main venue where HIV
prevention was being promoted throughout the country. Likewise, many
INGOs working on HIV and AIDS issues in the rural areas were targeted for
the same reason and had to close their projects under threats of the Maoists.
Fearing forced conscription by the Maoists or by the police, many young
men, including those who normally attended school, fled the rural areas,
which made them more vulnerable to the normal temptations of migrants
(a high risk group). And with these young men gone and the economy in
shambles, poverty increased, leading many women to turn to prostitution
out of sheer necessity. Lawlessness abounded in many rural areas as police
abandoned their posts, while the army, unconcerned with enforcing civil
laws, allowed traffickers and women abusers free reign during the conflict.
And perhaps most significantly, young people were taken away from their
families (their social structure) by the Maoists and put into coed bands of
warriors that traveled together for months or years. These young people,
who were ripped out of school, had little formal education, particularly on

---

[11] At the Nepal hospital where we serve we often encounter malnourished elderly
patients. They have encouraged their youth to depart for the cities to seek education and development, thus leaving the elderly to work the steep hillsides alone.
As a result, many are unable to tend their family plots except those closest to the
homestead, which does not provide enough income or nutrition. Meantime we find
their educated youth sitting in the city unemployed, refusing to return (and not
encouraged to do so by the elder generation that sent them). This is a counterproductive custom for Nepal's future. Who will grow the food?

[12] I have documented these factors elsewhere (see Beine 2006).

the behavior risks associated with HIV and AIDS—and they were in a ripe environment for risky sexual behavior, particularly without social reinforcement against any such behavior that they would have received from their families.

So, as demonstrated, many aspects of Nepal's educational system have had negative repercussions upon the spread of HIV and AIDS in Nepal. And despite the progress of the past ten years, Nepal still has a long way to go.

1.7 Medical systems

Nepali illness beliefs and practices have been influenced by many different sources throughout history. Most of the modern inhabitants of Nepal trace their ancestry to various waves of migrants, who brought with them, from their origins, many beliefs and practices regarding illness. The influence of these illness beliefs and practices is still evident in the various medical systems in use today throughout Nepal. For instance, the original Bodic-speaking peoples, of pre–fourth century Mongolian origin, brought with them central-Asian shamanistic practices that are still evident in some of the healing practices observed among shamans today (Gaenszle 1994; Streefland 1985; Watters 1975). Likewise, the Khas tribes, who started settling in Nepal around 2000 B.C., brought with them ancient Ayurvedic traditions from India that are still widely practiced today (Dhungel 1994; Streefland 1985). Waves of Muslims brought with them Greco-Arabic medical beliefs and practices that are evident in modern-day homeopathic medical practices (Blustain 1976). Later, waves of migrants from Tibet brought with them Tantric Buddhist ideas about healing (which combine elements of ancient Chinese medicine and shamanistic practices of the early Bon and Lamism religions) that are still popular today (Durkin 1984; Streefland 1985). And recently, the allopathic ideas of Western medicine have been introduced and well accepted (Dhungel 1994; Pigg 1995a; Streefland 1985). Acharya (1994), Durkin (1984) and Streefland (1985) have provided particularly good descriptions of the interface between the various medical systems in use today in urban Nepal.

One characteristic feature of the Nepali medical system is its pluralistic or eclectic nature. Although each system might be associated (originally) with a certain group (or religion), modern Nepalis easily incorporate ideas and utilize treatments from the various medical systems. Stone (1976:77) suggests that "in several contexts of illness treatment, [Nepali] villagers easily combine Western medicine with traditional practices" and "such observations suggest that villagers have little difficulty integrating Western medicine with their own traditions on an ideological level." Pigg (1995a) demonstrates that the way people determine which systems they will employ is dependent upon (1) their perceptions about which is most effective for particular illnesses and (2) their access to the various treatments. It seems that Nepalis have no problem integrating the ideas of the various systems into a new hybrid medical system.

Foster and Anderson (1978:53) dualistically divide non-Western medical systems into a "personalistic" and "naturalistic" dichotomy. In a personalistic system, illnesses are believed to be caused by the intervention of a sensate agent: supernatural beings (gods or deities), other nonhuman beings (ancestors, ghosts, or evil spirits) or human beings (sorcerers or witches). Sickness is often viewed as a punishment for some wrong committed. Naturalistic systems attribute disease causation to natural, impersonal phenomena, such as the disruption of the body's equilibrium. Disruption of the body's equilibrium can be caused by such things as an imbalance between the various humors of the body, the improper mixing of hot and cold foods, the imbalance of yin and yang, etc. When equilibrium is disrupted, illness occurs. Disease causation in naturalistic systems is impersonal, the result of more or less natural causes rather than a sensate agent.

Interestingly, both systems are practiced in Nepal. In many cases, demons or witches (personalistic) are believed to be the cause of illness. In other cases, sickness is interpreted as the result of the improper mixing of foods. Some individuals may consider certain classes of illness to be spiritually caused (personalistic) and others naturally caused, while another's belief about illness causation (whether personalistic or naturalistic) may be informed by the traditional healer or astrologer and shift from illness episode to illness episode. In some cases, an individual can even attribute naturalistic and personalistic causes to the same illness episode. Again, this displays the pluralistic nature of the Nepali medical system.

Various authors have studied different groups of Nepalis and have described diverse beliefs and medical practices among Buddhist Nepalis (Adams 1988; Holmberg 1989), Hindu Nepalis (Blustain 1976; Stone 1976; Stone 1988), Muslim Nepalis (Blustain 1976), and mainly animistic groups (Allen 1976; Gaenszle 1994; Watters 1975).[13] Although the medical practices of each group may focus mainly on the specifics of a particular system, influence of the various other systems is evident as well. Again, various authors have demonstrated that medical pluralism is well utilized throughout the various groups in Nepal (Acharya 1994; Blustain 1976; Dhungel 1994; Durkin 1984; Pigg 1995a; Streefland 1985; Stone 1976). Although there are

---

[13]I use the phrase "mainly animistic groups" to describe groups that, although they present a veneer of Hinduism (i.e., one would find a Hindu temple in their village), the bulk of their religious practices revolve around ideas of animistic shamanism rather than classical Hinduism. For instance, Gaenszle (1997:361) suggests that rather than becoming Hindus, the Mewahang Rai "have integrated parts of it [Hindu culture] into their own tradition by translating them into their own familiar idioms." Further, he suggests that "these modifications remained quite superficial as they did not really change much of the indigenous traditions" (1997:362).

differences between the various groups, some common features emerge.[14]
For instance, for all of the groups listed, disease etiology can be either single
factorial or multiple factorial, and disease can be either physically caused or
spiritually caused. Many of the other features common to the various groups
of Nepalis will be discussed further in chapter five.

Recently, authors have focused on the impact of "modernization" and
paradigms of Western development upon the Nepali medical systems
(Adams 1998; Justice 1986; Pigg 1992, 1995a, 1995b, 1996; Stone 1976).
Focusing on the impact of the application of Western paradigms for primary
health care programs in Nepal, Stone (1992) describes how Nepal has begun to favor a "community participation" approach to primary health care.
The result has been a shift from curative services to an emphasis on health
education. Although many aspects of this shift have been positive for Nepal,
Stone illustrates that it is actually the underlying development discourses
rather than issues of efficacy that have informed the community health
program in Nepal. She cites critics that contend that the new approach
(community participation) is simply another hegemonic Western device,
which "promotes current political and economic structures of inequality"
and she concludes that "the current focus on community participation appears to be an attempt to promote the Western cultural values of equality
and self-reliance (values not shared by the local population), while ignoring
alternative values and perceptions of how development might work in rural, non-Western societies of developing countries (Stone 1992:412)." Stone
(1986, 1992) also demonstrates how, ironically, this new mode of thinking
(with its emphasis on community participation) actually stifles the voices of
the local people rather than taking them into account.

Likewise, Pigg (1995b:47) demonstrates how many principles inherent
in Western development paradigms and discourses being deployed in Nepal
"systematically dismantle and decontextualize different sociocultural realities in the course of taking them into account." Similarly, Justice (1986)
demonstrates how Nepali health planners, even if they have social and cultural information available, do not use it in health planning. She suggests
that this is largely due to deference on the part of national health planners
toward the favored paradigms of international aid bureaucracies.

Pigg (1996:161), further illustrating the impact that Western development discourses (which dominate health development approaches in
Nepal) have had, demonstrates how traditional healers (shamans) have
been "caught up in the meanings of modernity." *Bikaas* 'development' is
perceived as good and anything traditional (such as shamanism) is seen
as backward. Likewise, Adams (1998) demonstrates how Nepali doctors,

---

[14]Gaenszle (1994:257) makes the point that for the Tibeto-Burman groups the
shamanistic journey *to* their deities is a prominent feature while for the Indo-Aryan
groups, the coming of the deities to humans (possession) is the norm.

favoring a paradigm of Western modernity, were instrumental in the recent democracy movement. According to Adams, Nepali doctors, who see themselves as modern individuals (which implies an understanding of modern medical science as objective "truth"), have served as harbingers of Western epistemological hegemony in the politicization of medicine in Nepal. She contends that the democracy movement was a product of individualism, which itself was largely the result of Western paradigms implemented by health planners in Nepal.[15]

All of these authors illustrate the impact that Western discourses of development have had upon the Nepali medical systems. This issue will be revisited in the following pages as we consider the impact of the concept of *bikaas* upon the HIV and AIDS epidemic in Nepal.

Topography and economy (which are related) combine to make health care services generally poor in rural Nepal. Add to this the pluralistic nature of the Nepali medical systems and one is left with a system that has affected, and will continue to affect, the spread of HIV and AIDS in Nepal. This will be discussed further in the coming chapters.

1.8 Religion

As can be seen, there is a strong tie between medical practices and religion in Nepal. The current census of Nepal (NPHC 2012) lists 81 percent of Nepal's population as Hindu, followed by 9 percent claiming Buddhism, 4 percent Islam, 3 percent Kirat, 1 percent Christian, and less than 1 percent each following Prakriti, Bon, Jainism, Bahai and Sikhism.[16] These figures are often debated and it is suggested that the numbers of non-Hindus is actually much higher (Pfaff-Czarnecka 1997). Many of the mountain populations counted as Hindu actually practice a "Hinduized" animism or shamanism, which is heavily influenced by the ancient Bon religion of early Tibet.

A key feature of the dominant Hindu philosophy is the caste system. Modeled on the orthodox Brahmatic caste system of India, this system creates social classes and social stratification throughout all of Nepali society.

---

[15]Adams suggests that (1) the emphasis placed on the individual as the unit of responsibility, rights and duties, is a construction of modernity; (2) this philosophy is inherent in Western development paradigms but not natural to Nepali culture; (3) Nepali doctors indoctrinated in Western philosophies, such as the Alma Ata agreement (basic health for all [individuals]), pushed this agenda; (4) the Alma Ata philosophy "formed a constitutive basis for medicine in Nepal, taking individual responsibility as a key to modern development" (1998:18); and (5) "many of these assumptions were shared by Nepal's revolutionaries, who saw individualism as a basis for social equality" (1998:17).

[16]Nepali Christian leaders dispute these census figures, claiming that there are now 2.5 million Christians in Nepal (BarnabasAID 2013), which would make Christians just over 9 percent of the population.

According to Stone (1997:86), Nepali castes are "ranked status groups, with the ranking sanctioned by religion. The whole system is expressed through Hindu religious ideas concerning purity and pollution: Higher castes are considered more pure than lower castes."

Stone presents a model of Nepali caste that posits sacred thread-wearing priests (Brahmans) at the top, followed by the sacred thread-wearing non-priests, the liquor drinking castes and the untouchable castes (fig. 1.2). Each of the castes has strict dietary and behavioral rules and interaction between castes is sanctioned by these rules (Stone 1997:86). And the most important rule is dietary: higher caste members cannot eat rice (or any food) cooked by persons of a lower caste (although the reverse is allowable). Many of the Tibetan, Tibeto-Burman and Muslim people groups of Nepal (all non-Hindu groups) also practice their own caste hierarchies.

Pure	Sacred thread–wearing	Priests	Brahmans
		Non-priests	Chetris, etc.
	Liquor drinking	Matwalis	
Impure	Untouchables	Various castes	

Figure 1.2 The Nepali caste system (adapted from Stone 1997).

The concepts of purity and pollution (which are at the core of the caste structure) will prove an integral part of cultural schemata (which underlie cultural models), as we will see in later chapters. As mentioned earlier, one's caste standing has traditionally determined access to education and employment, which has implications for the spread of HIV and AIDS. AIDS is viewed by some as a problem only for the impure low caste. In chapter three we will be introduced to other aspects of religion that may also prove detrimental to the spread of HIV and AIDS in Nepal.

1.9 Conclusion

Many aspects of Nepal's history, economy, geography, education and religion are linked to HIV and AIDS in Nepal and have played a part in fostering the spread of the disease. The impact of these various societal features will become evident when we consider the HIV and AIDS situation in Nepal further in chapter three. We will also see in later chapters that many of these same societal features have been influential in shaping cultural models of HIV and AIDS and their underlying illness schemata. Before we address HIV and AIDS specifically in Nepal, it will be helpful first to examine the topic of HIV and AIDS generally. This will be the focus of the next chapter.

2

AIDS

Nobel laureate David Baltimore, in a statement made at the American Academy of Arts and Sciences, said, "AIDS is a medical problem: The only issue is when we will solve it."[1] This represents one extreme view of AIDS, namely that it is purely a medical problem. At the opposite extreme there are those who suggest that the concept of AIDS is purely invented (Duesberg 1996). Others, taking a middle ground, recognize the biomedical reality of HIV (the virus that causes AIDS) but also recognize the social aspects involved in the construction of cultural meaning that is associated with the worldwide pandemic known as AIDS.

The one extreme position claims that AIDS is not real: it is a total "cultural construction," the product of Western modernity wrapped in the narratives and discourses of the science of the modern era, only a "fact" as viewed through the narrow epistemology of Western medicine. I do not go this far. Although this type of Foucaultian postmodern analysis has its value in challenging the over-reified view of all science as "truth" (i.e., objectively removed from all social influence), for the people of Nepal, AIDS is a reality—a terrifying reality. I take the middle ground: AIDS is a combination of biological reality (the HIV virus) and social construction (the meanings associated with AIDS). Or, as Treichler (1992) has aptly put it, the problem is medical, the drama is human.

Human beings view disease in the context of biological and social conditions (Fee and Fox 1992:9). AIDS is a particularly good example of the social construction of disease. In the process of defining both the disease and the persons infected, politics and social perceptions have been embedded in scientific and policy constructions of their reality and meaning.

The purpose of this chapter is to briefly introduce the reader to the biomedical "facts" about AIDS, including its causes, history and treatments, as well as to discuss AIDS as a social construction. Much has changed in the

---

[1]Fee and Fox 1992:10.

realm of HIV and AIDS since the first edition of this book appeared in 2003. Beyond the change of vocabulary (from HIV/AIDS to HIV and AIDS), new treatments are now available and there is even talk of a potential "cure" on the horizon. At the time of the first edition of this book, due to the emergence of antiretroviral therapy (ART) treatments and the subsequent first-time declines in associated death rates in the late 1990s—at least in the West—many (including myself) were just beginning to challenge the popular "dire predictions" narrative of the preceding decade.[2] Because of the unequal access to these drugs, however, and with no foreseeable cure in sight, many (again including myself) expected the AIDS epidemic to continue relatively unabated outside the west, and certainly in Nepal, into the foreseeable future. What we couldn't see at that time was the possibility of treatment as prevention and the emergence of possible "functional cures" that lay just around the corner. Given the recent developments of ART treatment as prevention and perhaps "functional cures," many scholars believe we may be at a significant "turning point" in the HIV and AIDS epidemic. These recent developments will be discussed further in this chapter.

2.1 AIDS as biomedical fact

AIDS is the acronym used for the medically defined acquired immuno-deficiency syndrome. In lay terms, the acronym can be explained in this way:

Acquired: the virus is non-hereditarily transmitted[3]

Immunodeficiency: the virus weakens the immune system, resulting in greater susceptibility to various opportunistic infections[4]

Syndrome: a collection of common symptoms or signs (usually opportunistic infections) appears, which are fairly typical in infected persons.

AIDS is caused by a group of related viruses referred to as HIV (human immunodeficiency viruses).[5] HIV, like most other viruses, requires

---

[2]"ART" stands for antiretroviral therapy while "ARV" is short-hand for antiretroviral drugs. "ART" is the more common nomenclature for the therapy protocol among international HIV and AIDS researchers while "ARV" has become the common nomenclature for both the therapy and the drugs in Nepal.

[3]This does not mean, however, that a child cannot be born with AIDS. Mother-to-child transmission is known as vertical transmission. The transfer, however, is through the blood, not through the genes, and therefore it is non-hereditary.

[4]Opportunistic infections are those which take advantage especially of a person's depressed immune system.

[5]There are two independent types of HIV: HIV-1 (with its various strain known as "groups" and now multiple subtypes) and HIV-2. Each is believed to have begun

reproduction within the cells of the body. Once inside the body, the virus attaches itself to the surface of T-cells (T-lymphocytes), commonly referred to as white blood cells. The virus then enters the host cell by attaching itself to a protein known as a CD4 receptor in the plasma membrane of the cell. When HIV comes in contact with the CD4 receptor, the cell opens up, letting the virus enter the host cell.

A defining characteristic of retroviruses (which include HIV) is that they are able to transcribe RNA into DNA (through the use of a special enzyme called reverse transcriptase), allowing the virus to integrate into the host DNA of the cell nucleus.[6] Thus, HIV becomes resident in the cell nucleus by inserting itself into the infected person's own DNA and grows in the body as cells divide and multiply. Cell reproduction takes place in the normal way (divide and multiply), but the newly emerging T-cells, which usually are involved in fighting infection, are compromised. T-cells are involved in attacking infected cells in our bodies. The HIV-infected T-cells, however, lack this ability, reducing the effectiveness of the body's immune system. As the number of these HIV-infected T-cells increases in the body, the immune system becomes more and more depressed, allowing foreign bodies to enter the body and survive. In this weakened state, the body finally succumbs to the "invaders" and the result is death.

According to AmfAR (2012), over 60 million people have contracted HIV since the beginning of the epidemic, and nearly 30 million of these have since died. It is estimated that there are currently 34 million people living with HIV or AIDS around the world (USAID 2012). In 2011, 2.5 million people became newly infected with HIV (UNAIDS 2012) and 1.7 million died from AIDS (AmfAR 2012). Each day nearly 7,000 persons contract HIV worldwide (AmfAR 2012) at a time when it is known how to prevent the infection by the virus that causes AIDS. By 1997 AIDS had been reported in over two hundred countries (Frumkin and Leonard 1997:117) and today it would appear that there is not a single nation remaining untouched by the epidemic.[7]

While these numbers are certainly daunting, recent advances in prevention and treatment are decreasing the infection rate around the globe. According to the latest figures from UNAID (2012), twenty-five countries have seen a 50 percent (or greater) drop in new infections since 2001. The

---

as simian immunodeficiency viruses (SIV)—the former in association with chimpanzees and the latter with the sooty mangabey or white-collared monkey—and then transferred to humans (a process known as zoonosis), although the exact process for how cross-species transmission might have occurred is hotly debated. Untreated, both HIV-1 and HIV-2 lead to clinically indistinguishable AIDS.

[6]HIV is further sub-categorized as a "lentivirus," a slow moving type of retrovirus.

[7]*The CIA Factbook* (2012) lists Svalbard as the only country with no recorded HIV cases. Svalbard, however, has officially been a territory of Norway since 1925 and is thus not an independent country.

Caribbean region (which ranks second behind sub-Saharan Africa as the most affected region of the world) has seen a 42 percent reduction in infections, and over the past two years, half of all reductions in new HIV infections have been among newborn children, demonstrating that elimination of new infections in children is possible. It would appear that, likely owing to the new ART as a prevention strategy now being employed around the world, globally the epidemic has actually leveled off and is now beginning a decline. According to UNAIDS (2010), the number of new HIV infections peaked globally in 1996 and the number of AIDS-related deaths peaked in 2004.

The latest data from UNAIDS (2012) also suggests, however, that new HIV infections have increased in East and North Africa by 35 percent or more for the same period (since 2001) and that Central Asia and Eastern Europe have also seen increases in HIV infection rates in recent years. This same data elaborates on the worrisome connection between HIV and tuberculosis (TB), concluding that TB remains the leading cause of death among People Living with HIV and AIDS (PLWHA). Furthermore, it concludes that although ART can reduce the risk of contracting TB by PLWHAs by up to 65 percent, fewer than half of those infected with both HIV and TB were receiving ART treatment as of 2011. And as is the case in Nepal (and likely elsewhere as well) there is certainly still a disparity between the availability of and access to ART treatments. So it would appear that the gap between rich and poor nations in regard to AIDS (noted in Beine 2003:56) remains true today, despite the progress noted above.

2.1.1 The history of AIDS

Although the term AIDS was not coined until 1981, and HIV, the virus which causes AIDS, was not "discovered" until 1983 (Frumkin and Leonard 1997:1), recent evidence suggests that HIV was already present in the West as early as the 1950s (Frunkin and Leonard 1997:7), and new evidence suggests that HIV may have had its origin among humans in Africa possibly as early as the period between the 1880s and 1920s (Worobey 2008). There is much controversy and continued debate about the origin of HIV and its subsequent transfer from simians to humans.

By the early 1980s the infection had become widespread enough to gain popular attention. Physicians were seeing multiple patients with strange symptoms. It wasn't so much that the symptoms were unusual, but the diseases identified were being diagnosed in populations not normally associated with these diseases. By 1981, the Center for Disease Control (CDC) had over one hundred reports of young, healthy, gay men who had contracted diseases such as Kaposi's sarcoma, a type of cancer that usually affects elderly men of Mediterranean descent, and Pneumocystis carinii pneumonia (PCP), an unusual lung infection in young, otherwise healthy men. When this phenomenon grew large enough, it caught the attention of the CDC, a government-funded agency whose job it is to study such anomalies. On the basis of their findings, scientists at the CDC hypothesized an immunodeficiency syndrome but still hadn't discovered the causative virus, HIV[8]. The link between HIV and AIDS would not be made definitively for another two years.[9]

Because the first cases noted were mostly in gay men, the disease was first termed gay-related immunodeficiency (GRID) (Flynn and Lound 1995:11). Fed by media reports of the new "gay disease," the first cultural model of AIDS—as it would later be called—began to emerge, namely that AIDS was a "gay" disease and a "death sentence."

During the next few years many immigrant Haitians were also found to be infected with GRID, as were hemophiliacs and even newborn infants (AmfAR 1999:370–374). Because the scope of the disease had now moved well beyond the initial community, GRID was renamed AIDS. The new findings began to modify the new cultural model of AIDS that was emerging among the general public. AIDS was still very much considered a "death sentence" but no longer understood as just a "gay" disease.

It has long been suspected that HIV had its origin as a zoonotic disease. Because HIV is so similar to simian immunodeficiency virus (SIV), a virus that causes AIDS-like symptoms in some kinds of monkeys, the link between HIV and SIV was hypothesized (Frumkin and Leonard 1997:13). New research (Gao, Bailes and Robertson 1999) has confirmed this hypothesis, suggesting the common chimpanzee (Pan troglodytes troglodytes) as the origin of HIV-1. Tests carried out on strains of SIV suggest that HIV-1 arose first in this species (as a related SIV). The natural range of this species also corresponds with the areas where HIV-1 is endemic, suggesting that the chimpanzee is the main reservoir for HIV-1. The research also postulates that chimpanzees have been the source of introducing SIV into human populations on at least three separate occasions.

2.1.2 Treatments, treatment as prevention, and "functonal" cure

It would seem we are at a pivotal turning point in the fight against HIV and AIDS. Although there is no true cure for AIDS at this time and no vaccine yet to prevent it, the development of several ART regimens has changed the

---

[8]HIV was being discovered in two places at once. In America it was being termed human T-lymphotropic virus (HTLV), while in Europe it was known as lymphadenopathy associated virus (LAV) (Flynn and Lound 1995:11). Later, the term HIV was agreed upon as a compromise by both the American and French scientists who had made the discovery (Giblin 1995:159).

[9]A few AIDS researchers—the most famous being Dr. Peter H. Duesberg, a well-respected virologist at UC Berkeley—have recently offered dissenting opinions to this well-accepted view linking HIV and AIDS (see Duesberg 1996 and Newton 1992:31).

course of the epidemic (Dieffenbach and Fauci 2011), lowering the death rate of PLWHAs around the world.[10] Further, it seems that using these same regimens prophylactically with the non-infected partners of HIV-positive persons (i.e., preventively) can actually decrease the new infection rate (by blocking transfer) dramatically. And it looms hopeful that certain uses of ART might actually provide a functional cure for many in the future.

2.1.2.1 *Early ART therapies*

Antiretroviral therapies first began to be developed for use against HIV between 1985 and 1990 (Broder 2010). The discoveries led to multi-drug therapies (often referred to as cocktail therapies since they involve the use of various drug combinations), which began to significantly lower the death rate from AIDS in the places where they were being used. With the advent of highly active antiretroviral therapy (HAART), mortality among patients with AIDS who were under ART treatment was nearly half what it was prior to the "HAART era" (Rathbun 2012), and life expectancies for those with HIV rose from months to decades (Dieffenbach and Fauci 2011). Many of these new treatments were successful at reducing the amount of HIV in the blood to an undetectable level. However, these drugs were found to control the virus but not to eradicate it. Once a person stopped treatment, HIV again began to grow in the body. The new treatments began to shift the cultural model to understanding AIDS as a chronic, manageable condition. "Living with AIDS" rather than "dying from AIDS" became the new model.

In the early years of antiretroviral drugs (ARVs) these new medical advances had little impact on the spread of HIV worldwide.[11] At that time, 95 percent of HIV infections occurred in the developing world and the developing world also experienced ninety-five percent of all deaths due to AIDS (UNAIDS 1999). There was a large gap between East and West (what I termed "the West and the rest" in the earlier edition) in their ability to access these new treatment possibilities. Many of these treatments at that time cost over one thousand dollars a month per person—an unrealistic hope for an AIDS sufferer, for instance, in Nepal, a country of socialized medicine, where the government then allocated the rupee-equivalent of seven dollars

---

[10]Since scientists began working on finding an AIDS vaccine in 1983, only three have made it to final clinical trials. The first failed, the second actually increased infection (to everyone's surprise) and the latest (2009) provided protection for only one third of its recipients, though it is unknown how (Washington Post 2012). At present there is a fourth vaccine in development that looks promising; it is currently in phase 1 clinical trials in Canada (Western News 2012). So far, perhaps because of the constantly changing nature of the virus, an effective vaccine has proven elusive.

[11]The problem was that these drugs (while under proprietary ownership) were very expensive. They were just not a reality for all but the wealthiest countries.

(US) per person per annum to health care and where the underlying trend was an annual decrease in health expenditure (Smith 1996:140). The cost of these treatments made them impossible for developing nations to ever consider. So, while the cultural model began to shift to "living with AIDS" in the West (for those who had access to ART), it remained "dying with AIDS" in the rest of the world (for those who did not have access to ART). In the next section, I will discuss the socioeconomic implications that these changing cultural models have had and will continue to have in the future.

In recent years an effort has been made to make these life-saving drugs more widely available to all. Today ART is considered "standard fare" in HIV treatment and is often made available for free (via a grant from the Global Fund to Fight AIDS, Tuberculosis and Malaria). Even so, by 2008 only 13 percent of those who needed it had access to ART in Nepal (USAID 2008). So, even though ART is now "available" free of charge in Nepal, there are still structural problems preventing access for all. And in 2011 the Global Fund announced an acute funding crisis, which may limit the fund's ability to continue providing these ART drugs free of charge in the near future (Boseley 2011).

2.1.2.2 ART as prevention

In 2011, a study conclusively confirmed what had long been suspected: that treating HIV-positive persons with ART would significantly reduce their chances of transmitting HIV to their sexual or drug-using partners. This landmark study (Cohen et al. 2011) concluded that ART treatment of an HIV-infected partner reduced the risk of transmission to the uninfected partner by 96 percent. Thus, the study definitively proved that early HIV treatment with ART has a "profound prevention benefit" (CDC 2013). The practice of treating HIV-infected persons as a method of reducing transmission came to be considered "treatment as prevention" (CDC 2013). *Science Magazine* hailed the discovery as the "breakthrough of the year" (Cohen 2011:1628).[12]

The discovery instantly worried some that it might be hailed as a kind of "magic bullet" and that future prevention efforts might therefore favor an overdependence on treatment-based prevention efforts (to the exclusion of all other prevention efforts). Soon after the announcement, well-known HIV and AIDS researchers Edward Green, Allison Herling Ruark, and Norman Hearst commented:

> This week, the United Nations General Assembly meets to discuss progress against the HIV and AIDS epidemic amid news that antiretroviral drugs can drastically reduce HIV transmission from

---

[12]Actually this same practice had been in use to prevent mother-to-child transmission since the mid-1990s.

infected to non-infected partners. The U.N.'s AIDS agency, UNAIDS, has already called this news a "game changer" and at this week's meeting will doubtless call for massive infusions of donor funding in order to implement this treatment-as-prevention approach.

Nearly as certain is that little will be said about investing in programs to encourage the kind of fundamental behavior change, particularly faithfulness between sexual partners, that has already saved millions of lives worldwide. Serious investment in such programs would cost a tiny fraction of the vast sums required for HIV treatment. Yet there is a serious lack of political will to invest in simple, low-cost programs which address the real drivers of the HIV epidemic, such as multiple sexual partners. (Green et al. 2011)

It seems that these words were almost prophetic as the discovery was "translated rapidly into policy for the global response" (Cohen et al. 2012:1439). The announcement created a firestorm of debate among HIV researchers, which is still raging as of this writing. At the heart of the debate seems to be a concern over resources. Some fear that already-limited resources (currently thinly spread over a variety of non-treatment prevention approaches) will be further appropriated from these approaches (such as behavioral change), to be spent more heavily on this new "treatment as prevention" drug-based method. And the concern seems warranted. In 2003, U.S. President George W. Bush initiated the President's Emergency Plan for AIDS Relief (known as PEPFAR), a program that committed 15 billion dollars over five years (2004–2008) to be used globally to fight HIV and AIDS. The plan allocated 80 percent for treatment and care (e.g., ART delivery) and 20 percent for prevention (e.g., sexual behavioral change efforts). In 2008, PEPFAR was renewed by Congress, shifting emphasis toward "expanding existing commitments around service delivery" (i.e., treatment) and removing the 20 percent funding allocated for prevention altogether (Moss 2008). The debate, pitting behavior-change prevention efforts against other methods (e.g., treatment as prevention, condom distribution, etc.), is not new and it seems to be indicative of a possible ideological divide among HIV and AIDS researchers.[13] And it is difficult to assess what the final repercussions of this funding shift will produce.

---

[13]This resembles the ABC debates of the 1990s when some suggested A (Abstinence) only, others suggested AB (Abstinence and Be faithful) only (promotion of sexual behavior change), while others suggested C (Condom) only was the best use of money. The best comprehensive approach over time has proven to be AB and C in an even and comprehensive prevention strategy.

2.1.2.3 Limitations of ART

One of the first limitations to ART as prevention is that subsequent studies have shown far more modest results. A study published in *The Lancet* in 2012 (Jia et al. 2012) found that ART used to prevent HIV transmission in serodiscordant couples in China produced a far more modest reduction of 26 percent.[14] While certainly significant, the results are far from the 96 percent findings of the earlier study, suggesting that while ART as prevention is a positive step forward, it alone may not be the silver bullet researchers had hoped it would be.

Many field-based anthropologists working in developing countries seem to have a less-than-optimistic view about the ability of ART (i.e., treatment as prevention) to completely solve the AIDS problem. Fauci, in an earlier article (Fauci 2011), had conveyed great optimism that ART would be the final answer to the pandemic. In a follow-up to the article, Jonathan Imbody, the Christian Medical Association Vice President for Government Relations, asked Fauci directly about the remaining barriers to ART delivery and compliance (Christian Medical and Dental Association 2011). When questioned about the challenge of getting AIDS patients to adhere to their medicines, Fauci "acknowledged the need noting, 'we have to do behavioral intervention along with the biological.'" Imbody then went on to list various reservations that a number of individuals and organizations working with AIDS patients in developing countries had expressed to him. These included issues related to (1) motivation. "Those who haven't yet experienced the symptoms may be less motivated and disciplined in treating the disease"; (2) stigma, which inhibits some from seeking treatment; (3) money. Because of cutbacks, some who began receiving treatment free under PEPFAR have now lost, or will soon lose free access as noted previously; (4) adherence. Non-adherence can create future drug resistance, which could be disastrous; and (5) mistrust. Testing and treatment depend upon the acceptance of science and scientists, and many individuals in developing countries do not trust either.

Many of these same concerns are relevant to the Nepali context as well. And there are certainly many other structural issues still inhibiting ART delivery in Nepal (even though it is, for now, still free). These will be elaborated on in the next chapter. So while the amazing development of ART as treatment and prevention is obviously very substantial in the global fight against HIV and AIDS, it may not be the panacea that some have made it out to be. Given the new emerging data, coupled with the limitations noted above, it would seem prudent (and responsible) for HIV researchers and the

---

[14]A serodiscordant couple is one in which one partner is HIV positive and the other HIV negative. A seroconcordant couple, on the other hand, is one in which both are either HIV positive or HIV negative.

media to curb their excitement and communicate publically that, in light of the new studies and the remaining identified barriers, our approach to HIV prevention needs to remain "both/and" (i.e., treatment as prevention and behavioral change), not "either/or."

Fortunately, there seems to be an emerging understanding concerning the limitations of any future total dependence upon treatment as prevention.[15] The CDC (2013) concludes, "treatment by itself is not going to solve the global HIV epidemic" but that "controlling and ultimately ending the epidemic will require a combination of scientifically proven HIV prevention tools." And in a recent review of its current PEPFAR plan, the Institute of Medicine (IOM) concluded the following:

> To contribute to the sustainable management of the HIV epidemic in partner countries, PEPFAR should support a stronger emphasis on prevention. The prevention response should prioritize the reduction of sexual transmission, which is the primary driver of most HIV infections, while maintaining support for interventions targeted at other modes of transmission. (IOM 2013:723)

It would seem that another pendulum shift may be close at hand. It is critical to once again reassert the importance of prevention in the overall equation in order to eliminate HIV and AIDS. Such a shift would be an important and necessary correction on the part of policy planners.

2.1.2.4 A "functional" cure?

The first hope of a cure for HIV came in an anomalous case when an HIV-infected man living in Berlin was being treated for acute leukemia, which he had developed subsequent to his HIV infection. He was given a bone marrow transplant from a donor whose cells were genetically resistant to HIV. Following the procedure, he stopped his HIV drugs and ART treatments and his HIV remained undetectable in his body (NPR 2012) (Salter 2012).

In a second case, an HIV-positive baby born in Mississippi was treated aggressively with ARVs just after birth. Even after the cessation of ARVs there was no remaining trace of HIV in the baby's body (Pollack and McNeil 2013a). This is thus the second documented "cure."

In a third recent case, French doctors reported fourteen HIV-positive patients whose bodies seemed to be controlling their HIV without further medication (Pollack and McNeil 2013b). Like the Mississippi baby, they had

---

[15]Even UNAIDS (2012) acknowledges the limitations of ART in their 2011 fact sheet. They note that although the number of people accessing HIV treatment increased by 63 percent between 2009–2011, there are still roughly 7 million people eligible for HIV treatment who still do not have access to it. And that 72 percent of children living with HIV who are eligible for treatment do not have access.

been aggressively treated with ARV medications soon after their infection. Unlike the baby, they still had traces of HIV but their own immune systems seemed to be keeping the virus at a near-undetectable level. The researchers consider these patients "post-treatment HIV controllers" in "long-term remission," and "functionally cured."

The indications of the French patients may be that early aggressive ART may be effective at preventing the HIV virus from creating a reservoir of HIV-infected cells, thus giving the patient's own body the chance to control the virus naturally. This form of cure is sometimes termed a "functional cure" because the body's own defenses seem to control the virus even after the suspension of medication. A month later, AmfAR published an article in which a further distinction was made (Johnston 2013). A "sterilization cure" is considered such because it eliminates all traces of the virus from the body rather than merely controlling the virus. According to Johnson (2013), the man known as the "Berlin patient" and the baby "may be as close to a sterilizing cure as we will ever come." Johnston states, however, that there is still much that is not well understood about these cases, and it must be noted further that they are confined to the West.[16] It seems likely that due to the various limitations noted above, cures for "the rest" are probably a long way off.

The discovery and success of new AIDS treatments, treatments as prevention, and possible functional cures, also have implications in that they have changed and will further change the face of AIDS. A key element in the social meaning attributed to AIDS (a product of a shared cultural model) in the early years was the infectious and fatal nature of the disease (i.e., AIDS as a death sentence). With the advent of new treatments and the widespread use of these combination-drug therapies, however, the cultural model of AIDS then shifted to being understood as a manageable chronic disease, much like diabetes (the idea of "living with AIDS"). And with a potential cure in sight (i.e., a functional or sterilization cure), the cultural model of HIV and AIDS is likely to shift again—at least in the geopolitical areas where functional cures are available. This will be discussed further in the next section.

2.2 AIDS as social construction

As discussed above, AIDS is a biomedical reality, but it is also a reality as a social construction. As Fee and Fox (1992:9) claim, "AIDS is a particularly

---

[16]In two other cases in Boston, two men who were HIV-positive underwent bone-marrow transplants and then discontinued use of antiretroviral drugs, without any signs of HIV for months; however, their infections have recently reappeared. On the other hand, Ray Brown, the "Berlin patient," and the HIV-positive baby are still thought to be cured." http://www.pbs.org/newshour/rundown/2013/12/hiv-reappears-in-two-boston-patients-thought-to-be-cured.html.

good example of the social construction of disease." Further building on this hypothesis, they contend that AIDS, the syndrome associated with the HIV virus, is more of a social construction than a biomedical reality (Fox and Fee 1992:10). Various other authors, making this same claim to varying degrees, also allude to this social side of AIDS. Schoepf, for instance, commenting on her research in Zaire, states that "AIDS may be usefully viewed as socially produced" (1992:260). Farmer (1992:xi) contends that "the world pandemic of AIDS and social responses to it have been patterned by social arrangements." Herdt (Herdt and Lindenbaum 1992:3) claims that "culture shapes our response to the disease." And Susan Sontag (1988) demonstrates that people used familiar metaphors to make meaning of AIDS when it first emerged.

Medical anthropology has recognized that cultural models of health and illness are strongly influenced and shaped by cultural factors. AIDS is no exception. It has been said of the Western medical model that a patient comes to the doctor's office with an illness but departs with a disease (Treichler 1992:75). Thus, illness is "the culturally defined feelings and perceptions of physical and mental ailments and disability in the minds of people in specific communities," while disease is recognized as the "formally taught definition of physical and mental pathology from the point of view of the medical profession" (Pelto and Pelto 1996:302). It seems that both the illness of AIDS and the disease of AIDS (as defined above), at least in part, are culturally informed.

As alluded to previously, however, one must make a distinction between illness and disease as pure cultural construction (i.e., no "truth" behind the biomedical model) and illness and disease as a product of the interaction between natural law and culture. John Gagnon (1992:33) makes a useful distinction between "epistemological doubters" and "methodological doubters" when it comes to the evaluation of science, whether hard or soft. The former (the epistemological doubters) argue that researchers do not discover facts; rather they participate in their production and reproduction. He characterizes this as the position of Foucault and others who express an extreme postmodern position of social constructionism. For those in this camp, scientific "facts" are purely the product of social construction. The latter (the methodological doubters) recognize the limitations of theory, the imperfection of techniques and the often error-laden nature of data, but also recognize that there is, indeed, an underlying natural order in the universe that scientific tools can help at least approximate.

Methodological doubters, of which I am one, recognize the role of culture in shaping our perceptions but hold that through refinement of theories, improvement of techniques, limitation of bias and reduction of data error, we, in our human effort called "science," may at least approximate some of the true parameters of nature. For epistemological doubters no such thing as objective truth even exists. For methodological doubters, the discovery of approximate objective truth, while embedded in human culture, is at least attemptable.

There is also a danger, however, in minimizing the role of culture in the production of scientific fact. Farmer (1992), for instance, demonstrates that the construction of the biomedical model of AIDS in America in the early years of the epidemic was strongly influenced as much by the North American folk model of Haitians (which posited certain Haitian voodoo practices as the cause of AIDS) as it was by biomedical science.[17] One must strive for reason in the balance between these two positions.

Whether or not one stands in the first camp (of epistemological doubt- ers), or, as I do, the second (of methodological doubters), both groups ac- knowledge that culture shapes our perceptions of illness and disease. This is true of AIDS as well.

2.2.1 Various cultural models of AIDS

There are various socially constructed cultural models of AIDS around the world.[18] Paul Farmer (1994), for instance, traces the development of a cultural model of AIDS in Haiti. Farmer's research illustrates a widely shared representation of the new disorder that has developed over time. To the Haitian, AIDS (known as SIDA in Haiti) is conceptually understood as (1) a new disease; (2) strongly associated with skin infections, "drying up," tuberculosis, and diarrhea; (3) can be caused "naturally" (via sex) or "unnaturally" ("sent" to another through a kind of witchcraft); (4) caused by a microbe; (5) transmitted by contact with "dirty blood;" and (6) is viewed as a product of a larger problem of North American imperialism, lack of class solidarity among the poor, and corruption among the ruling elite (Farmer 1994:805–806).

Although not explicitly identified as a cultural model of AIDS, various widely shared conceptions about AIDS have existed in America since the in- ception of the disease. Using several recent histories about AIDS, a cultural model can be posited which developed during the early years of the epi- demic here in America. As mentioned previously, the first component of this cultural model was that AIDS was a "gay disease" (American Foundation for AIDS Research 1999:376; Flynn and Lound 1995:11; Giblin 1995:197).

---

[17]Farmer suggests that a newly-emerging American folk model of Haitians (that was strongly influenced by the U.S. daily press reports about Haitian immigrants) informed the developing cultural model of AIDS, which early on posited a Haitian origin for the disease. This North American cultural model of Haitians imagined all Haitians as "ragged, wretched, pathetic, superstitious, disease-ridden, backward peasants (Farmer 1992:4).

[18]By "cultural model" Farmer means "some sort of consensus," or "collective representation" of what is meant by AIDS.

This concept soon widened to include other marginalized "bad people" such as intravenous drug users (Flynn and Lound 1995:14; Herdt 1999:3). This, coupled with the second element of the early model that AIDS is infectious, resulted in stigmatization toward the disease and anyone associated with it. The final, and perhaps most powerful element of the newly emerging cultural model, was that AIDS was fatal (Flynn and Lound 1995:55). This recognition often led to irrational fear. People feared touching HIV positive persons (Flynn and Lound 1995:55) or even sitting near them (Giblin 1995:135). We feared using utensils that AIDS infected persons might have used (Flynn and Lound 1995:56; Giblin 1995:135). We even feared getting AIDS by sitting on public toilet seats (American Foundation for AIDS Research 1999:376; Giblin 1995:134). These were all elements of the early cultural model, or what meaning people associated with AIDS during the early years of the epidemic in America.

While the average American (following the early cultural model) took refuge in AIDS only being a gay disease, the early cultural model developing in Britain focused on AIDS as a life-threatening heterosexual disease of epidemic proportion which was a "danger to the general population rather than a specific 'risk' group" (Berridge 1992:52). This is not to say that there were not some in Britain who associated AIDS with the gay community, but those who were involved in early education, and therefore the formulation of a wider cultural model, focused their efforts on the "need for public education to stress the heterosexual nature of the disease rather than the 'gay plague' angle of the popular press" (Berridge 1992:59). This had its impact upon the resultant cultural model of AIDS in Britain. Like in America, fear was a major early reaction to the newly emerging life-threatening disease, but the use of public policy to construct a cultural model that considered such fear as unwarranted "moral panic," had a positive impact upon popular views in Britain. So, although the early British cultural model shared some features with the American model (fatal and infectious), it also differed in significant ways that lead to the formulation of a different cultural model of AIDS in the two countries.

If one were to analyze in the same way the countries of Africa, where the infection attacks men and women equally, other cultural models of AIDS would emerge. Cultural models are a unique combination of factors. There may be shared elements in the cultural models of AIDS in many cultures, but the unique situations specific to each culture may also affect the construction of various unique cultural models of AIDS, as has been demonstrated. Nepal has yet different cultural models of AIDS; cultural models based on her unique culture, history (including political structure), economy, geography, and religion. Having made the point that different cultures construct different cultural models of AIDS, however, we will see in the next section that one characteristic of a cultural model is its ability to change over time.

2.2.2 The changing face of AIDS

One major feature of cultural models is that they are dynamic. Farmer (1994) and Berridge (1992) have both traced the change of the dominant cultural model of AIDS through the years in Haiti and Britain, respectively. The "face of AIDS" in America has also changed through time. In the early years, AIDS was perceived to be a fatal, infectious disease. Then with the advent of the newly available ARTs in the mid to late 1990s, the image of AIDS in the USA, as in the rest of the developed world, began to be modified from understanding AIDS as an "acute" problem to more of a "chronic" condition (Herdt 1992:11). Even though the numbers of new HIV infections was on the rise in the USA at that time, the death rate for AIDS related deaths dropped in 1996 for the first time since the advent of the epidemic (The Register-Guard 1997:1). The American media then boasted that "AIDS has been contained."[19] Furthermore, it proclaimed that the once certain "death sentence" had then become a "chronic manageable condition" (Treichler 1992:88).

A National Public Radio story (NPR 1999) at the end of the century even featured HIV positive couples having children, an idea that was once taboo for HIV-infected persons. This trend illustrated the shifting cultural model of AIDS in America. With improved prospects for longevity provided by the new drugs—life expectancies had increased from months to decades—many couples with HIV wanted to start families. New technologies, such as a new method of *in vitro* fertilization that included "sperm washing," were also reducing the risk of passing the virus to unborn children. The available new drug therapies began changing the cultural model of AIDS for those who were HIV positive. On the radio program, one HIV positive interviewee commenting on his improved health said, "For ten years we had been waiting for an illness that would be the final one. Now we say, dammit, let's start living." Another HIV-positive interviewee added:

> If you asked me five years ago whether people with HIV should have children I would have said no. Medicine is so improved now that I've gone from close to death—very sick—to undetectable levels of the virus in my system. I am able to work and function normally. And that's something I couldn't do five years ago.

This man's wife, also HIV positive, speaking about HIV in the past said, "It was definitely a death sentence then. You were given your diagnosis and out into the world you went. And you waited like a time bomb for the bomb to explode." This couple's nine-year-old daughter, also HIV positive from birth, commented that her friends at school considered her "lucky" to have HIV. She said that her friends didn't make a big deal of her HIV status and

---

[19]This comment was made by a commentator of the Voice of America Radio Service in discussing the recent therapies now available for AIDS sufferers.

that they even considered her lucky because she got to go to special camps and do other neat things that her friends didn't get to do. In response to her comment, the commentator asked in surprise, "Do you feel lucky to have HIV?" The girl responded in the affirmative, echoing the response of her friends regarding the "neat opportunities" and also added that her trips to the doctor had been fun. She was also on the new medications and hadn't yet been sick. It is clear that the cultural model of HIV and AIDS had begun to change dramatically for these people. The motif of the AIDS sufferer went from "dying from AIDS," to "living with AIDS."

Around this same time there was another interesting and dangerous phenomenon that began to take place in the American and other nations' cultural models of AIDS. What some researchers refer to as "AIDS fatigue" had set in. Singer (1999) reported the words of one of Thailand's leading AIDS workers: "We've become used to AIDS because someone is dying here every day…today no one is afraid." It seems that the message had become so prominent that many were just getting tired of hearing about AIDS and being afraid of it. Couple that with the cultural model change of AIDS as a deadly, infectious disease, to a chronic manageable condition, and you have a problem. *Time* magazine then reported that although death rates were lower, "the numbers of new HIV infections is holding steady at over forty thousand per year, and researchers reported a surge in unsafe sex practices" (*Time* 1998). This was a stark contrast to a report published in Time magazine in 1994 which cited fear of contracting AIDS as the biggest concern of youths between the ages of nine and seventeen (Giblin 1995:184). It seemed that fear of contracting AIDS was just not as strong of an issue anymore. This AIDS fatigue trend began in the late 1990s and continues to the present. It is so prevalent today that Wikipedia (2012) dedicates a page to discuss the topic, AIDS activists blame it for decreasing contemporary media coverage of related issues (Bjerk 2012), and Peter Piot (the former head of UNAIDS) accuses it of affecting ongoing AIDS funding (Bloomberg 2010).

At the thirtieth anniversary of HIV and AIDS we can clearly define two specific cultural models evenly dividing the thirty-year span. According to Dr. Michael Saag:

> If we divide the 30 years in half—literally, 15 years—the first half was death, dying, huge stigma, isolation and, to some degree, hopelessness. Through this remarkable investment—in particular, by the NIH and our government and pharmaceutical companies working together—within a very short period of time, the virus was discovered, drugs were identified that actually worked dramatically well, such that by 1996, we had what we now call HAART or triple drug therapy that totally transformed the face of AIDS. Such that over the last 15 years, HIV has been converted from a death sentence to a chronic manageable condition that

someone diagnosed today can live a normal lifespan if they take the medicines regularly and they get the virus in check. That's remarkable. (NPR 2011)

So the evolution of this cultural model is clear—from AIDS as a death sentence, characterized by death and dying (1981–1986)—to the time of ART, where AIDS is viewed as a chronic manageable disease (1997–2012), and is perhaps best characterized as a time of hope.[20] One must wonder, with the possibility of a cure at the doorstep, if another shift in the cultural model of AIDS is just around the corner; a cultural model of "being cured of AIDS," or of the possibility of the elimination of the AIDS epidemic altogether?

2.2.3 Aids as socioeconomic disease—the continuing gap

As we have seen, AIDS is a biomedical reality and it is a sociocultural construction. Because of the statistics, we must conclude that AIDS is a socioeconomic disease as well. At the time of the first edition of this book, the inner cities of the U.S. as well as the African American and Hispanic populations had been hit hardest by the epidemic (Flynn and Lound 1995:56; Singer 1999) and it had been predicted that the world's underdeveloped nations would likely bear the brunt of the AIDS epidemic in the future (Flynn and Lound 1995:60; Singer 1999). Prospects of declining interest in the subject (due to the advent of new treatments and the phenomenon of AIDS fatigue) in the West had AIDS experts worried that there would be a growing gap between the rich and poor nations of the world in regard to AIDS. This "growing gap between rich and poor nations" was even the focus of the World AIDS conference held in Geneva (1998). In Europe and North America, AIDS treatments (ART) were developed that cut the death rate significantly, but the spread of HIV and AIDS in the third world continued unabated. It seemed that AIDS was quickly becoming a disease of the poor, both internationally and within nations. Merrill Singer (1999) asked the appropriate question: "How do we ensure that the new AIDS treatments are not the exclusive property of people in rich countries and rich people in other countries?" As I alluded to earlier, the cost of AIDS treatment was outside the realm of possibilities for many third-world governments and individuals at that time. The Economist reported (1997) the expectation that these new therapies would cost over ten thousand dollars yearly, and that "nine out of ten people who contract AIDS live in countries where $10,000 a year exceeds by many times the gross domestic product per head."

A newspaper article from that time (The Register-Guard 1997) demonstrated another facet of this socioeconomic issue: profits. In a South African court, U.S. pharmaceutical companies (with U.S. government assistance)

---

[20]Although this cultural model would also include the problem of AIDS fatigue.

were seeking to block a new law that allowed generic versions of AIDS drugs (generic copies of those that were available in America) to be manufactured locally or imported without permission of the patent holder. The U.S. companies challenged the law on the grounds of patent infringement. The goal of the law was to reduce the cost of the AIDS-fighting drugs, making them more affordable for their populace. The drug companies argued that the law "undermines their industry's multibillion dollar research efforts and could hinder the development of new AIDS-fighting medicines." Critics charged that the move was all about profits, a charge that seems warranted. The companies claimed sensitivity to the dire epidemic in the third world, but insisted that the pharmaceutical industry "must protect the rights of its companies to profit from their research."

So ten years later where do we stand? Around the world overall HIV infection rates are mostly in decline (as noted previously).[21] Despite that fact, it was acknowledged recently at the International AIDS Conference (2012) that hunger and malnutrition are now significant obstacles to the global fight against HIV (World Food Program 2012).[22] And hunger and malnutrition are generally problems of poverty. Likewise, the Center for Disease Control (CDC 2012) continues to report that "Poverty can limit access to health care, HIV testing, and medications that can lower levels of HIV in the blood and help prevent transmission. In addition, those who cannot afford the basics in life may end up in circumstances that increase their HIV risk."

So on the global level, socioeconomic disparity would seemingly still play a role in the unequal success of treatment. And if cuts to global ART subsidies spoken of earlier become a reality, only the rich countries and the rich in poor countries will continue to benefit from the medical advances available.

And even in the developed world, socioeconomics still creates an obvious divide in the epidemic as well. In Washington D.C., America's capital, the HIV prevalence rate is higher than the third world countries of Gambia, the Democratic Republic of Congo, and Senegal (Boseley 2012a).[23] If the

---

[21]According to UNAIDS (2012) the number of people newly infected in the Middle East and North Africa increased by more than 35% (and is "concentrated among injecting drug users, men who have sex with men, and sex workers and their clients") and there have also been increases in new HIV infections in Europe and Central Asia (associated with the surge in injecting drug use in 2000 and mainly concentrated among injecting drug users, sex workers and their clients and partners, and men who have sex with men) and an associated increase in AIDS-related deaths in Eastern Europe and Central Asia (21%) and the Middle East and North Africa (17%). I have seen no clear connection made yet between socioeconomic factors and the particular drivers noted for the epidemic in these regions.

[22]A new emphasis in HIV prevention has to do with keeping people healthy. Poor nutrition and hunger weakens the body, making ART less effective overall.

[23]In 2009, Washington D.C. had an estimated HIV prevalence rate of 3.2% (CIA 2012).

city were its own nation it would tie with Togo as the twenty-second worst nation in the world in regard to its estimated HIV infection rate; this at a time when the nation's overall infection rate (0.6%) would place it at number sixty-four overall in the world.[24] So, what explains the discrepancy? Poverty (*The Guardian* 2012). And in 2011 Dr. Michael Sagg, Director of the Center for AIDS Research at University of Alabama was asked, if despite the progress mentioned earlier, there was still any particular American population remaining in the "bulls-eye" of the epidemic. Dr. Sagg responded, "It's mostly people of lower income and especially minorities. And in Alabama, in rural areas, there is a large number of people who are HIV-infected and don't know it, and that's the tragedy" (NPR 2011). So, even with the ability to treat HIV and AIDS in the West, it is the poor, mostly minorities who continue to suffer the most. It seems as if the socioeconomic gap noted ten years ago remains a reality even into the present.

2.3 Chapter conclusion

Between the time of the first discovery of a handful of AIDS cases in the USA (1981) and the early 1990s, AIDS had become one of the worst epidemics the world had ever known. By then over four million people had died, several million more were living with HIV, and it seemed as if AIDS was spreading like "wildfire."[25] Prevalence rates in some countries of Southern Africa were estimated to be near 30–40 percent and predictions for the future were dire (Knight 2008). In response, the United Nations established the Joint United Nations Programme on HIV and AIDS (UNAIDS) in 1996 in an effort to more effectively deal with the growing pandemic. However, by the early 2000s, mostly due to better surveillance, the original figures for Sub-Saharan Africa began to be revised downward (Asamoah-Odei et al. 2004). And since 70 percent of the cases presumed to exist at that time were in that region, the prediction for the overall size of the epidemic was adjusted significantly as well. Although still very significant—nine of forty-one countries in the region still list prevalence rates of between 11 percent and 25 percent as of 2010 (UNAIDS Global Report 2010)—prevalence rate figures are now half of what they once were. The overall prevalence for the region is now listed at around 5 percent (UNAIDS 2011).

As estimates were modified downward and our understanding of the epidemic grew, fear lessened that AIDS around the world would ever reach the

---

[24]Interestingly, Nepal with an estimated prevalence rate of 0.4 percent in 2009 (CIA 2012) would rank number 71 in the list of countries.

[25]There is a game by this same name still used by prevention educators in Nepal to graphically illustrate how HIV spreads. Unfortunately it assumes multiple concurrent partners, which is not the norm in Nepal. It can induce greater fear (and therefore stigma) toward AIDS than is warranted; therefore I have suggested it be discontinued in the prevention curriculum.

rates seen (or over estimated) in sub-Saharan Africa.[26] Prevalence rates grew only modestly among the general population of the world over the next few years, and then came the discoveries and application of ART in the mid to late 1990s. As the pandemic peaked and actually began to decline globally around 2000, some began to question whether AIDS still warranted an "exceptional status" (Smith and Whiteside 2010:47).[27] In response, the WHO and UNAIDS announced they would take a common stand against the three deadly communicable diseases of HIV and AIDS, tuberculosis, and malaria (WHO 2000).[28] Although political will to fight these epidemics had been established, in 2001 United Nations Secretary General Kofi Annan called for the creation of a global fund to channel additional resources, and in 2002 the Global Fund to Fight AIDS, Tuberculosis, and Malaria (known simply as "The Global Fund") was established and has become a major conduit for funding for the trio of remaining worldwide epidemics.[29]

Even though global prevalence rates are now lower than once thought and new HIV infections and AIDS-related deaths are down overall, HIV and AIDS still continues to warrant our attention. Three-quarters of AIDS-related deaths take place in the Sub-Saharan Africa region and the highest prevalence rates are among the productive age group, resulting in a missing generation, which in turn creates huge social issues (e.g., AIDS orphans, grandmothers having to raise their grandchildren, not enough "workers," etc.). The destruction of human capital retards economic growth in these already poor areas, intensifying poverty and resulting in a higher susceptibility to HIV, which has been linked to malnutrition, a byproduct of poverty. Also, in many of the third-world countries of the world, the co-infective relationship between HIV and TB is concerning (I will talk about this in relationship to Nepal in the next chapter).

Meantime in the West, the cultural model has shifted from a death sentence to a chronic manageable treatment, with a cure even possibly in sight

---

[26]For instance, an association was made between the cultural practice of multiple concurrent partners (MCP) in the countries where HIV prevalence rates were highest, thus although problematic (particularly among "high risk" groups), the prevalence rates in the general public were never expected to reach the levels where MCP was practiced.

[27]With the downward revisions of estimates and the reductions of deaths related to new available treatments it became apparent that nearly as many people die yearly of TB, yet there was not a specially designated UN program to fight this equally deadly disease. For instance, in 2009 there were 1.8 million reported AIDS-related deaths (UNAIDS 2011) and 1.7 million deaths attributed to Tuberculosis (WHO 2010) for the same period.

[28]In 2009, 781,000 deaths were attributed to Malaria (WHO World Malaria Report 2010).

[29]As of 2013, the Global fund was supporting more than 1,000 programs in 151 countries (Global Fund 2013).

(as noted previously). But even in the developed West there are problems with the increase in new infection rates among some populations as AIDS fatigue has set in and the poor have unequal access to ARVs and HIV education, as noted earlier. And new issues of medical complications associated with antiretroviral treatment and questions about quality of life for some even in developed countries have emerged, placing more realistic parameters upon our expectations for ART.[30] In response to the recent trajectory of HIV and AIDS worldwide, the Executive Director of UNAIDS, Michel Sidibé, expresses both hope and concern:

> Hope because significant progress has been made towards universal access. New HIV infections have dropped. Fewer children are born with HIV. And more than 4 million people are on treatment.
>
> Concern because 28 years into the epidemic the virus continues to make inroads into new populations; stigma and discrimination continue to undermine efforts to turn back the epidemic. The violation of human rights of people living with HIV, women and girls, men who have sex with men, injecting drug users and sex workers must end. (Sidibé 2009)

And UNAIDS and WHO in their combined AIDS Epidemic Update (2009:8) conclude:

> AIDS continues to be a major global health priority. Although important progress has been achieved in preventing new HIV infections and in lowering the annual number of AIDS related deaths, the number of people living with HIV continues to increase. AIDS-related illnesses remain one of the leading causes of death globally and are projected to continue as a significant global cause of premature mortality in the coming decades (WHO 2008). Although AIDS is no longer a new syndrome, global solidarity in the AIDS response will remain a necessity.

Since the first edition of this book (2003), the changing face of HIV and AIDS is certainly evident. HIV-related mortality rates have peaked and the total number of people living with the virus in 2008 was more than 20 percent higher than the number in 2000. At that same time the number of infections had fallen over the preceding eight-year period (and was 30 percent lower than at the epidemic's apparent peak in 1996). It is clear, however, that our work with HIV and AIDS globally is not done. In this chapter we

---

[30]Recent studies have indicated that there is an association between ART and premature cognitive aging in HIV patients under treatment (Deeks and Phillips 2009). Likewise, regarding quality of life, an article from the Guardian (Boseley 2012b) concludes that while HIV survivors in the West are alive, many are facing poverty, loneliness and prejudice.

have looked at AIDS from a biomedical, social and socioeconomic view. We have examined the construction of various cultural models of AIDS around the world noting that each is specifically unique to the social and cultural factors that have influenced their formation. We have also examined the new treatments which are changing the face of AIDS around the world and have also considered the various social and socioeconomic factors that are continuing the gap between the rich and poor and between the West and the rest in their fight against AIDS. Next, we will examine more specifically AIDS in Nepal.

3

AIDS in Nepal

At the time of the first edition of this book (2003) there were some pretty dire predictions being made regarding the HIV and AIDS epidemic in Nepal. The number of AIDS cases had increased fifteenfold over a three-year period (1990–93) and was expected to reach 100,000 cases by the year 2000 (Suvedi et al. 1994). The total number of HIV-infected persons in South and Southeast Asia had surpassed the total number of infected persons in the industrialized world (Dhalburg 1994), and at the 1996 worldwide conference on AIDS it was estimated that India, Nepal's giant neighbor, had more HIV-infected persons (3-5 million) than any other country in the world (Spaeth 1996). Given the geographical proximity and historical relationship of trade between India and Nepal, it was expected that AIDS would grow at an alarming rate in Nepal as well. There was also frequent travel of both tourists and nationals between Thailand and Nepal, and Dixit (1996:50) suggested that "Nepal's overwhelming reliance on tourism for foreign exchange also increases the possibility of easy access for the virus. Nepal has direct links (through sex workers and businessmen) with the two cities with highest and second highest prevalence of HIV infection in Asia—Bangkok and Bombay."

In 2003, Thailand had one of the highest incidences of HIV infection in Asia (World Health Organization estimated two to four million by year 2000) and migration between Nepal and Thailand seemed likely to further facilitate the spread of HIV and AIDS into Nepal. As one author warned, all of these factors pointed to an expected "coming crisis" for Nepal (Seddon 1995:2).

Ten years later, HIV and AIDS has not become the crisis we had once expected it to become. As mentioned previously, estimates for nearby India were revised downward and the current estimates for Nepal place the prevalence adult rates among the general population at just 0.3 percent (NCASC 2012), well below even the United States. This is better news than the earlier predictions. However, HIV and AIDS in Nepal still warrant our attention. HIV remains a concentrated epidemic among several high risk groups, and the connection in Nepal between HIV and drug resistant [1] tuberculosis is very concerning for the future. So, while there has been progress, many of the factors that influence the discrepancy between the west and the rest (spoken of earlier) still impact Nepal as well.

The purpose of this chapter will be to examine in-depth the current HIV and AIDS situation in Nepal. This will include a presentation of the most current epidemiological information as well as a critical examination of the literature published on HIV and AIDS in Nepal. I will discuss the various HIV and AIDS prevention models that have been promoted in Nepal and introduce the major Nepali discourses on HIV and AIDS that have emerged since the AIDS epidemic arrived in Nepal. I will also introduce the key ideas associated with AIDS in the literature—ideas, which we will see in later chapters, have been influential in the creation of a dominant cultural model of HIV and AIDS in Nepal.

3.1 The epidemiological "facts"

The first case of AIDS was identified in Nepal in July 1988 (Suvedi 1998:53). Since then, the numbers have grown slowly but steadily. Or at least we think so. When talking about numbers in the context of Nepal, it is important to make a distinction between estimated HIV cases and reported cases of HIV and AIDS. Figures 3.1 and 3.2 display the latest cumulative estimates reported by Nepal's National Center for AIDS and STD Control, the agency responsible for tracking such statistics nationwide (NCASC 2012a). Figure 3.3 displays the cumulative reported (i.e., "tested and confirmed") number to date (NCASC 2012b).

---

[1]An HIV epidemic is considered "concentrated" when the HIV infection prevalence rate is above 5% in any high risk group while at the same time the overall infection rate for the general population is less than 1%. An epidemic is considered "generalized" when more than 1% of the general population is infected (UNICEF 2008).

Government of Nepal
Ministry of Health and Population **National Centre for AIDS and STD Control** Teku, Kathmandu

Factsheet N°1: HIV Epidemic Update of Nepal, As of July, 2012

Facts about HIV Epidemic in Nepal

- The first HIV infection was detected in 1988 in Nepal. Since then HIV and AIDS epidemic has evolved from low to concentrated among **High Risk Groups:**
  - Injecting drug users (IDUs),
  - Men who have sex with men (MSM),
  - Female sex workers (FSWs),
  - Clients of female sex workers, and
  - Seasonal male labour migrants.
- Heterosexual transmission is dominant.
- HIV prevalence in general population is <1%.

Situation of HIV in Nepal, 2011

- Estimated number of HIV infections (2011) by age groups:
  - Children (0-14 years): 3,804
  - Adults (15-49 years): 43,239
  - Adults (50+ years): 3,244
- Adult (15-49) HIV prevalence: 0.3%
- Adult women (15-49) living with HIV: 28%
- Young people (15-24) living with HIV: 10.2%
- Estimated newly infected in 2011: 1,437

Source: NCASC, 2012

Table 1: Estimated HIV Infections by Risk Population Groups, 2011

Population sub-groups (15-49 years)	Total infections	% share
Injecting drug users	939	2.2
MSWs, transgender and clients	3,099	7.2
Other MSM who do not sell and/or buy sex	6,245	14.4
Female sex workers	647	1.5
Clients of sex workers	1,915	4.4
Male labour migrants	11,672	27
Remaining male Population	6,914	16
Remaining female Population	11,808	27.3
Total	43,239	100

Source: NCASC, 2012

Figure 1: Adult (15-49) HIV Prevalence, 2011

0.3%

1980 1985 1990 1995 2000 2005 2011 2015

Source: NCASC, 2012

Figure 2: Estimated HIV Infections vs. Estimated HIV Prevalence in 2011

	Injection Drug Users (IDUs)	MSW, TG and Clients	Other MSM who do not sell and/or buy sex	Female Sex Workers (FSWs)	Clients of FSWs	Male Labour Migrants	Male Remaining Population	Female Remaining Population
Infections	1,367	3,345	6,724	650	2,440	13,219	7,378	12,522
Prevalence	4.4%	4.5%	3.8%	2.5%	0.3%	1.0%	0.2%	0.2%

Source: NCASC, 2011

Figure 3.1. 2012 Estimated HIV infections in Nepal: Part one. (Source: NCASC, 2012 [as of 15 July 2012], used by permission)

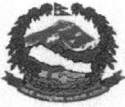

Government of Nepal
Ministry of Health and Population **National
Centre for AIDS and STD Control** Teku,
Kathmandu

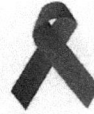

Figure 3: Distribution of Estimated HIV Infections by Sub-Population Groups, 1980-2015

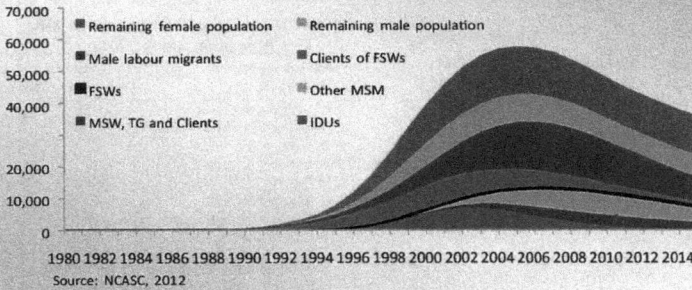

Remaining female population   Remaining male population

Male labour migrants   Clients of FSWs

FSWs   Other MSM

MSW, TG and Clients   IDUs

1980 1982 1984 1986 1988 1990 1992 1994 1996 1998 2000 2002 2004 2006 2008 2010 2012 2014

Source: NCASC, 2012

- Heterosexual transmission is the major route of spreading HIV in Nepal. About 80% infections are through sexual transmission.
- Injecting drug users, female sex workers and their clients, men who have sex with other men and male labour migrants (primarily to high HIV prevalence areas in India) are the key high risk groups driving the epidemic.
- Further intensifying the effective targeted quality interventions for high risk groups with improved coverage is critical to contain the epidemic among high risk groups and to prevent spread into general low risk population.

Table 2: Key Indicators of HIV and AIDS Situation in Nepal, 2011

Indicators	Value (2011)
Adult (15-49) HIV prevalence	0.3%
Proportion of women 15-49 living with HIV	28.2%
Proportion of women and girls 15-24 living with HIV	4.2%
Average number of new infections per year (% male newly infected)	1,437 (65%)
Average number of new infections per day	4
Average number of new infections amongst children (0-14) per year	378
Average number of AIDS deaths in year 2011	4,722
Average number of AIDS deaths among children (0-14) in 2011	277
Average number of AIDS deaths among children (0-4) in 2011	157
Total number of AIDS orphans till 2011	12,904
Average number of AIDS orphans in 2011	713

Source: NCASC, 2012

Figure 3.2. 2012 Estimated HIV infections in Nepal: Part two.
(Source: NCASC, 2012 [as of 15 July 2012], used by permission)

Ministry of Health and Population
National Centre for AIDS and STD Control

Cumulative HIV and AIDS Situation of Nepal
As of Asad 2069 (15 July, 2012)

Total HIV infections reported	Male	Female	TG	Total	Cases Reported in This Month
	13,157	7,417	9	20,583	216

Cumulative HIV infection by sub-group and sex

Sub-groups	Male	Female	TG	Total	Cases Reported in This Month
Sex Workers (SW)	27	997	0	1,024	15
Injecting Drug Users	2,750	70	3	2,823 *	7
Men having Sex with Men (MSM)/TG	250	-	6	256	7
Blood or Organ Recipients	49	19	0	68	3
Clients of Sex Worker	8,651	121	0	8,772	35
Housewives	-	5,331	0	5,331	33
Male Partners	97	-	0	97 **	9
Migrant Workers	376	22	0	398	53
Spouse of Migrant	19	250	0	269	26
Prison Inmates	-	-	0	-	0
Children	829	543	0	1,372	19
Sub-group NOT identified	109	64	0	173	9
Total	13,157	7,417	9	20,583	216

* Mode of Transmission – IDUs or
Sexual
** Male Partners of FSW/Female IDU/Female Migrant

Cumulative HIV infection by age group and sex

Age group (Years)	Male	Female	TG	Total	Cases Reported in This Month
0 - 4	325	193		518	10
5 - 9	359	244		603	6
10 - 14	153	104		257	1
15 - 19	306	334	1	641	6
20 - 24	1,461	1,105	2	2,568	17
25 - 29	2,703	1,693		4,396	30
30 - 39	5,341	2,617	5	7,963	86
40 - 49	1,962	880		2,842	45
50 - above	547	247	1	795	15
Total	13,157	7,417	9	20,583	216

Source: NCASC, 2012 [as of 15 July 2012]

Figure 3.3. 2012 Cumulative HIV and AIDS infection reported in Nepal.
(Source: NCASC, 2012 [as of 15 July 2012], used by permission)

According to the estimated figures (fig. 3.1), just over fifty thousand persons are thought to currently be living with HIV in Nepal (0.3% prevalence among the general population). Of this number, 86 percent (43,239) are estimated to be adults aged fifteen to forty-nine, 8 percent (3,804) children aged zero to fourteen, and 6 percent (3,244) adults over fifty. According to these estimates, heterosexual transmission is still the dominant form of HIV transmission and HIV infection rates remain at "concentrated epidemic" levels among several high-risk populations, such as injecting drug users (IDU), men who have sex with men (MSM), female sex workers (FSWs), clients of female sex workers and seasonal migrant laborers. The NCASC concludes that "further intensifying the effective targeted interventions for high risk groups with improved coverage is critical to contain the epidemic among high risk groups and to prevent spread into large general low risk population" (NCASC 2012a). Likewise, USAID claims that due to targeted prevention interventions among these key population groups, new infections rates have decreased significantly over the past five years and that Nepal is "on track" to achieve the sixth Millennium Development Goal.[2] They acknowledge, however, that "it is critical to improve coverage in order for HIV and AIDS programs to reach the national target of halving new HIV infections by 2015. In addition, despite continuous efforts to combat stigma and discrimination, such barriers have remained major impediments to open access to information and services"(USAID 2013a).

According to the reported figures (fig. 3.2), the numbers for the same period are less than half of the estimated number. Interestingly there is clear continuity (and even verbatim language) between the National Center estimated statistics (figs. 3.1 and 3.2) and UNICEF, UNAIDS, USAIDS, and WHO estimates. The "HIV epidemic update of Nepal," provided by the National Center, cites "NCASC 2011" and "NCASC 2012" for its data, but there is no explanation about how the National Center derives their estimates. It is hard to tell whether these organizations mentioned earlier get their estimates from the National Center or vice versa? As one who has studied HIV and AIDS in Nepal for well over a decade, I am always mystified as to how these estimated numbers are derived.[3]

To be fair, it has always been difficult to accurately assess HIV numbers in Nepal. In the early years of the epidemic, reporting of AIDS was thought to be very low (Suvedi 1998:53). At that time, Dixit (1996:46) concluded that "there can be no doubt that there have been deaths in Nepal from AIDS which were not recognized" and that "there are probably people ill with AIDS today whose condition has not been diagnosed." Often times, people died in a village and the actual cause of death was never actually determined. Also, because of the nature of AIDS, often the cause of death was reported (if at all) simply as an opportunistic infection and no association with AIDS was ever made. In most places in Nepal, HIV tests were then unavailable. Even if they were available, many were not interested in determining if they were HIV positive, either because of lack of awareness about HIV, prohibitive cost involved in getting such a test, or desire to avoid the social stigma then attached to HIV positive persons in Nepal. Measuring prevalence (known as "sentinel surveillance") was initiated among the general public but was far from successful due to various logistical problems (Maskey 1998). And

[2]The Millennium Development Goals (MDG) are a set of eight international development goals established by the United Nations in 2000, which are intended to "end poverty by 2015." MDG number 6 addresses HIV, with the target of having reversed and halved the spread of HIV by 2015.

[3]There are also other anomalies in the data from the National Center. For instance, if one totals the numbers listing all estimated infections by age categories it equals 50,287, while grouping by risk-group categories totals 43,239, and when all the numbers listed for figure two on that same page are added the total is 47,645.

today many of these factors still prevent accurate counting. According to the Director of the NCASC, the biggest barrier to accurate numbers today is that little headway has been made in testing (Sharma 2010). Dr. Rai admits that Nepal still "lags behind" in identifying infected cases who remain "hidden" in "fear of exposing themselves to the public" and concedes "the unidentified infected cases are exactly the reason why Nepal will not be able to meet the Millennium Development Goal (MDG) of halting and reversing the spread of HIV and AIDS by 2015" (Sharma 2010). So while various international agencies working from estimated numbers are touting Nepal's success for meeting their goals, given the real numbers and the concessions by those leading the efforts in Nepal, it makes one wonder how we can be so certain of the progress?

Despite the discrepancy between estimated and reported numbers there are a few epidemiological "facts" that seem certain. By 1998, HIV infection had been reported in fifty-eight of Nepal's seventy-five districts and the main concentration of cases was in the central and eastern regions, namely, the capital and surroundings areas (Suvedi 1998:54). Early studies focused mainly on high prevalence rates which had reached and surpassed "concentrated epidemic" levels among those practicing high risk behaviors in the city regions. Several authors presented papers concerning HIV prevalence among these various groups at the Second National Conference on AIDS held in Kathmandu in 1998. Shrestha and Gurubacharya (1998) found the prevalence of HIV among female sex workers (FSWs) in the capital city to be 20 percent. In another study, Gurubacharya (1998) found the prevalence rate among non-migratory FSWs in Kathmandu had increased from 0.66 percent to 8.66 percent over a three-year period. The significance of this second study is that it was limited only to FSWs who had never been to India, thus suggesting that HIV infection had moved into, and for the first time was being spread by, the local FSW population rather than being limited to those coming from the outside.[4] Among injecting drug users (IDUs) the prevalence rate was found to be 48 percent (Shrestha 1998). Interestingly, these earliest studies seem to be the basis for much "recirculation" of data that continues to be cited (as "current estimates") throughout the most current literature.[5] Since the publication of these original articles, it would appear that there has been a dearth of primary biomedical studies on these

[4]A large number of CSWs in Nepal were formerly in India and were deported back to Nepal once they tested positive for HIV. For further details see Seddon (1995:7).

[5]Nepal and Ross (2010) citing the 2006 Joint United Nations Program on HIV AND AIDS for Nepal and *estimates* published by Family Health International in 2004 (which likely are based on the earlier studies) report that 40% of IDUs and 20% of CSWs are infected. Likewise, Pokheral, Regmi and Piedade (2008) cite UNAIDS data from 2006 and FHI data from between 2000 and 2004 that estimate HIV prevalence rates between 13–17% among female sex workers in Kathmandu,

topics and some follow up studies are needed for comparative purposes. Once again, estimates can be deceiving.

In recent years, the epidemiology of HIV in Nepal has begun to shift. HIV has now been detected in all regions of Nepal (Sharma 2008) and the largest numbers of HIV sufferers are to be found in the west and midwest of Nepal where out-migration rates are the highest. Male migrant laborers and their wives now make up the largest group of infected persons. According to Dr Krishna Kumar Rai, Director of the NCASC, by 2010 this group made up 45 percent of the total number of infected persons (Sharma 2010). Further, Rai admitted that by that same year prevalence rates in the midwest and far west regions had reached "generalized epidemic" levels with between 2–3 percent of the region's population infected with HIV (Sharma 2010). So while it is difficult to discern between the rhetoric of estimated and re-ported numbers it would appear that there is still work to be done.

There have been four proposed worldwide patterns of HIV spread. According to Gurubacharya (1996), in pattern one countries, HIV spread mainly among homosexual males and IDUs beginning in the late 1970s and early 1980s. This is the main pattern initially identified in the United States, Europe, Canada and Australia. In pattern two countries, HIV affected the general population beginning about the same time period, but mainly spread heterosexually and in the prenatal period. This is the main pattern found in sub-Saharan Africa, Latin America, and the Caribbean. Pattern three, identified as beginning in the late 1980's, is characterized by HIV in-fection generally being "contained" within "high risk groups" such as FSWs and IDUs. This is the main pattern identified in Asia, Eastern Europe, some Pacific countries and the Middle East. In the mid 1990s a fourth pattern (pattern four) was proposed for parts of Asia (Brown and Xenos 1994). Pattern four is comprised of five waves of infection. The first of these was among homosexual or bi-sexual men having contact with foreigners. The second wave was among IDUs. The third was among FSWs and their clients. The fourth wave was among the girlfriends and wives of the FSW clients. And the final wave was among the children of these women. Smith (1996:8) suggests that this new pattern most closely fits (with a few modifications) the situation in Nepal.

Dixit (1996:15) reported that the first wave of HIV and AIDS in Nepal was among Western tourists and FSWs returning from India. The second wave spread to the clients of these FSWs (the largest group being truck drivers and soldiers), mainly Nepali men, and to the population (many who were concurrently clients of FSWs) and spread rapidly among this most-ly male population. Since then, the third wave, which began in the early 2000s, dominated with the highest numbers of HIV cases among migrant

---

3–4% among CSWs nationwide, 68% among male IDUs in Kathmandu and 22–35% among IDUs elsewhere in Nepal.

males, who have been bringing HIV home and transferring it to their wives and unborn children. And recently the fourth wave has begun; as of 2010, housewives of these men have become the single largest group accounting for nearly 45 percent of all new infections (Sarkar 2010). This assertion is confirmed by the estimates given in figure 3.1. It is also likely, given the numbers of HIV positive children reported (1,372 in fig. 3.3) and estimated (3,804 in fig. 3.1), that the final fifth wave (noted by Smith above) is also well underway in Nepal.

Although these types of epidemiological studies are a crucial part of a deeper understanding of the complexities of HIV and AIDS in Nepal, they often ignore the complex social issues involved in the spread of the disease. These issues will be the focus of the remainder of this chapter.

3.2 Nepali HIV and AIDS literature

The HIV and AIDS literature reviewed from Nepal generally falls into three broad categories: strict bio-medical and epidemiological profiles (e.g., those from which the above data is derived), literature that focuses primarily on the structural factors contributing to the HIV and AIDS problem in Nepal, and literature that focuses mainly on aspects of individual agency or various cultural traditions. Factors in each of these categories contribute to the spread of HIV and AIDS in Nepal. I have already addressed the epidemiological literature. In this section I will focus on the literature which addresses the social side of HIV and AIDS in Nepal. In each section I will first address the early years of the epidemic and then address the newer literature.

3.2.1 Structural issues

The dominant discourse in Nepal during the early years of the epidemic (and still a prevailing discourse today) goes something like this: Commercial sex work has been identified as the main route through which HIV infection has entered the general population (Cox and Suvedi 1994; New Era 1997; Sattar 1996). This happened through three main channels: (1) Nepali women are "trafficked" to India (usually Bombay) where they work as FSWs for some years.[6] Then, either after "retiring" or being repatriated for being HIV positive (Dixit 1996:52; Smith 1996:10), they return to their homeland of Nepal, where they continue to work, thus spreading the AIDS virus to the remotest corners of Nepal (Sattar 1996). (2) Nepali men in search of work migrate in large numbers to India and further abroad where they subsequently obtain the services of HIV-infected FSWs (Cox and Suvedi 1994; Smith 1996). They then return home, transmitting the virus to their unsuspecting wives, who subsequently pass the virus to their unborn children (Poudel 1994). (3) Truck drivers and soldiers are well known for their promiscuity and

---

[6]For a good discussion on the discourse of girl trafficking see Fredrick (1999).

preference for unprotected sex (Sattar 1996). These factors, coupled with the transient nature of their occupations, make soldiers and truck drivers natural conduits for the spread of HIV and AIDS along the roads and trails and into the remotest corners of Nepal.

Because commercial sex work has been identified as a primary factor in the spread of AIDS in Nepal, the discourse on HIV and AIDS has subsequently been subsumed within the wider discourse of commercial sex work and other related discourses such as "girl trafficking." Those analyzing the issue of HIV and AIDS in Nepal from a critical medical anthropology (CMA) perspective or a political economy medical anthropology (PEMA) perspective, tend to focus on the underlying causes of commercial sex work in Nepal. Prostitution and occupational migration are viewed as the result of deeper economic and political problems. David Seddon, for instance, suggests:

> There has been, and remains, a tendency...to focus attention on women, both as sources of infection (prostitutes) and as the main victims. While understandable, this tends to result in an under emphasis of other factors which contribute to the spread of infection and the development of the epidemic. The economic and social pressures which force women into prostitution, and men to make use of commercial sexual services, and the economic rewards which lead men to organize the sex trade as a source of profit, also need to be analyzed and understood. (Seddon 1995:4)

So, for Seddon, the root of the problem of HIV and AIDS is not commercial sex work, rather it is the economic and social pressures which push women into this profession, and which push men abroad where they are vulnerable to the use of commercial sexual services.

Likewise, Meena Poudel (1994:10–11) suggests that rural women are the most adversely effected by poverty in Nepal and that poverty is, in turn, "the principle cause of the greater risk of HIV infection in Nepal." Poverty, according to Poudel, is mainly a result of "resources being whittled away by multinational companies" that leads women to pursue prostitution because of a lack of viable alternatives. Poudel claims that "the main reason for this situation among women can be ascribed to widespread poverty, low status, lack of decision making rights, lack of access to time for education and information, rural-urban imbalances, inability to assert their rights, and so on" (1995:11).

Dixit (1996:50) also reflects this political economy approach when he concludes that in Nepal, "poverty is the root cause of the problem of AIDS," and that prostitution and migration, "two processes that expose the Nepali population to the HIV virus," are "the result of an attempt at poverty alleviation."

Another study of STD and HIV infection among prostitutes in Calcutta (based on self-reporting) found that extreme poverty, illiteracy and family disturbances were among the factors most responsible for leading FSWs into prostitution (Chakraborty et al. 1994:165).[7] The authors claim that economic necessity was the most important reason for entry into prostitution and that "illiteracy was probably the main reason why they could not struggle to find some other means of livelihood and resorted to sex trade as the best alternative." Again, economic necessity is stressed as the structural factor contributing most greatly to the spread of HIV and AIDS. Various other authors who note poverty as a key factor strongly linked to the spread of HIV and AIDS in Nepal are Sattar (1996), Keyser (1993), Nigam (1994), Smith (1996), Dixit (1996), and Suvedi, Baker and Thapa (1994). And more recent studies on HIV and AIDS in Nepal continue to address the epidemic from this perspective (e.g., Poudel and Carryer 2000, Sarkar et al. 2008, Rodrigo and Rajapakse 2010).

Although a CMA or PEMA perspective is useful and adds another dimension to the earlier epidemiological perspective, this structural approach tends to ignore the agency of the individual in making his or her own decisions. For instance, in the Calcutta survey (Chakraborty et al. 1994), the authors found that 39 percent of the women who had turned to prostitution claim they did so of their own volition, yet they don't address this issue anywhere in their findings. The focus of the article is only upon the structural factors influencing the 61 percent who claim to have been forced into prostitution through economic necessity. In a study of 289 FSWs in Nepal, 66.7 percent cited "necessity" while 21.4 percent cited "pleasure" as their reason for entering the sex trade (Karki, Geurma, and Suvedi 1995). Although 51 percent of FSWs in another study (Bhatta et al. 1994) listed "economic hardship" as their main motivation for entry into the sex trade, "enjoyment," "separation from husband" or "husband's long absence from home," and "husband's polygamy" were other reasons given. In a third study of FSWs in Pokhara, Nepal, the authors found that many women self report that they have chosen this profession of their own volition. The authors quote one woman as saying:

> I do not care what people say but I am happy to be earning money in such an easy way. I can feed my child, have a place to live, eat good food, wear good clothes, move around in taxis… it gives me great relaxation when I have sex! Any ways nobody will give me any other job and I do not want my child and myself to starve. I saw my friends earning and I did not find it wrong and I started working too. (Baral 1999)

I imagine many CMA or PEMA advocates would argue that these women's own words do not fully represent the "whole picture" (and they are right). It

---

[7]This study was categorized with the articles from Nepal because although Calcutta is in India, a large number of the sex workers in the survey were Nepali women.

is clear, however, that in some cases, individuals can and do (at least in part) manipulate the system, and this perspective is completely absent in the CMA or PEMA analysis of the HIV and AIDS situation in Nepal. Poverty certainly explains why many women enter the sex trade, but it does not explain why all do so. A study from 2008 (Sarkar et al.) might provide a healthy middle ground between these two seemingly polar positions. In this study the authors note that 68 percent had joined prostitution "voluntarily" (meaning that they were not "trafficked" in the traditional sense), thus, they had exercised a degree of personal agency in their decision to become a CSW, but perhaps they had done so ultimately for structural reasons (i.e., poverty).

Migration has also been a factor identified as contributing to the spread of HIV and AIDS in Nepal (Seddon 1995). As mentioned previously, it is believed that many migrant laborers are bringing the HIV virus home with them when they return to Nepal. In 1994 it was estimated that there were up to 200,000 Nepali women involved in the sex trade in India (Poudel 1994). There are also many Nepali men working abroad. In 1981, it was reported that over one-half million Nepalis were working away from home and that the majority of these migrants were from the mid-hills region (Savada 1991:72). By 1981 that number had grown to more than 762,000. And by 2011 that number had grown to 1.9 million. Today, one out of every four households reports one or more members of the household absent. The highest proportion (42%) of those absent is in the fifteen to twenty-four age group and the absentee rates were still highest in the middle-hills regions of the Western and Mid-Western Development Zones (NPHC 2012). In a family planning survey conducted in Gorkha District in 1995, I found that of the women surveyed, 40 percent of their husbands were working abroad (Beine 1996). Likewise, in my research in the village of Saano Dumre in the late 1990s, 56 percent of the men were reported to be working either in India or further abroad. The implications of such large migrations are obvious. Migrant laborers and their wives now make up over one half of the current HIV infections in Nepal.

Besides those mentioned above, there are also other semi-migratory groups not usually considered in the migration figures, whose practices are also cited as contributing to the spread of HIV and AIDS in Nepal. Seddon includes the following groups:

> Truck drivers taking loads to and from India; smugglers operating across the borders; officials making formal visits; merchants and traders traveling on business; small farmers involved in seasonal or temporary labor migration—all of these are internationally mobile—and have become increasingly so—and may contribute to the spread of HIV infection into Nepal. (Seddon 1995:5)

Seddon, focusing on structure, views most of these occupational choices as strategies necessitated by the economic pressures of poverty.

Many other authors also cite poverty as the main factor contributing to migration in Nepal. Smith (1996:139) comments that among the populations of the middle hills, there is an ever increasing need for farming families (90% of Nepal's population) to supplement their income through migratory labor. Sattaur (1993:15) reports that 6 percent of Nepal's population owns 46 percent of the cultivatable land and that 75 percent of the population own less than one hectare (2.74 acres) of land. Sattaur (1993:15) also reports that the average family of five requires one hectare of hill land for subsistence. The average size of a Nepalese family sharing one hectare of land is well beyond five members. Beside this, heavy deforestation is creating loss of precious topsoil and is further reducing agricultural productivity. The result is that most families raise only enough food to support their needs for part of the year and then must rely upon supplemental income from family members who migrate to the city or abroad in search of work. The United Nations Children's Fund cites increased population pressure, scarcity of arable land, limited food production, underemployment, debt, exploitation, and hunger as the main "push" factors for migration in Nepal (UNICEF 1992:14).

Nepal's insufficient infrastructures (poor roads and communication systems) are also believed to structurally contribute to the spread of HIV and AIDS. Poor infrastructure begets poor education and illiteracy, which in turn, facilitates low awareness, which then cultivates the spread of HIV and AIDS. Likewise, as mentioned earlier, these same issues create structural barriers to HIV treatment; availability does not necessarily mean access. The wider world's cultural model of ART (solving the HIV crisis through treatment rather than prevention) is just not a reality for Nepal at this time. Even if available free, many barriers to HIV treatment remain: physical barriers—frequent strikes make travel impossible and bad weather often closes roads for days at a time; financial barriers—patients have to pay to travel to distribution centers and require food and lodging while there (they are taken away from work for the time required and cannot leave unattended children at home, etc.); and the stigma associated with HIV. Many of these barriers will be evident as I discuss newly emerging HIV narratives in chapter six.

Conflict or war should also certainly be considered as a structural issue. The impact of war upon healthcare is well documented in the literature. Various authors have noted the direct and lingering effects of war on healthcare and healthcare delivery. Paul Farmer (2006) has commented that political instability and violence has had similar effects in Haiti. According to Farmer, "the deaths from Haiti's cycles of violence do not all come by gunfire. Riots and revolutions, and lawlessness have also interrupted the healthcare that Haitians receive." According to Farmer there are the obvious, directly related results of conflict that impact healthcare delivery, such as treatment of gunshot wounds, low blood supply, destroyed medical facilities, etc., but there are other more pernicious ways that disruptions in political systems can disrupt entire healthcare systems. He points out that treatment of chronic illnesses (such as HIV and AIDS) require a stable health provision system and this is severely impacted by conflict. War often means no functioning laboratories (due to destruction of facilities, disruption in power supply, etc) and lack of services and lack of equipment to treat people. And many health care providers, facing this lack of facilities and shortages of essential supplies, often depart in frustration. Likewise, many health care providers, fearing for their lives or the lives of their families (and because they have the financial resources to do so) will often depart these war zones for safer ground. The lack of necessary supplies and essential healthcare workers means the cessation of essential services vital in the ongoing treatment of chronic illness. Farmer has concluded that "you can't do public health in a war zone. You can do your best to patch people up but you can't really do good public health in the middle of political violence. It's just not possible." In relation to Nepal, several authors have noted the toll that the ten year long civil war has had upon the spread of HIV and AIDS in Nepal (e.g., Singh et al. 2005, Beine 2006, Karkee and Shrestha 2006, Pokhrel et al. 2008, and Ghimire 2010). In one of the most poignant examples, Ghimire (2010) illustrates how "social separation" precipitated by war led both men and women of rural Rolpa District into behaviors that exposed them to the risks of contracting HIV.

David Seddon has also suggested that environmental degradation, a byproduct of poverty, has played a role in the spread of HIV and AIDS in Nepal:

> The resources of the hill areas in the hinterland of the Kathmandu Valley urban centers, perhaps more than anywhere else in the country, have been progressively degraded and depleted as demand for wood fuel has increased over the past decades. With increasing land degradation and inadequate access to forest resources or land for agricultural production, the inhabitants of these areas have become increasingly reliant on selling their labor and their bodies to provide their families with a living income. (Seddon 1995:7)

Between 1950 and 1980, Nepal's forest cover was cut in half and deforestation continues to occur at an alarming rate. Savada (1991:125) suggests increased demands for grazing lands, farmland and fodder for animals, combined with the growth of human population and people's dependence upon firewood for energy, as the major factors inciting deforestation in Nepal. In turn, major deforestation has caused erosion that limits the future productivity of agricultural lands. Savada (1991:72) also suggests that the large migration figures from the mid-hills are "an unmistakable indicator of the region's deteriorating economic and environmental conditions."

We have seen that many authors have made a strong link between poverty and commercial sex work, migration, war and even environmental degradation, and that this factor (poverty) is facilitating the spread of HIV and AIDS in Nepal. These authors contend that the search for alternative forms of employment is most often a response to dire economic situations. Again, Seddon concludes:

> The clear implication is that it is the degradation of resources and poverty that creates vulnerability and drives the rural poor, particularly from certain identifiable regions, into economic survival strategies that take them away from their homes to work elsewhere; migration is a necessity, and as far as employment is concerned, "beggars cannot be choosers." (Seddon 1995:7)

It is not difficult to understand why such focus has been placed on Nepal's poverty as the root cause of HIV and AIDS. Nepal is one of the world's poorest nations as noted earlier. We have also seen, however, that there is a growing awareness that personal agency (including various cultural practices) is also involved in the spread of HIV and AIDS in Nepal. This will be the focus of the next section.

3.2.2 Issues of agency

As opposed to the focus on the structural factors pushing people into lifestyles that facilitate the spread of HIV and AIDS in Nepal, many authors have focused more on the personal choice (agency) involved, as individuals or communities adopt lifestyles or strategies that are contributing to the wider problem. Bhatt, Gurubacharya and Vadies (1993), taking an agency approach, studied a unique cultural group in the southwestern part of Nepal that relies exclusively on prostitution for economic security. This group, known as the Badis, was interviewed about its sexual practices and was tested for VDRL and HIV positivity.[8] Although 70 percent were found to be VDRL positive, none tested positive for HIV. The article focuses upon the Badis' choice of prostitution as an economic strategy enabling them to own lands and houses, something unusual for a low-caste group such as the Badis. The authors trace the unique history of the Badis.[9] They conclude:

---

[8]This test was developed by the Venereal Disease Research Lab (thus, the name VDRL) and tests for syphilis seropositivity.

[9]This same author makes the point that the Badis were involved in a number of other activities (not prostitution) until the end of the Malla Dynasty in 1769 (Bhatt 1993:280). Historical changes, however, coupled with their status as an untouchable caste made economic survival very difficult and they turned to prostitution. Thus, we can see the role of history and religion (the caste system is a product of the Hindu religion) in the spread of HIV and AIDS in Nepal.

> Like Gypsies, [the Badis] would travel and provide musical enter-
> tainment for hire...and would entertain at the homes or estates
> of wealthy landowners in the region. Probably some landowners
> began paying young Badi girls' high fees for sexual favors, in addi-
> tion to the other entertainment being provided. This was probably
> very tempting to Badi girls as well as the family and the commu-
> nity, which were always economically deprived as part of the un-
> touchable caste. This caste is the lowest caste, lower than even the
> fourth caste in the traditional Hindu caste system. More recently,
> income primarily from prostitution has enabled some Badi families
> to own land and homes, something normally unheard of for most
> members of an untouchable caste. (Bhatt et al. 1993:280)

The first point I would make about the above quote is that it illustrates
the highly speculative nature of this piece. "Probably" is overused and de-
serves the criticism of CMA advocates who would accuse these authors of
blaming the victims. On the other hand, moving beyond this weakness, the
authors do acknowledge the political economy involved in the caste system
but choose to focus further upon the personal agency behind the Badis'
choices. The article describes a sliding fee scale developed by the Badi (politicians are charged the most), the 'marriage' ceremony at which a Badi girl
is initiated into the sex trade, and their preference not to use condoms.
Concerning the latter, the authors write:

> When questioned about the non-use of condoms, Badi women again
> stated the desirability of pregnancy and the resulting possibility
> of more female sex workers within the family...family planning
> is not a priority. This is because the Badi view female offspring
> as future economic security as prostitutes. Male offspring are still
> accepted but are not considered as desirable as females. (Bhatt et
> al. 1993:282)

The article concludes that although the Badi are currently uninfected
with HIV and AIDS, their practices and choices put this group at the highest risk of HIV infection in the near future. The authors suggest that "there
is some evidence that counseling alone may have little or no effect in getting prostitutes to leave their profession, even after they have become HIV
infected. There is also some evidence that despite efforts at training and
providing alternative employment to Badi prostitutes, they return to their
practice in a short time (1993:282)."

Bignall (1993), in a review of Bhat, Gurubacharya and Vadies (1993), for
the British journal *The Lancet,* focuses further on the agency of the Badi that
is exacerbating the epidemic. These two articles clearly reflect a focus on
the personal choices (agency) of the Badis in manipulating the system and
in determining their own future.

Near the turn of the century, various writers began to challenge the traditional girl trafficking discourse (which was the main discourse at that time).[10] John Fredrick (1998) asserted that much of the discourse was, in fact, myth. The consensus view, he contended, was that a majority of women trafficked to India were being abducted and sold into sexual slavery as prostitutes mainly in the brothels of Bombay. Fredrick termed this sort of trafficking "hard trafficking." The reality was, he suggested, that much of Nepal's girl trafficking was actually done with the families' own complicity. He termed this form of trafficking "soft trafficking" and suggested that in most of the cases of girl trafficking, the families' own agency was involved. Many more women actually were going of their own free will; or at least with their families' firm encouragement and blessings. Prostitution, as it was among the Badi, was more of an economic strategy to address the growing problems of providing dowries, paying off generational debts from an established bonded-labor tradition, or providing a better quality roof (tin) for the family home. Fredrick (1998:19) claimed that this "family-based" prostitution in Nepal was "an increasingly common response to poverty and a significant source of rural income." [11] Likewise, Campbell (1997:220) suggested that prostitution was simply the "latest form of commoditizing Tamang[12] labour power."

It seems clear that there are both issues of personal choice (agency) as well as wider socioeconomic (structural) factors that underlie commercial sex work in Nepal. Economic pressures are pushing people into commercial sex work in one of two ways: either as an economic strategy needed to survive absolute poverty (structural), or as a way to provide extra income for luxuries that could otherwise not be afforded (agency). Either way, as the earlier statistics reveal, commercial sex work puts one at highest risk for HIV infection, so both structure and agency are important factors to be considered.

---

[10]This discourse is still popular today, but is only one of many HIV discourses heard today. At that time it was one of the only public discourses.

[11]In a published response to his article (http://www.himalmag.com/component/content/article/2180-.html) I applauded Fredrick for challenging us to critically consider the over-simplified discourse of trafficking then being offered us by NGOs, various governments, and the media. At the same time, however, I warned him against replacing one myth with another; I encouraged him to seek conclusions based on actual research rather than speculation (which his conclusions relied heavily upon).

[12]The largest number of women seems to be coming from the Tamang area (Seddon 1995:5). The Tamang are an ethnic group in Nepal that have historically been used by the elite class to serve as a major source of labor. The early rulers of Nepal even prohibited recruitment of Tamang men to the Gurkha regiment in order to protect this "labor source."

3.2.3 Cultural issues

Besides issues of personal choice, there are also many widely held beliefs and cultural practices (usually considered issues of agency) that are contributing to the spread of HIV and AIDS in Nepal. The following list is a summary of widely held beliefs elicited from HIV positive persons at a local non-governmental organization (NGO) sponsored education class held in Kathmandu. These are all related to folk beliefs about prevention and cures for HIV and STDs.

1. Having sex with 108[13] virgins will cure AIDS and STDs.
2. Cleaning the penis with urine, Detol soap[14], or Coke, will cure AIDS and STDs.
3. Naag[15] Puja will cure AIDS and STDs.
4. Anal sex will cause HIV.
5. HIV is prevalent only in Bombay. 6. A *tika* from Sai Baba placed on the penis will cure STDs and AIDS.[16]

As one can see, there are many widely held beliefs reported by these HIV positive persons that would actually advance the spread of HIV and AIDS.

According to Ghimire (1997:8), "There are certain cultural traditions in Nepal that approve the sale of girls and prostitution." The Badi tradition spoken of earlier is one such case. The Deuki tradition is another. Smith (1996:27) explains that in the Seti Zone of far-western Nepal, parents offer their daughters to a temple deity in order to improve health, acquire a new job, get a son, or a number of other such reasons. The girls remain at the temple and are held in high esteem. Although the girls are unmarriageable, sex with a Deuki is said "to insure eternal bliss." The similar Devidasi

---

[13]The number 108 came up over and over in my research. I am told that the number is significant in Hindu mythology. Most directly, it relates to a story in which the Pravati offends her husband Shiva by requesting the dominant position during one sexual encounter. Shiva submits, but during intercourse, his penis grows tall sending Pravati into the heavens from where she is unable to come down. Once there, she seeks advice from Brahma about how to remedy her situation. He suggests that she begin to cut her way down piece by piece. In the end, 108 pieces of Shiva's penis remained. Interestingly enough, Pashupati, Nepal's most holy temple, is said to contain 108 lingams (phallic symbols). It is also notable that Tibetan prayer bead necklaces contain 108 beads. Fredricks (1999:13) also cites the common folk belief that sex with a virgin will cure AIDS. Chhetri (1998) also asserts that this is a belief found in Africa as well.

[14]Detol is a well-known brand of soap in Nepal. The use of Detol to avoid STDs was also reported by New Era (1997)

[15]Naag is the snake god. *Puja* 'worship' done to him is commonly believed to cure STDs.

[16]A *tika* is the small dot usually placed on the forehead. Sai Baba is one of India's most famous gurus.

tradition is yet another. Chhetri (1998) explains that the Devidasi (which literally translates as 'slaves of God') tradition is "a distorted legacy of a seventh century religious practice in which girls were dedicated to temples to live as dancers. Today, the girls pledge fealty to the goddess Renuka, and then—with the full knowledge of their parents—are spirited off to brothels" (1998:3).

Several other authors also cite the sub-continental preference for Nepali girls as FSWs (Dixit 1996:52; Brewer 1995:4; Chhetri 1998), because of their "fair skin" and "oriental features," an appearance found "so exotic" by Indian men (Chhetri 1998).

Another interesting belief about sex, which may contribute to the spread of HIV and AIDS, is held by truck drivers, one of the largest groups frequenting FSWs (Cox and Suvedi 1994:6). This common fallacy held by truck drivers is that long hours spent behind the truck's engine "heats up the body" and that they can rid themselves of this harmful heat through frequent sex (Brewer 1995:6).

As mentioned earlier, there is a strong connection between migration and the spread of HIV. Nepal has a long tradition of migration. Seddon (1995) claims that the "search for employment abroad has always been an important feature of Nepalese economy and society." In the 1950s, the government encouraged resettlement to the newly mosquito-eradicated Terai region of Nepal. And for at least 180 years the British Army also has been hiring Nepalis to fill its famous Gurkha regiments (Savada 1991:199). Likewise, Nepali watchmen have a positive reputation and can be found all over the subcontinent. In short, Nepal has a historical tradition, or culture, of migration. Although this tradition has always been rooted in the search for better financial opportunity, it would be a mistake to assert that poverty has been the catalyst for all people to migrate. Much of this migration has traditionally taken place from areas that were self-sufficient and where poverty was not a severe problem as it was elsewhere in the country. Many Nepalis have found a way to fill a foreign niche that has boosted their families' economies tremendously. Unfortunately, this culture of migration results in faithful housewives (now the largest category of HIV suffers) bearing the brunt of the remaining epidemic in Nepal (as earlier statistics reveal) as well as facing the strong stigma that still remains associated with HIV and AIDS in Nepal (Beine 2011).

Many of the Tibeto-Burman cultures of Nepal's mountainous regions also have traditionally practiced a semi-nomadic lifestyle. Seasonal migration has traditionally been a major feature of their culture as they brought salt from Tibet and traded it in India. Savada (1991:70) claims that these groups "historically were deeply engaged in interregional as well as cross-border trade with Tibet as their principle economic activity." Again, for many of these groups, migration is a historical, chosen economic strategy that provides an above-average standard of living rather than a supplemental income-generating strategy designed to alleviate poverty. Dahal (1994) makes this assertion among the Byansi, a semi-nomadic group in far-Western Nepal. Nepal's indices for measuring poverty usually include such features as land ownership, development of infrastructure, and availability of basic social services. Using this standard, the Byansi people are very poor. Dahal (1994:37), however, contends that they are actually one of the most prosperous peoples in the whole region. He claims that this is because "the conventional measurement of 'income' is unable to capture the diversity of local resources and their cultural modes of exploitation" (1994:36). Although it is clear that for many, migration is an economic strategy necessitated by low yields and growing populations, for others it is a tradition that has supplied economic abundance.

There is also a cultural tradition of drug use in Nepal. Shrestha focuses upon elements of Nepali culture that facilitate the use and abuse of drugs and alcohol. These include a historic cultural acceptance of alcohol use, recreational cannabis use by the elderly, and religious cannabis use by holy men (and distributed by the government for this purpose) (1992:1241–1242). IDUs have been identified as the second largest risk group for contracting HIV and AIDS in Nepal and although the issues need to be examined more closely, poverty does not seem to be the main cause pushing people into drug use. In a recent study among IDUs it was determined that the majority were highly educated and financially self-sufficient, earning well above the national average (Maharajan et al.1994).

Except for cases in Nepal where HIV is transmitted through drug use, HIV is spread mainly as a result of sexual transmission. In the earlier edition of this book I wrote much about the public or conservative versus the supposedly private or promiscuous nature of sex in Nepal. I concluded (based mainly on the existing literature) that "there has long been a tradition of premarital and extra-marital sex in Nepal" (2003:87). I used the writings of authors such as Cox and Suvedi (1994) who have "noted that 'among young unmarried men the use of FSWs is well accepted'" and authors such as Smith (1996) and Gurubacharya and Suvedi (1994) to conclude that, "contrary to the portrayal of Nepali society as sexually conservative, premarital and extramarital sex is not uncommon." I added anecdotal evidence from my own informants (all HIV positive): one who told me, for instance, of the "'custom' of being taken (by older friends) to a prostitute when 'coming of age'" in a kind of "'sexual initiation'" that is "not uncommon among Nepali boys"; and another who said that "promiscuity is expected among young men—Nepali men are assumed to be unfaithful," to strengthen this working hypothesis. I concluded that "sex may be a taboo topic in Nepal..., but, as various authors have demonstrated, just because people are not discussing it doesn't mean it's not happening" (Beine 2003:87).[17]

In recent years, however, because of my studies and experience in Nepal, I have begun to doubt the veracity of such claims being normative among the wider society. Green, Farley, and Ruark have concluded that "national surveys in Africa and Asia repeatedly show that a majority of unmarried teenagers practice abstinence and that a majority of adults practice faithfulness to one partner in any given year (Green et al. 2009). Nepal seems to be no exception to this. For example, in a study of 573 male college students in Nepal, 61 percent report being abstinent (Adhkari and Tamang 2009). In a study of young factory workers in Kathmandu, 80 percent of young boys and 88 percent of young girl factory workers report being abstinent (Puri and Cleland 2006:237). In a seven district survey of Nepali teenagers done by UNAIDS and UNICEF, 78 percent of the boys reported no premarital sexual experience. And in another study of male adolescent students, 53 percent reported intent to remain abstinent until marriage (Iriyama et al. 2007:64). Interestingly, each of these studies (except the last) were all framed in the negative rather than the positive (as I have done above); that is, they only reported the percentage of sexually active (which was 39%, 20%, 12%, and 22%, respectively) and made comments regarding this data, such as, "These studies indicate a growing trend toward premarital sexual activities among adolescents," "showed risky behavior especially among boys," etc., and yet no comparative data is given to support these claims (Adhikari and Tamang 2009:242). Another study (Puri and Cleland 2006) states that "despite religious and cultural restrictions, one in five boys and one in eight unmarried girls reported experience of sexual intercourse," and that "early sexual experimentation and low and irregular use of condoms are not uncommon." Don't these numbers actually show that the majority of unmarried adolescents are practicing abstinence? I don't know how these authors would define "uncommon," but if only two in ten boys is sexually active (which actually seems low to me), then early sexual experimentation is not common, although I am left with the impression that it is, based on the use of this negatively framed language. The same trend continues in the literature today. Regmi, Simkada and van Teijlingen (2010:61), citing many of these same sources, similarly concluded that "despite these generally traditional views [regarding sex] a significant proportion of young people are engaged in premarital and high risk-sexual activities." Is there an ideology undergirding these perceptions? This is an issue I hope to address in a forthcoming publication. So while premarital sex is certainly not unknown, neither is it "common." As I have reassessed, I would take a more middle

---

[17]Others citing many of these same sources, recently similarly concluded that "despite these generally traditional views a significant proportion of young people is engaged in premarital and high risk-sexual activities (Regmi et al. 2010).

ground position. It is not as conservative as publically presented and not as promiscuous as other authors would suggest. There also seems to be a growing rural and urban divide (including western sexual values) that accompanies urbanization. I will talk more about the implications of this later as I address prevention strategies.

In conclusion, it seems clear that the spread of HIV and AIDS in Nepal is due to a combination of complex factors. Structural factors, issues of agency, and culture are all involved in creating casualties and have extracted a high price.

3.2.4 KAP studies

Much of the social research conducted on HIV and AIDS in Nepal has been in the form of knowledge, attitudes, and practices or behavior (KAP or KAB) studies.[18] The majority of the findings above (concerning the cultural factors that contribute to the spread of HIV and AIDS) are, in fact, the result of such KAP or KAB studies. This type of study is a product of the Health Belief Model[19] and the Theory of Reasoned Action (Tones 1994) that posits lack of awareness as the primary factor contributing to the spread of disease, and education as the primary weapon to fight it. As will be seen later, Nepali policy planners, informed by this Western applied anthropology perspective, made "awareness-building" the major focus in Nepal's first prevention strategies and programs. Since lack of awareness is reasoned to be the primary factor contributing to the spread of disease, and education is viewed as the primary weapon to fight the spread of disease, resultant prevention programs developed from this theoretical paradigm tend to give primacy to "awareness-building." For instance, one KAB study done in Nepal concluded that "the most effective strategy to reduce the spread of the epidemic in the short term and protect women is to raise the awareness amongst the men" (Smith 1996:i).

It cannot be denied that increased awareness is an essential component in the fight against HIV and AIDS in Nepal. It is encouraging that several studies have reported success in awareness building among certain populations. Among certain groups of FSWs, for instance, it has been determined that "HIV messages have been successfully disseminated and understood by target populations" (New Era 1997:xiii). Among IDUs, "all but three (1.5%) had some knowledge of HIV and AIDS and the majority of the respondents were aware of the routes of HIV transmission" (Maharjan et al. 1994). And in an awareness study done among adolescent students in Chitwan District,

---

[18]Allen and Fischer (1994:xvi) suggest that this is because most of the anthropology done in Nepal has been of an applied nature. The KAP/KAB studies are a favorite tool of applied anthropologists.

[19]For a good description and overview of the Health Belief Model see Feldman and Johnson (1986:131).

100 percent had heard of HIV and AIDS and 95 percent "had correct knowledge about causative agents" (Shilendra Kumar Singh et al. 2005). Having said this, however, increased awareness doesn't always mean changed behavior. Although these examinations of knowledge, attitudes and practices or behaviors are absolutely essential to a fuller understanding of the HIV and AIDS situation in Nepal, they are not enough. Smith has made this point adequately herself. In the context of HIV, she cites Meadows, Catalan, and Gazzard (1993), commenting that "it has been shown that the possession of 'adequate knowledge' about HIV does not in itself predict the intention to comply with preventative health recommendations" (Smith 1996:32–37). This same phenomenon has certainly been confirmed in the Nepal context as well. Erpelding and Bista (1997) (using a KAP format) demonstrate that although over half of the male students in their study acknowledged avoidance of multiple partners as a means of avoiding STDs, 15 percent had more than two partners in the last four months. Their study revealed that although 81.6 percent of their student sample was aware that the use of condoms prevents STDs, more than a third of the sample (indicating multiple partners) did not use condoms. Another KAB study targeting people under the poverty line concluded that although people have increased access to AIDS information, their attitudes have not changed significantly. And even those who have changed their attitudes haven't changed their behavior (Roy 1998). Another study indicated that increased education was not an inhibitor to promiscuous behavior (Puri et al. 1998). A fourth study demonstrated that despite the public awareness campaign regarding safe sex, there has been no significant increase in condom use by FSWs or their clients (Gurubacharya 1998). And in perhaps the most recent poignant example of this phenomenon, Nepali nursing students' knowledge and attitudes regarding HIV and AIDS were assessed (Mahat and Eller 2009), revealing that although knowledge of HIV and AIDS differed statistically significantly between students, their attitudes were universally negative (despite differences in knowledge), resulting in "stigmatization and unwillingness to care for patients with HIV and AIDS." This gap between knowledge and behavior is often referred to as the "KAP gap" and it provides the main criticism to the Health Action Model and the Theory of Reasoned Action. According to the critics, the belief that if we just educate people (raise their awareness) then their behavior will change, has been proven wrong in many situations. "Awareness-building" is clearly not enough.

KAP and KAB studies have also been challenged on a methodological basis. Stone and Campbell have demonstrated the limitations of using KAP and KABs in the Nepali context. They conducted an experiment in Nepal in which they used qualitative methods to cross-check the findings of an earlier KAP study regarding fertility issues. The KAP study data had been collected using quantitative methods. According to the authors, "the experiment uncovered severe problems of data validity" (Stone and Campbell 1984:28). Far from advocating the abandonment of the use of KAP studies, however, the authors support the supplemental use of qualitative methods along with quantitative methods in social science research.

3.2.5 Other recent literature

In recent years, others have done a marvelous job of covering the HIV and AIDS epidemic in Nepal from a variety of other angles and critical perspectives.[20] Although these do not fit "cleanly" into any of the categories noted above, I list them here topically and will refer to them again more in depth as their content becomes relevant to other issues I will subsequently address. Various authors have conducted bio-medical studies, focusing on the relationship between HIV and other opportunistic infections (Dhungel et al. 2008; Paudel et al. 2008a), HIV prevalence rates in Nepal (Banerjee 2008; Silverman et al. 2007; Paudel et al. 2008a), and HIV and migrant labor (Nepal 2007; Paudel et al. 2008b; Paudel et al. 2008c). There have also been articles which focus on the remaining stigma associated with HIV and AIDS in Nepal (Beine 2011; Jha and Madison 2009; Nepal and Ross 2010 and Pokhrel, Regmi, and Piedade 2008), and those which focus more on cultural aspects of HIV and AIDS, such as providing training about HIV and AIDS to traditional healers (who then can become the conduit of this information to the masses they treat [Poudel et al. 2005]), or using traditional entertainment forms, such as drama and dancing, to send linguistically and culturally appropriate HIV and AIDS prevention messages (Dahal 2008; Family Health International 2010; Desh Pradesh 2010; Beine 2011).

In concluding the discussion of the AIDS literature in Nepal, I must address what some once considered the most comprehensive work published about AIDS in Nepal. In 1997 the American Foundation for AIDS Research (AmfAR) published a book by the same title (*AIDS in Nepal*) that addressed many important issues related to HIV and AIDS in Nepal. Although the author (Hannum 1997) did provide a good cursory look at AIDS in Nepal, critics of her book suggested that it fell well short of its intended goal of providing a comprehensive examination of many of the deeper issues. In reviewing the book, Stacey Pigg (1999) wrote:

> *AIDS in Nepal* is the first comprehensive published work on the
> AIDS issue in South Asia to describe these challenges [various

---

[20]In 2006 a systematic review of electronic databases was conducted to determine the number of documents focusing on HIV and AIDS in Nepal. According the report (Nepal 2007) 116 documents were retrieved from the Medline database, another 120 article abstracts regarding HIV and AIDS in Nepal were archived at the International AIDS Society's website, and the websites of various other national and international agencies "housed a number of reports on qualitative and qualitative studies, estimates of HIV cases, policy analysis, and government strategies."

AIDS issues in Nepal]. At first glance, however, the book appears to be a promotional piece for AmFAR, written in a relentlessly optimistic tone of American can-do-ism. Author Jill Hannum spent only a month in Nepal, rushing from place to place. For Nepalis and other readers familiar with Nepal, her trite clichés about beautiful, remote, impoverished Nepal are tiresome. The Nepali situation is packaged for international consumption through the eyes of a naïve witness, fresh to the scene, recording what she is told.

Although dated, and despite its weaknesses, *AIDS in Nepal* offers a major contribution especially in that it condenses many of the issues raised by various authors into one volume and packages it for the international community. It provides, at least, a cursory look at the face of AIDS in Nepal. And that is an important first step in understanding the deeper issues. More up to date perspectives have been presented since then (Wasti et al. 2009 and Pokhrel et al. 2008), which when combined with Hannum's treatise, provide a thorough (and more contemporary) overview of HIV and AIDS in the context of Nepal.

3.3 National HIV and AIDS awareness and prevention programs

Although the first case of AIDS was not identified in Nepal until 1988, prevention efforts (in response to the growing global AIDS epidemic) were begun in 1986 with the formation of an STD/AIDS Control Committee (Suvedi 1999:9).[21] The first short-term plan (1987–88) of the National AIDS Prevention and Control Program was to encourage individual behavior change among highest risk persons by: (1) promoting consistent condom use, (2) stopping needle sharing, and (3) providing ART to pregnant women in order to prevent mother to child transmission (Bastola 2011:16). After a two-year continuation of the first plan beyond its original operational dates, the first medium-term plan (modeled on the first short-term plan, which focused on highest-risk groups) was developed and implemented from 1990 to 1992. In 1992, however, after the results of an external review, a multisectoral National AIDS Coordinating Committee (NACC)—with the Minister of Health chairing the committee—was established to encourage more multisectoral involvement and to oversee that the review findings were being implemented; thus, the second medium term plan was launched in 1993 and in effect until 1997 (Fursad 2013). In 1995 the Nepali Parliament adopted the National Policy on AIDS and STD control to "address all the major components of AIDS and STD prevention efforts accepted globally" (Suvedi

---

[21]The National Center for AIDS and STD Control was established (under the Ministry of Heath) as the main government agency tasked with HIV and AIDS prevention efforts in Nepal.

1999:10). The first National Strategic Plan (NSP) of this National Policy was implemented from 1997 to 2001 with goals to develop the participatory process and to expand multi-sectoral involvement beyond the health sectors (Bastola 2011:18). During this time (1999) the National Center for AIDS and STD Control (NCASC) conducted its first HIV prevalence survey.

In 2002 the National AIDS Council (NAC) was created. According to the World Bank (2008:2), the NAC was established to "raise the profile of HIV and AIDS" and "set overall policy, lead national level advocacy, and provide overall guidance and direction to the program." With oversight of the NAC, all AIDS prevention activities are now coordinated through the National AIDS Coordination Committee (NACC), which is chaired by the Health Minister and comprised of representatives from various NGOs, international non-governmental organizations (INGOs), key ministers, donors, and others involved in the fight against AIDS. District AIDS Coordination Committees have also been formed to carry out major AIDS prevention activities at the local level. According to CARE (2011:18), "the multi-sector composition of the council was expected to allow for greater involvement of different ministries, the private sector, and civil societies, including PLHIV, in the response to the HIV epidemic."[22] And the NCASC, now under the Ministry of Health and Population, is responsible for "framing HIV & AIDS & STI [Sexually Transmitted Infection] Policy" (Bastola 2011:iv). The World Bank, in its 2008 report on HIV/AIDS in Nepal, stated the goals of the NCASC:

> The NCASC should focus on the health sector response to HIV, specifically delivery of public health services..., continuing to serve as the lead technical agency for surveillance, policy and technical guidance, capacity building of the health sector, and monitoring and evaluation of the health sector response. It will also assist with the mainstreaming of HIV- and STI-related activities within the sectoral programs of the MoHP and other line ministries. (World Bank 2008:3)

In 2002 the NCASC, "in response to the loopholes of the first national mid-term and short-term program and the first National Strategy Plan," developed the Second NSP (2002–2006). This plan included a five year (2002–2007) operational work plan, known as the National Action Plan (NAP), which outlined detailed activities and implementation plans that "catered to the needs of various high risk groups" (Bastola 2011:18). The NCASC then developed the third NSP (2007–2011) and associated NAP (2008–2011) in response to "the lessons learned from the implementation of the second NSP 2002–2006,"

---

[22]In 2007 the Government of Nepal established a third entity, the HIV and AIDS and STI Control Board (HSCB), a semi-autonomous entity (SAE) tasked with "developing appropriate policies, strategies and plans, strengthening multisectoral coordination, overall monitoring and evaluation and mobilizing national and international resources for the effective response to HIV and AIDS in the country." I am not sure who this board is, what they do, or how their aims are different from the other two entities.

and "the low coverage and access to services, insufficient focus on treatment, care and support, and the inadequate link between prevention and treatment, care and support that resulted" (Bastola 2011:18). The goal of the third NAP was to expand universal access "to reach 80 percent coverage of prevention, treatment, care and support services to Most at Risk Population (MARP) and PLHIV" (Bastola 2011:18). How did the third plan fare? Care (2011) concluded that "despite such efforts, studies show that the HIV epidemic is concentrated among MARPs." The fourth NSP (2011–2016), revised from the third, is now in operation and focuses more heavily on mobile populations. Likewise it is coordinated closely with the United Nation's Millennium Development Goals, particularly goal number six, which vows to reverse the spread of the epidemic by 2016. And an associated NAP (2010–15), which now also includes the spouses of most at risk migrants, is also now in operation.

So how effective has the national strategy been to date? Each of the early short and mid-term plans had weaknesses (that have been noted), but each subsequent plan attempted to address these weakness and were adjusted accordingly. Then various bureaucracies, such as the NACC and NAC, were created to develop and operationalize National Strategic Plans intended to lessen the impact of AIDS on Nepal. However, due to "political turmoil and changes in government leadership," the NAC did not meet once between 2002–2008 (Bastola 2011:18). And according to the World Bank (2008), both the NAC and the NACC were essentially "non-functional" as of that time. In 2008, the World Health Organization (WHO 2008), which probably has the best handle on the real situation in Nepal, noted that a number of "health systems challenges and issues" and "structural weakness" remain as barriers to making Millennium Development Goal number six a reality for Nepal.[23] And overall, the World Bank has concluded that "the lack of a suitable institutional mechanism with adequate capacity and an appropriate mandate, effective multi-sectoral involvement, and strong public-private partnership, has been a key impediment to mounting an effective response to the epidemic thus far" (2008).

As mentioned previously, lack of surveillance and testing (self admitted) has led to gross under-reporting (Sharma 2010) and even leaders in the effort concede that "the unidentified infected cases are exactly the reason why Nepal will not be able to meet the Millennium Development Goal (MDG) of halting and reversing the spread of HIV and AIDS by 2015" (Sharma 2010). In evaluating the current strategy of the NAP 2011–2016, CARE (with its emphasis on migrant laborers) has concluded that "the magnitude of the epidemic among mobile populations in Nepal may be underestimated due to inadequate surveillance mechanisms and poor record keeping. The risk imposed by migrants to housewives, their offspring and others may further expand and generalize the epidemic" (Bastola 2011:19).

---

[23]This WHO report contains the most comprehensive (and from my perspective, realistic) critique of the current National response to HIV and AIDS in Nepal.

In concluding the discussion on Nepal's national response to HIV and AIDS, Wasti, Simkhada, Randall, and VanTeijlingen (2009) have done a masterful job at addressing some remaining key challenges that the government of Nepal faces in successfully carrying out a national HIV prevention and treatment program in Nepal. These authors provide a good summary overview of the government HIV and AIDS prevention programs through the years, concluding that the remaining challenges are "shaped mostly on cultural and managerial issues from grass roots to policy level." This finding corresponds closely with my own experience in Nepal and I would encourage any reader interested in better understanding the unique issues involved in HIV and AIDS prevention in Nepal to consult this resource.

Looking back at the trajectory of Nepal's first responses to HIV and AIDS, Suvedi (1999:9–13) has identified three main strategies of the initial AIDS prevention model implemented in Nepal. These were: (1) multi-sector involvement, (2) targeting of specific "high risk" groups, and (3) awareness raising. Multi-sector involvement seeks the active participation in planning, implementation, and evaluation of AIDS prevention programs by local bodies in cooperation with national planners. This is a "grass roots" approach rather than a top down model. The goal is capacity building and sustainability of prevention activities at the local level. Examples of this strategy are income-generating projects for women (to keep them from going to India in search of work), FSW "rehabilitation" activities (like sewing classes), AIDS education camps held for local kids, and local adult literacy classes, which build practical skills while introducing AIDS education. Suvedi (1999:10) reported that by 1999 only six out of seventy-five districts in Nepal were actually implementing these types of multi-sector programs.

The second strategy of this AIDS prevention model is the targeting of specific "high risk groups."[24] In Nepal, these groups were first identified (via the studies presented previously) as (1) FSWs and their clients and (2) IDUs. Because the prevalence rates had grown to "concentrated epidemic" proportions within various populations practicing high risk behaviors, attention during the early years of the epidemic seemed to focus on these groups. The reasoning here was obvious; if the epidemic could be contained within these groups it would not spread to the general population (as is made explicit in fig. 3.2). Therefore the early targeted interventions focused primarily upon IDUs and FSWs, most of whom resided in the capital city and urban centers.[25] This also had the effect of framing the cultural model of HIV and AIDS in the early days, as we will see shortly.

---

[24]These days it is more politically correct to speak of "high-risk behavior" or "at risk populations" rather than "high-risk groups."

[25]According to Suvedi (1999:11), by 1999 this strategy was only being implemented in the central region of Nepal (comprising nine districts) mainly along the highway routes.

The third strategy, awareness building, was the most visible in Nepal during the mid to late 1990s. The National Center for AIDS and STD Control, under the direction of the NACC, implemented many national programs designed to increase public awareness. These included a mass media campaign in which AIDS awareness messages were dispersed widely across the country via signboards, newspapers, radio, and TV; the production of AIDS awareness pamphlets distributed to the local level health posts; the sponsoring of public events, such as the Second International AIDS Day celebration held in Kathmandu (fig. 3.4); and inclusion of information about AIDS in the national education curriculum as part of the eighth grade health reader. Studies support the fact that Nepalis were then becoming more aware of AIDS—a change I also observed in my own visits to various rural locations. AIDS information was seen and heard along the highways, miles off the road in the rural Chepang area, in Gorkha District, and even along the trekking route in Langtang National Park. Suvedi (1999:11) suggests that the awareness-raising model "assumes that creating awareness and knowledge among the general population will greatly reduce the vulnerability to high risk behavior activities and thereby help in reducing transmission of HIV infection" (Suvedi 1999:11). As we have seen, however, this isn't always the case.

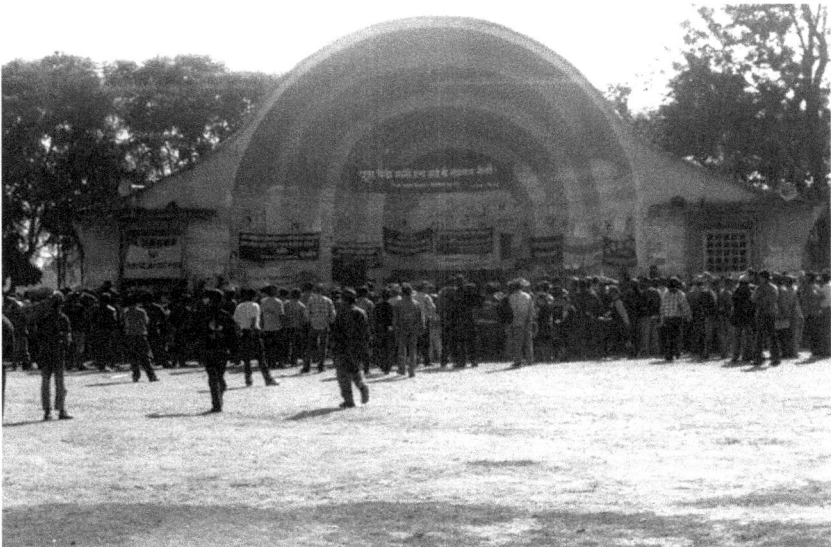

Figure 3.4 World AIDS Day celebrated in Kathmandu
(Photo © David Beine, used by permission)

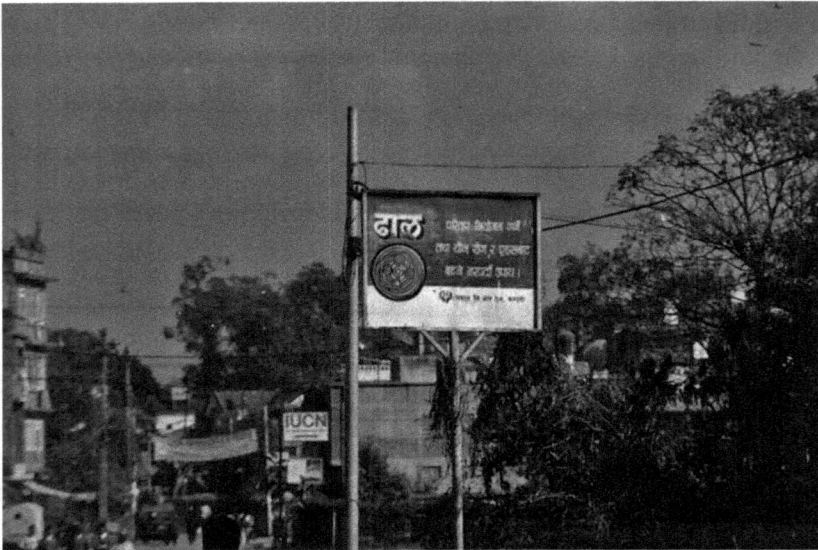

Figure 3.5 One of many condom billboards around the city
(Photo © David Beine, used by permission)

The national campaign against HIV and AIDS has been most strongly influenced by models and methods from the West. The KAP or KAB model has been the most often used model to determine the factors contributing to the epidemic and, not surprisingly, "awareness-building" has risen to the top as the most preferred prevention strategy in the national AIDS prevention program. In a letter welcoming participants to the Nineteenth All Nepal Medical Conference, for instance, Nepal's Honorable Health Minister commented that "lack of awareness is the major factor facilitating the transmission [of HIV and AIDS]" (Hissaria 1999). This was a strikingly similar conclusion to that of several KAP studies financed and directed by various Western INGOs a half decade earlier. For instance, Cox and Suvedi (1994) have concluded that "a low level of public awareness contributes to the growing AIDS problem in Nepal. This lack of awareness relates to the country's low rates of literacy, a shortage of appropriate AIDS education messages, and strong cultural prohibitions against the public discussion of sex" (1994:2).

In the beginning, Nepal leaned heavily upon the West for help in fighting the newly emerging epidemic. One Nepali doctor working on the prevention side of the epidemic in Nepal told me that "when AIDS first came we didn't know what to do, so a Western dominated approach was used" (personal communication). Funding was from the West, AIDS prevention ideas (including the manuals used) were from the West, and prevention workers, who really didn't want to take sexual issues to the public, were "forced" to do so "by the donors." Further, he stated, "We did this because in the beginning we didn't know what to do, so we followed the manual [Western]. At the time, we felt it worked out. But slowly, we have discovered that it has had another impact" (personal communication).

The "impact" he was referring to was various misnomers about AIDS that were to develop as a result of the AIDS awareness-building campaign. For instance, the traditional health belief model posits gods or "ill fate" as a fundamental cause for illness, not germ theory. He commented:

> We came presenting a model that the people were not acknowledging; that microorganisms, not gods and ill fate, are causing disease. It's pretty difficult then to dodge that idea [gods and ill fate], but we came directly and started talking about the "virus." And the doctors didn't know how to translate that into the lay people's language. We tried to translate that [into the awareness-building literature] (because at that time the doctors were considered to be the most knowledgeable about the issue). And medical persons went into the villages to provide technical knowledge about HIV and AIDS. They talked about germ theory, something the people had never heard of. Then they tried to explain viruses and the HIV virus on top of that, and the complexity of it. They tried to explain the immune system. They tried to explain the immune system to lay people and it created a whole set of rumors. They tried to explain that only the antibody, and not HIV, is detectable—that created a whole lot of other issues. And the medical people are somehow responsible for that.
>
> We said that the virus is an obligatory parasite. It doesn't have life in itself. People understood it quite differently. When the testers came and said that we are not really testing for the virus but for antibodies, it was too complex for them and they understood that the virus doesn't really exist but there is instead, an AIDS disease. Then we began condom promotion. People came to believe that this was the Americans' way to sell condoms. This is because people cannot see the virus. This idea was too abstract. They got this concept from the doctors who were telling them that HIV could not be detected. They got the idea that even the scientist cannot see HIV and that we cannot test for it or detect it. They were thinking "now they're telling us that to protect [ourselves] from this disease, which cannot be detected or seen, we must wear a condom, and now they're selling it." They came to believe AIDS was an American program to sell the condom.

Likewise, this same doctor told of a martial arts instructor who called him, concerned that he would get AIDS because he had taught HIV positive persons judo. Since talking about sex is taboo in Nepal, prevention workers in Nepal decided to translate "intercourse" euphemistically as "physical contact" in the literature they distributed regarding AIDS. This instructor had read the material and was afraid since in teaching these people judo, he had had "physical contact" with them. In another instance, when it was discovered that there was an increase in HIV and AIDS among IDUs, the use of "disposable syringes" was promoted through an education campaign. People got the message that disposable syringes cannot transmit HIV. Therefore, they were using "disposable syringes" and sharing them, believing that they could not transmit HIV this way. And in a final example, the doctor told of rural people who had concluded that AIDS was a brand of beer because the AIDS ads (part of the awareness-building campaign) began to be aired on the radio immediately after the news, a time slot formerly filled with beer advertisements.[26]

The emphasis on awareness building has led to a nation-wide multimedia advertising campaign to promote condom use and discourage intravenous drug use. Upon my return to Nepal after a three-year absence, I was amazed to see the public display of topics considered too taboo to even speak of by the wider society: Billboards displaying condom ads on one side and drug awareness messages on the other, every tenth of a mile on the major road ringing Kathmandu (fig. 3.5); banners promoting Panther Condoms hanging over the street outside the local market in my quiet residential neighborhood; and, images of Dhaaley Dai[27], an animated condom character prominently displayed every few miles along the main highway—a full-size smiling condom encouraging us with the message, "Let's wear a condom and chase away AIDS!" (fig. 3.6). To the joy of the awareness-building advocates, the once taboo topic of sex is now prominently displayed throughout the country.

But what are the possible implications of such a public promotion of topics considered taboo by the society? Smith suggests that in Nepal, something is not wrong or "bad" until it is brought into the open. She asks the question:

> Could this also be true, then, of the open display of condoms and discussion of sex in public, as practiced by the HIV and AIDS campaign? It may be, that, far from liberating people to discuss sex more freely, the current approach actually makes sex appear sinful, reinforcing the perception that "bad people" get HIV and AIDS and that those teaching about it are also bad? If so, then this has serious implications for the HIV and AIDS education campaign. (Smith 1996:83)

---

[26]I also heard this same story from villagers (chapter five).

[27]*Dhaal* literally means 'shield' and it is the Nepali word and symbol chosen to represent the 'condom', a borrowed concept. We will see in later chapters that the application of a war schema to describe associations with disease, is also a borrowed feature. The verb chosen, *bhagaanu*, also has a military association, meaning 'to chase away' as you would do to an enemy. *Dai* means 'older brother'.

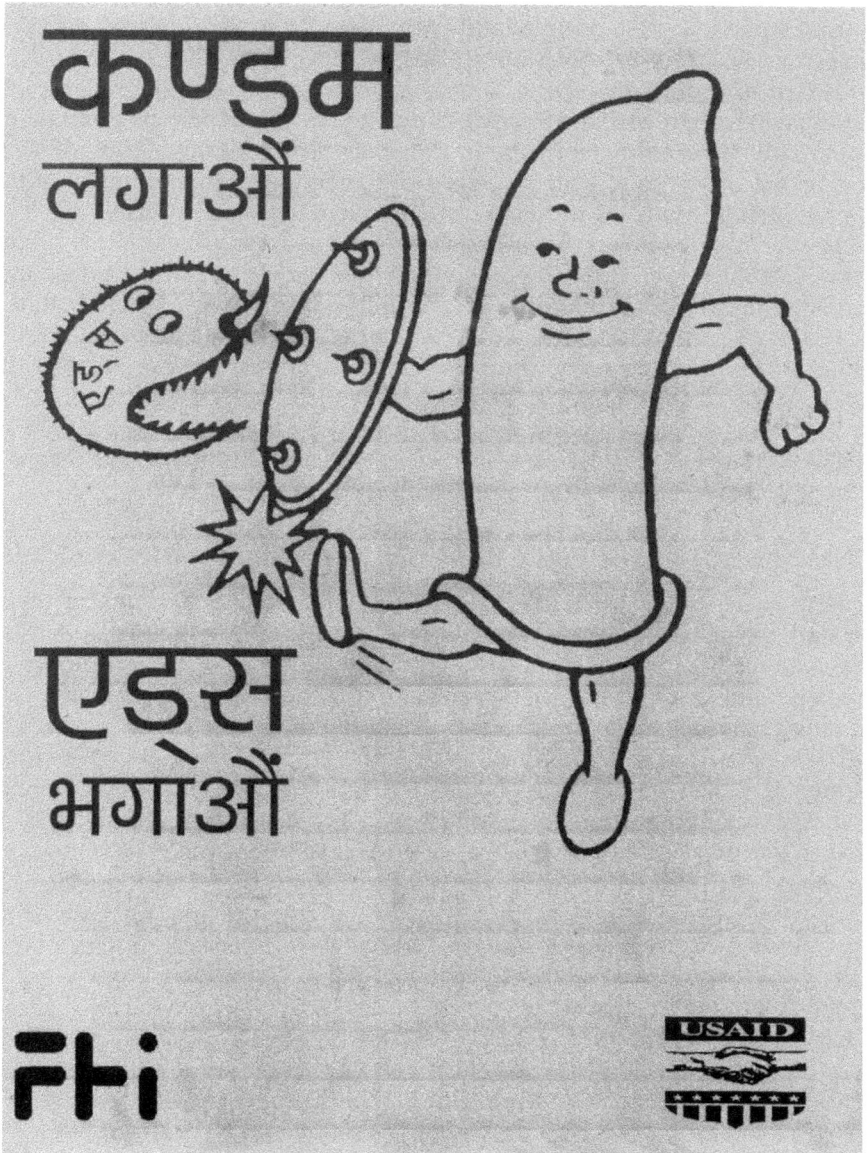

Figure 3.6. Dhaaley Dai, the animated condom.
(Photo © David Beine, used by permission)

Further, Smith, who has a good handle on Nepali culture, suggests that the use of a condom as a "campaign symbol" has the negative repercussion of "alienating certain groups" and further "fuels the idea that AIDS is bad" (Smith 1996:84).

And what about the prominent display of anti-intravenous drug use messages on the billboards as well? It has been reported that the campaign launched to promote injecting drug abstinence in Nepal actually led to "a rapid switch from oral to injecting drug use" as the advertising campaign apparently "peeked the curiosity of oral drug users" (Mangla 1993:684). It seems that many prevention strategies designed to lessen the impact of the spread of HIV and AIDS in Nepal actually had deleterious effects.

In recent years many have begun to question the effectiveness of the "standard fare" prevention approaches in the Nepali cultural context and are beginning to advocate for approaches that take culture seriously in the equation (Beine 2003; USAID 2004; Poudel et al., 2005; Wasti et al. 2009; Beine 2011) and provide culturally informed prevention models (USAID 2004; Wasti 2009; Poudel et al. 2005). Even so, "awareness-building," a product of the West, remains a major strategy in the fight against AIDS in Nepal.[28] One must wonder what ideologies underlie this approach? This is a topic I will take up in a subsequent publication.

3.4 Emerging HIV and AIDS discourses and cultural models

Much of the focus of the early public discourses on AIDS in Nepal revolved around the blame of certain "high risk groups."[29] As mentioned earlier, the major AIDS discourse was first subsumed primarily under the wider discourses of commercial sex work and intravenous drug use. We will see in later chapters that the discourse and earliest emerging cultural model of AIDS as a "bad peoples" disease was, in part, a product of the prevention strategies which 1) targeted high risk groups and (2) created a national awareness-building campaign. And in part, the cultural model of AIDS as a "bad peoples" disease was created when traditional ideas were applied to what was then the new disease known as "AIDS." Once the disease was associated with groups that the culture traditionally categorizes as "bad people," a stigma was created and blame and societal hate has been expressed toward those with AIDS.

FSWs and IDUs (often referred to as "AIDS junkies") were the two groups most often "blamed" for the spread of AIDS in Nepal in the beginning. At that time, Pigg (1999:59) wrote, "Though few officials will publicly admit it, AIDS is thought of as a distasteful problem of prostitutes, perverts and

---

[28]These days fewer billboards are seen across the country, but the pamphlets and educational materials of the various NGOs and the national curriculum still prominently display these same sexually explicit and drug-related images, which we will see later play a role in instantiating indigenous cultural schema.

[29]It is interesting to me that medical professionals do not consider themselves a "high risk" group in Nepal. This will be discussed at length in the coming chapters as well.

drug addicts, of 'bad people' who are not worthy of the scarce public resources available for public health."

These "bad people" were viewed as both the reservoir of the disease as well as the vectors of transmission through which the disease threatened the general public. Even though the number of infected men (clients of FSWs) was twice that of infected FSWs, little was ever mentioned in the media about the male clients of these women, and when it was, they were assumed to be "greasy old men with STDs or sex-starved construction workers" (Fredrick 1999:19).

Cultural models do not change overnight. More accurately they do not change at all, but embedded elements are added or subtracted as culture changes. While these "bad people" might have been the first face of AIDS to the Nepali public, today that face is in transition. Migrant laborers and their spouses are now the most affected population. As the demographic shifts, the discourses will begin to shift as well. And as the discourses shift, the cultural model will be modified. But as of today, much of the "awareness building materials" still focus on these original vectors of spread, which reinforces the cultural model. So while beginning to change, this initial element is still a central element in the Nepali cultural model of HIV and AIDS. Likewise, as the introduction of ART has its impact upon Nepali perceptions of HIV and AIDS (from "death sentence" to "living with HIV"), we will see an associated modification of cultural model taking shape as well.

In this chapter, we have examined the issue of AIDS in Nepal from the epidemiological and social perspectives. We have seen how factors as disparate as poverty, culture, and even AIDS awareness programs have facilitated the spread of HIV and AIDS in Nepal. We have cursorily examined the AIDS discourse in Nepal and have caught a glimpse of how borrowed prevention models have reinforced traditional ideas and have been influential in the emergence of a cultural model of hate and blame toward those with AIDS. We have also begun to see how underlying illness schemata have been borrowed from the West to represent the newly emerging disease of HIV and AIDS in Nepal. We will return later for a much deeper look at this newly intimated cultural model of AIDS in Nepal and its underlying illness schema.

4

Cultural Models, Schema Theory, and Cognitive Methodologies

Cultural models have been defined most simplistically as "shared cognitive schemas through which human realities are constructed and interpreted" (D'Andrade and Strauss 1992:i). In this chapter I examine the theoretical concept of cultural models more closely, discussing the history of the development of a theory of cultural models and schemata, as well as discussing the various types of cultural models and schemata proposed. I also introduce the cognitive methodologies employed in the research and discuss the implications of understanding cultural models of AIDS and underlying illness schemata in Nepal.

4.1 Cultural models—what are they?

The term "cultural model" gets used quite loosely in the literature these days. Paul Farmer (1994) uses the terms "cultural model" and "cognitive model" synonymously throughout his article on the constitution of cultural models of AIDS in Haiti. In discussing Farmer's work, Mattingly and Garro (1994:772) use the terms "explanatory framework" and "cultural models" interchangeably. Holland and Quinn (1987:ix) also use the terms "folk model" and "cultural model" interchangeably in their treatise on cultural models in language and thought. Filmore terms them "frames" (cited in Holland and Quinn 1987:23), Caws calls them "explanatory models" (cited in Holland and Quinn 1987:23), and D'Andrade equates them to a "general folk theory" (1995:130) and "cultural schema" (D'Andrade and Strauss 1992: 34). Keesing (1987:370) suggests that many of the earlier concepts such as "folk models," "prototypes," "schemas," "instantiations," and "conventional metaphors," all products of cognitive anthropology and psychology, have been "recast" today as "cultural models." So, what exactly are cultural models?

4.1.1 Cultural models as "product"

It seems as if the term "cultural model" is being used in two different ways in the literature, both as product and producer. Holland and Quinn define cultural models as presupposed models of the world that are widely shared (although not necessarily to the exclusion of alternative models) by the members of a society and which play an enormous role in their understanding of that world and their behavior in it (1987:4).

In another article, Holland has suggested that cultural models are "shared, conventional ideas about how the world works that individuals learn by talking and acting with their fellows" (1992b:86). Here we see cultural models as collective and shared understanding (product). For instance, Quinn (1987) has demonstrated a cultural model of marriage among Americans; Farmer (1994) has outlined a cultural model of HIV and AIDS among Haitians; and Fillmore (1977) has demonstrated a shared understanding of events we interpret as commercial transactions. I have also alluded to a changing cultural model of HIV and AIDS among Americans (chapter two).

As Keesing (1987) has suggested, the idea of cultural models appears similar to earlier concepts of "folk knowledge." However, cultural models differ from folk knowledge in that they generally center on the ideational mechanisms (schemata) believed to produce "folk" or "cultural" models, while folk knowledge focuses on the ideas themselves. The second part of Holland's quote from above continues, "Defined cognitively, cultural models consist of 'schemas' that guide attention to, drawing inferences about, and evaluation of, experience. These schemas also provide a framework for organizing and reconstructing memories of experience" (1992b:86).

So, we see the concept of cultural model as a product, but it is closely tied to the examination of the producer of the product, schemata, which some authors (as we will see below) also refer to as "cultural models." Keesing (1987:378) has suggested that we distinguish between the two. Cultural models (I) as collective and shared models about the way the world works (product) and cultural models (II), those models (or schemata) that are located in the individual and are used in forming the cognition of the individual (producer). I find this distinction quite useful. Although a major goal of this research will be to examine cultural models (I) of HIV and AIDS that currently exist in Nepal, I am also interested in the schemata (cultural models [II]) that have been influential in the production of these cultural models (I).

4.1.2 Cultural models as "producer" (schemata)

As suggested above, cultural models (II) have also been defined as a type of schemata. Strauss (1992:3) has defined cultural models as "culturally formed cognitive schemas" that are "learned, internalized patterns of thought-feeling that mediate both the interpretation of ongoing experience and the reconstruction of memories." To put it more simplistically, cultural models (II) are types of schemata we use to make sense of things. What makes them "cultural" is that many of the schemata used to produce the models are culturally formed and the resultant models (a product of the application of these various schemata) are more or less "shared" by a group.[1] D'Andrade (1995:132) considers these schemata "culturally shared mental constructs." It is these cultural models (II) that we use to produce meaning associated with any given phenomenon. An understanding of cultural models as schemata requires a better understanding of schema theory in general, as discussed in the next section.

4.2 Schema theory

The idea of schemata as organizing mechanisms for human cognition is not new. Brad Shore (1996:44) credits Immanuel Kant (1929 [1781]) with coining the term "schema." Kant, he suggests, proposed that schema underlie and guide our human understandings of particular experience. Shore then traces the the schema idea through its further development under Bartlett (1932), who proposed that cognitive schemas structure memory, and under Piaget (1932), who "employed schema theory as the basis for a developmental view of human intelligence" (Shore 1996:46). Today, schema theory remains a central theme in cognitive psychology (Fiske and Taylor 1984; Mandler 1984; Rumelhart 1980), cognitive linguistics (Lakoff 1987; Langaker 1987; Tannen 1993), and cognitive anthropology (Atran 1990; Boyer 1990; Casson 1983; D'Andrade 1995; D'Andrade and Strauss 1992; Dougherty 1985; Fiske 1991; Hirshfield and Gelman 1994; Holland and Quinn 1987; Schwartz, White and Lutz 1992; Shore 1996).

Schema theory in anthropology has developed mainly within the rubric of cognitive anthropology. Cognitive anthropology was born during mid-century (1950s), a time when the materialist view of culture was central in anthropology.[2] Discoveries in psychology[3] and

---

[1]This is not to suggest that biologically based schemata are not involved in the process of cultural model construction. They certainly are. I will address this issue later in this chapter and in the concluding chapter I will attempt to identify some of the biologically based schemata that are embedded within cognitive models of HIV and AIDS in Nepal.

[2]Much of the cognitive anthropology presented in this chapter was culled from D'Andrade (1995) and Tyler (1969).

[3]By the 1920s B.F. Skinner's Behaviorism paradigm had replaced Freudian theory as the dominant paradigm in psychology. Skinner's Behaviorism had reduced humans to simple stimulus-response animals. Then Tolman demonstrated that rats have in their minds a complex map of their environment that they use to make decisions. Likewise, Piaget proved that as children develop they construct more and more complex models of their world and Bruner demonstrated that students employ a variety of strategies in concept attainment tasks. All of these findings challenged

linguistics[4] fueled the "cognitive revolution" and these ideas soon led anthropologists to rethink their understanding of culture as material phenomenon as well. Goodenough (1956) soon redefined culture as a mental phenomenon. Although the school of anthropology known as "ethnoscience" (which was most active at Yale) had been interested in cognition since early in the century, interest in ideational systems had remained a minority interest in anthropology until this point. Goodenough (1956) applied the etic/emic (distinctive features) linguistic principle introduced by Pike (1956) to kinship in order to understand how people classify kin. Soon other anthropologists were applying the same "feature analysis" principles to areas as diverse as ethnobotany (Concklin 1954) and color classifications (Berlin and Kay 1969). Cognitive anthropology soon became a major paradigm in American anthropology.

Other anthropologists extended the "feature analysis" model to behavior that leads to classification. James Spradley (1972), for example, attempted to discover major "themes" which are prevalent throughout multiple "domains" of culture. The goal was to discover "cultural grammars," or the underlying rules which control our behavior. Or as Goodenough (1957:167) put it, "whatever it is that one needs to know or believe in order to operate in an acceptable manner within their given culture." Various methods (such as taxonomic and componential analysis) designed to match the rigors of linguistic science were developed for discovering these underlying themes and rules.

It was soon recognized that although the feature analysis model was useful to examine how people organize knowledge (categorically), it had many limitations as well. For example, feature analysis was unable to reveal anything about the apparent relationship between categories. It was also unable to tell us anything about the cognitive distance between categories or between members of any one class. Emphasis began to shift from the emic categories to the relationships (connectionist networks) between these categories. Semantic networking models were proposed (D'Andrade 1995:63) and various methods such as free-listing, sentence framing, triad tests, pile sorting, paired comparisons, and multidimensional scaling were developed for assessing saliency within categories as well as the relationship between cognitive categories. Even given the improvements of techniques, limitations of this type of research still remained. This type of analysis works well

---

the dominant paradigm by demonstrating that cognition (a complex cognitive process) underlies behavior (D'Andrade 19956–9).

[4]Bloomfeild's descriptive linguistic model (which also took a behaviorist approach) was the dominant linguistic paradigm of the day until Chomsky (1957) posited a deeper psychological process behind language learning. Chomsky's discoveries suggested that people have a complex map in their heads that they use to construct language and it is impossible to account for this process using the Bloomfield's model of language (D'Andrade 1995:10).

for "natural kinds" (Atran 1990), but not for other types of data. It is descriptive but not predictive. Feature analysis provided us a good look at the mental maps people draw, but it could take us no further. Interest shifted from what we order to how we order (the process).

In the late 1970s psychologist Eleanor Rosch, theorizing about the nature of categories, proposed that a "prototype" represents a category in our mind and that these prototypes are perceived or remembered not simply as a list of features, but as a configuration (gestalt). For instance, a person's prototype for the concept 'bird' is actually a configuration (gestalt) that consists of feathers, wings, a bill, and the ability to fly. One type of bird does not represent the "prototype" exactly, but the more features shared with the prototype, then the more salient the class member is considered. Robins would appear at the top of the category called "birds" while ostriches and penguins would be less salient members of the class. D'Andrade (1995:120) suggests that Rosch's work synthesized the findings of the research on folk taxonomies. Cognitive differences were discovered between different hierarchical levels. Upper-level terms are comprised of a smaller number of features that are usually more formal and "schematic in nature" (D'Andrade 1995:120). This provides an effective means for making broad distinctions between items. Rosch effectively demonstrated the human ability to create configurations of features (like "birdness"), which then serve as the cognitive representation for a category. D'Andrade (1995:120) concludes that "[Rosch's] work on taxonomies shifted cognitive anthropology from an exclusive interest in features to an interest in configurations of features, which create psychological objects."

Following the work of Rosch it soon became apparent that there are higher-level mental structures that produce the categories that those using feature analysis had been discovering. Emphasis quickly turned to an investigation of these higher-level mental structures that came to be known as "schemata."

4.3 Schemata—what are they?

Schemata are conceptual abstractions proposed to be "the building blocks of cognition" (Casson 1983; Rumelhart 1980). These abstract knowledge structures are hypothesized to serve as the basis for all human information processing, including perception and comprehension, categorization and planning, recognition and recall, and problem solving and decision making (Casson 1983). Schemata are proposed as a kind of template that we hold in our heads that organizes the past (i.e., structures memory), orders the present (meaning construction), and predicts the future (makes inferences based on schemata) (D'Andrade and Strauss 1992; Fiske and Taylor 1984; Holland 1992a).

4.3.1 Kinds of schemata

Ronald Casson (1983), summarizing much of the earlier work on schemata, identifies three types of schemata. These are (1) universal schemata, (2) idiosyncratic schemata, and (3) cultural models. Casson describes the distinction between these schemata in this way:

> Schemata differ in their distribution in populations: some are universal, some idiosyncratic, and some cultural. Universal schemata are uniform in the human species because of innate faculties of the mind and/or inherent divisions in the natural world; idiosyncratic schemata are unique to particular individuals as the result of their personal histories and life experiences; cultural schemata are neither unique to the individual nor shared by all humans, but rather shared by members of particular societies. (1983:440)

Universal schemata, which Brad Shore (1996) calls "primitive innate mental schemas (PIMS)," are believed to be biologically innate schemata which structure all human learning in some domains due either to innate facilities in the human mind or inherent divisions in the natural world. PIMS would appear to be schemata that regulate such things as early childhood attachment with caregivers and the perception of facial gestalts. PIMS would explain such phenomena as the universal color categorization such as that described by Berlin and Kay (1969) and the early stages of childhood reasoning as described by Piaget. Shore (1996:10) suggests that PIMS may best be understood as a form of "species knowledge, learned and transmitted biologically through Darwinian selection."

The second type of schemata proposed is idiosyncratic in nature. Shore (1996:10) suggests that idiosyncratic schemata (IS) are "opportunistically constructed by individuals as a way of negotiating novel situations or environments." These become a part of an individual's personal knowledge. Dorothy Holland (1992b) suggests that one of the early limitations of schema theory is that it couldn't account for what she calls the "messy situation." Humans are believed to be "schema driven," yet two schema-driven individuals can arrive at different solutions to the same situation. This demonstrates that besides PIMS and cultural models (described below), there are also personal schemata (idiosyncratic schemata) that people quickly develop and employ to handle novel situations.

Between the two ends of the spectrum above (PIMS on one end and IS on the other) lay cultural models, those schemata which are neither universal nor idiosyncratic, but which are shared by members of a particular society. D'Andrade and Strauss (1992:3) define cultural models as "shared cognitive schemas through which human realities are constructed and interpreted." These cultural models are "culturally formed cognitive schemata" that "mediate the interpretation of on-going experiences and the reconstruction of memories" (D'Andrade and Strauss 1992:3). Or as Dorothy Holland (1992b:68) has put it, schemata "channel experience of the present, inform anticipation of the future, and play an important role in the (re)construction of memories of the past." These cognitive schemata are a kind of cognitive template built, in part, through social interaction, which produces a fairly similar understanding of experience when activated. Although these cognitive structures are formed through social interaction, they reside in the mind of the individual, and they function just like every other form of schemata. I will talk more about how schemata work in the next section.

Because cultural schemata are shared by members of a society, and because cognitive anthropologists are interested in the cultural part of cognition, the remainder of this section will focus upon cultural schemata, often referred to as cultural models (II). Ronald Casson (1983) proposes five types of cultural schemata. These are: (1) object schemata,(2) orientation schemata, (3) event schemata, (4) metaphor schemata and (5) narrative schemata.

The first type of cultural schemata, which is proposed to underlie object classification systems, is known as "object schemata." Object schemata are utilized with things that seem to fit quite naturally into taxonomies. Scott Atran (1990) calls these "natural kinds." Types of plants, animals, manufactured items (such as cars, furniture, clothes, etc.), occupations, emotions, illnesses, and kin would be examples of items for which object schemata seem to be employed. This process of class inclusion and classification seems to be the way we make sense of new "objects" that enter our experience. Using the schematic process we build hierarchical cognitive taxonomies based on perceived similarities and differences between items. "Vehicle," for instance, would be the prototype for the category that includes buses, cars, and trucks. Subordinate categories for bus would include city bus and school bus. Because classification of the same items can differ from culture to culture (i.e., a bullock cart is considered a type of vehicle in Nepal but not in America), object schemata are considered a type of "culturally formed cognitive schemata."

According to Casson, orientation schemata are another type of cultural model. Orientation schemata, usually referred to as "cognitive maps" in anthropology, "represent knowledge about spatial relations among objects and their relative positions in the physical environment" (Casson 1983:444). Cognitive maps can be small (such as the one you might use to explain to your spouse, over the phone, where in the house you left your checkbook) or large (such as the cognitive map you might draw upon when giving someone directions to your house from across town). Cognitive maps can also be quite complex. Gladwin (1970) has described a complex orientation schema traditionally employed by navigators in Oceania in order to travel long distances without the aid of compass or visual helps.

According to Kuipers (1978), cognitive maps contain three types of representational information: (1) the knowledge one has about his/her particular environments, (2) the understanding of one's current position in relation to where you want to be (a kind of "you are here" pointer), and (3) knowledge about the processes that will complete the task of traversing the map (i.e., a preferable route). Although the cognitive maps of individuals in every society contain these three types of representational information, the types of maps we "draw" may differ from culture to culture. I would also suggest that the cognitive maps of individuals within a culture vary. For instance, I have a way of giving directions that seems more akin with other males in my culture (such as using directionals—north, south, east, and west—and actual mileage), while my wife uses many more left-right directionals and landmarks (such as turn left at the park). We all use cognitive maps daily (most of us multiple times), but the content of these maps may be formed culturally as well as idiosyncratically.

The third type of cultural schemata proposed by Casson (1983) is event schemata. One example of event schemata is what many authors refer to as cultural "scripts." Fiske and Taylor (1984:167) define scripts as "structures that describe appropriate sequences of events in well-known situations." When "The Star Spangled Banner" begins to play at a baseball game, all Americans know to stand, remove their hats, and remain quiet in reverence, or sing along. Likewise, we all know the various steps of the restaurant script, from being seated, through paying the bill. These are all culturally formed event schemata, which define expectations and guide our behavior in scenes we interpret to require certain scripts.

Another example of event schemata is the "commercial event" schema made famous by Fillmore (1977). The commercial event (that our schema dictates) contains a buyer, seller, a product to be purchased, change of ownership, and money. Again, our understanding of the commercial event is the product of the application of a culturally formed cognitive schema. The expectations are defined by this schema and guide our behavior in situations interpreted to be commercial events.

The fourth kind of cultural model proposed by Casson (1983) is metaphor. Metaphor is often employed as a type of schema in which the meaning associated with one concept is understood to apply to another usually unrelated concept as well. Casson (1983:449) suggests that "a metaphor states an equivalence between two concepts from different domains." He uses as an example, the metaphoric phrase, *George is a lion.* In this example, the dissimilar characteristics (e.g., fir, paws, tail) are omitted from the schema and the similar characteristics (culturally defined) of courage, strength, and aggressiveness, are retained and are applied to our understanding of George. The "lion" schema is applied metaphorically and what we know to be true of lions (minus the dissimilar characteristics) we assume to be true of George. Thus, the lion schema is used to provide meaning to our under-standing about George. Other famous examples of this type of schematic application are "time as money" (*we spend it, buy it, save it,* etc.), "ideas as food" (*they are half-baked, we chew on them,* and sometimes *they are hard to swallow*), and "argument as war" (*we defend a position, attack a point,* and *win or lose*). We will also examine the idea of "illness as war" (*we fight colds, kill germs,* and *are losing the battle against AIDS*) more in depth later in this book.

Casson (1983:451) suggests that metaphoric schema (what Lakoff [1987] calls "image schema") can be broken into three main types: (1) ontological, (2) orientational, and (3) structural. Regarding the first of these, Casson states that "ontological metaphors are used in comprehending events, actions, activities and states. Events and actions are metaphorically con-ceptualized as objects, activities as substances, and states as containers" (1983:451).

The "ideas as food" metaphor is a good example of ideas as objects. "Vitality as substance" metaphors are represented by sayings such as *He's full of life* (full of vitality) or *I'm drained* (devoid of vitality). The container schema (life as container) is another popular ontological image schema. We say, "*He lived life to the full*" or "*His life was empty.*" According to D'Andrade (1995:133), "The container schema is used for a great variety of objects; one walks out of a room, puts milk in a glass, falls out of love, puts ideas into words, falls into a trap, etc."

The second type of image schemata is orientational metaphors. According to Casson (1983:451), "Orientational metaphors are used to structure ab-stract concepts that are not well grounded in experience in terms of con-crete concepts arising from experience with spatial relationships." Examples of orientational metaphors are, "happy as up" (*I feel really up today, I am in high spirits*) and "sad as down" (*I am feeling really down today, I'm down in the dumps*), "health as up" (*I'm in top shape*) and "sickness as down" (*under the weather*), and "control as up" (*I'm on top of it*) and "being controlled as down" (*I've got him under control*).

Structural metaphors are the third kind of metaphorical schemata, in which one complex concept is presented in terms of another concept:

> Structural metaphors are used in comprehending complex, highly structured concepts. While ontological and orientational meta-phors are basic in providing the means of referring to concepts, quantifying them, orienting them, and so on, structural metaphors provide the use of "one highly structured and clearly delineated concept to structure another" (Steiner 1974:61). In structural meta-phors, the constituent structures of complex object, orientation, and event schemata serve as the means of structuring other com-plex schemata. (Casson 1983:452)

Casson (1983:452) uses the "life as game" *(Life is a game, Life is a gamble)* metaphor as an example of a structural metaphor based on a complex event schema and "love as journey" *(This relationship isn't going anywhere)* as an example of a structural metaphor based on an orientation schema.

Casson's final proposed cultural models are narratives. Casson (1983:452) suggests that the aforementioned event, object and orientation schemata "provide the underlying organization for narrative discourse." Casson considers narratives to be a type of cultural model because cultural differences have been noted in story schemata in terms of how different cultural groups organize stories.

4.3.2 How schemata work

The "commercial event" example noted earlier provides a good opportunity to illustrate how schemata are proposed to work. The theory begins with the presupposition that "perceivers actively construct their own reality" (Fiske and Taylor 1984:139). We do this through the use of schemata. According to Piaget and Inhelder (1969), children pass through stages of development in which they construct increasingly complex models (schemas) of the world around them. The first stage, which they termed "sensorimotor" (0–2 years of age), is characterized by non-verbal individual learning that derives from their experience with concrete objects in the physical world. In the second stage, which they called "pre-operational" (2–7 years of age), children learn that words represent objects. In the third stage, which they dubbed "concrete operations" (7–12 years of age), objects are classified by similarities and differences. Later scholars (Shore 1996) proposed that during this stage, the primitive innate mental schemas (PIMS) would begin to be employed. The final stage (12 to adult), which Piaget and Inhelder titled the "formal" (or scientific) stage, was characterized as a period in which formal logic, propositional thinking, and deductive reasoning developed.

The main criticism of Piaget and Inhelder's theory was concerning their proposal that all of the stages were biologically determined. Vygotsky (1962), the first major critic of this theory, defended the primacy of culture in shaping development (Howe 1996). For Vygotsky, childhood development (especially in the later stages) was a product of culture, not biology. Piaget and Inhelder stressed the psychological underpinnings (biology) of children's behavior while Vygotsky stressed the role of culture.

Brad Shore (1996:75) describes the influence that Vygotsky's work has had on the development of schema theory:

> Vygotsky's approach to cognitive development influenced a number of cross-cultural psychologists who have studied how cultural models are learned by children and how cultural learning shapes cognitive development. Vygotsky turned developmental psychology

inside out, stressing the social and cultural origins of even the most intimate and private aspects of thinking. For Vygotsky, the social context within which cognitive development takes place is not just the local cultural setting but the entire historical context within which social relations are embedded.

Likewise, Holland contends that it is a neo-Vygotskian developmental approach that informs much of the modern work on cultural models. Holland (1992a:63), referencing the American cultural model of marriage, writes, "In the context of social interaction, the individual comes to internalize cultural resources, such as cultural models, language, and symbols, as means to organize and control her thoughts and emotions."

Cultural schemata are formed through a complex process that includes both biological and cultural influences. Although the following is a simplified example, the process that underlies the construction of schemata goes something like this: First, basic schemata (that include biologically based schemata as embedded elements) are experientially built (through, for example, the process of categorization of new items based on the principle of class inclusion spoken of earlier) and then are stored in memory[5] as a general case, abstracted from specific cases (Fiske and Taylor 1984:140).[6] As new information appears, certain stimuli automatically[7] trigger familiar schemata, producing meaning, which is attributed to the new situation. Using the earlier example of the commercial event, the schema (a prototype) includes various constituent elements such as buyer, seller, product, and exchange. When you look out the window and see a nicely dressed man carrying a briefcase walking to your door, he might be interpreted as a "salesman." This interpretation then turns on the commercial event schema. You know that he will be SELLING a PRODUCT and will want you to BUY it in EXCHANGE for your money. Fiske and Taylor (1984:142) claim, "The schema concept builds on the constructive or interpretive view of perception by positing that organized prior knowledge shapes what is perceived and recorded in memory."

The fact that we begin with biologically based schemata (PIMS) and the fact that the process of schematization seems to be the same for all human

---

[5]These stored schemata contain "both the attributes of the concept and the relationship among the attributes" (Fiske 1984:140).

[6]Schemata are stored in memory in an abstract form, as a simplified template rather than as a collection of all the original encounters that produced the schema. Schema theory advocates claim that this process "makes possible a certain efficiency and adaptiveness in social cognition" (Fiske 1984:139). If we were to actively store each experience in memory rather than storing information as simplified general schemata, it would require much more "space" (to use a computer analogy).

[7]Casson (1983:431) claims that schemata are "autonomous and automatic—once set in motion they proceed to their conclusion."

beings regardless of their culture, highlights the role of biology in the formulation of higher level schemata. The fact that the creation of higher-level schemata is dependent upon such things as categorization (which differs from culture to culture), highlights the role of culture in the process.

4.3.3 Characteristics of schemata

The "commercial event" example above also illustrates several of the characteristics of schemata. First of all, schemata are "embedded" structures which themselves can be made up of other lower level schemata as well as being constituent members of other higher level schemata. For example, "exchange" may include the subordinate concept of "money," which may, in turn, include the concepts of "currency," "coin," and "check." Casson terms these lower level schemata "subschemata":

> A schema generally includes a number of embedded subschemata as constituent parts, each which interacts in its own right with elements in the environment. A schema, in other words, is most often a complex structure in which variables are bound by subschemata. Overall, then, schemata are organized as hierarchical structures in which schemata at the higher levels represent the most general concepts, and at successively lower levels represent more and more specific concepts. Schemata at the lowest level are atomic, i.e., primitive concepts that are components of knowledge that do not break down into constituent parts or further subschemata. (Casson 1983:436)

Thus, schemata are constructed out of other schemata and it is probable that the "commercial event" schema is a constituent part of other even higher-level schemata.

Secondly, this example demonstrates the flexibility of schemata. When new information is encountered (such as the discovery of credit cards), the "money" schema can be modified to include the "credit card" concept as a constituent member. The schematic process has been equated (or analogized) with computer data processing models (D'Andrade 1995:136). The first computers used a "serial" data processing method that was characterized by a one-way flow of information. Today's computers allow for "parallel" data processing, the free flow of information in both directions, and parallel processing has served as the model to help us understand how schemata work (D'Andrade 1995:139). Although the higher level schemata which "direct the overall processing of information" are generally more "fixed and invariant" than the lower level schemata, they are "active processes...capable of evaluating their own goodness of fit to elements in the environment and of thereby accounting for them" (Casson 1993:439). Schemata are flexible templates that allow for a range of possibilities (D'Andrade 1992:52).

Another characteristic of schemata is that they include "default values." Once a schemata is employed these default values may be automatically "filled in" even if they were not present or perceived in the initial stimuli (D'Andrade 1992:52). As D'Andrade (1992:52) has aptly noted, "Rarely does one perceive a whole battleship—both sides, top and bottom, inside and out; most of the battleship one understands to be there is filled by default values." As has been demonstrated, however, new information can modify these default values, given enough cases. This characteristic of schemata demonstrates the obvious implications that schemata can have upon perception (e.g., what we think we see), memory (e.g., what we thought we saw) and inference (e.g., what we expect to happen next)—all created from activated schemata.

4.3.4 Modifications to the "cultural model"

Brad Shore (1996) offers an important refinement of the "cultural model" theory. Shore suggests that early theories about cultural models (among cultural anthropologists) implied that cultural models are the only mechanism through which people experience and make sense of their world (a position he characterizes as the "strong constructivist" view). He also suggests that the dominant anthropological idea about cultural models (that cultural models construct a shared reality), in turn, has overly reified the "shared" nature of culture in cultural models. Shore offers an important refinement to the cultural model concept. He proposes an adaptation to the model that also accounts for the place of human agency and historical contingency in the process of meaning construction (1996:317), something that had been lacking in earlier theoretical models.

According to Shore, cultural models (as anthropologists currently define them) are one way people go about making meaning, but not the only way:

> Cultural models are not the only way in which people experience the world. The view that cultural models "construct" reality has dominated cultural anthropology. But a closer look at what happens in the case of conflicting models suggests that the experience of confusion, ambivalence, and irony, which often accompany serious conflict in models, do not support the strong version of the constructivist view.

> Cultural models are better understood as one kind of necessary resource by which people make meaning in their lives. From a cognitive point of view, cultural models are salience-enhancing templates. They render certain kinds of experience perceptually significant and readily communicable within a community. But people may also have powerful experiences not directly predictable

> from any cultural model. And in the absence of a credible cultural
> model for making sense of a situation, individuals have the resourc-
> es for schematizing their own models on the fly. (1996:315)

This would seem to describe the "idiosyncratic" schemata as proposed
by Casson (1983). One must also wonder if, beyond what Shore has suggested, perhaps these "powerful experiences," which create variation within
a group, are possibly the result of the application by individuals of differing
personal "person," "self," and "role" schemata (social schemata identified
by Fiske and Taylor (1984) and described in 4.3.5)?

Much of meaning construction, however, does involve the application
of cultural models more widely shared by the community (many of which
have also developed into personal mental models for many individuals):

> Meaning construction involves the perceptual encounter of a
> meaning-seeking subject and an historically and culturally orches-
> trated world of artifacts. Meaning construction is a kind of learn-
> ing, but it is not by itself a complete account of how we learn.
> Specifically, meaning construction is a Piagetian "assimilation"
> process whereby people employ old cognitive models as resources
> for making sense out of novel experiences...Cultural meaning con-
> struction is a specific kind of assimilation requiring two distinct
> cognitive processes. First, a conventional form of a cognitive mod-
> el is derived from instituted models present in the social environ-
> ment. Second, a novel experience is organized for an individual
> in relation to this conventional cognitive model, providing a sig-
> nificant degree of sharing in the way individuals within a commu-
> nity experience the world. Cultural cognition is a special kind of
> meaning-seeking activity closely related to more general processes
> of meaning construction. (Shore 1996:319)

So, Shore is in agreement with the other authors regarding the first two
types of schemata (universal and idiosyncratic), but offers a further refinement to the general typology of cultural models. Shore proposes two types
of cultural models: (1) special purpose models (such as the invitation script
in Samoa), and (2) foundational schemata. Special purpose models are
basically the same as Fiske and Taylor's (1984) idea of script. "The Star
Spangled Banner" and the restaurant script would be other examples. These
are models that have relatively limited application (i.e., they can only be
applied to a limited number of situations). Foundational schemata on the
other hand are used to organize a large number of diverse models (Shore
1996:45). Shore points out the value of this distinction:

> Different cultural models may share a family resemblance because
> they are organized in relation to common foundational schemas.

> The distinction between a foundational schema and a cultural
> model is really extrinsic, since any model can serve to schematize
> lower-level models. But foundational schemas tend to be more ab-
> stract than models and not as committed to a particular form or
> genre. The value of the distinction between model and schema is
> clear from the great number of different American cultural models
> connected through the modularity schema. (1996:312)

An example of this would be the obvious similarity noted between airports, bus stations and train stations. Shore suggests that these transportation stations are all "instantiations" of the "hub and spoke architecture
schema." The similarity of architectural layout, therefore, is a result of the
application of a foundational schema (hub and spoke architecture). This
concept seems quite similar to Spradley's (1970) earlier ideas of "cultural
themes" which he proposed could be discovered running through various
"domains" in every cultural "scene."

Shore also distinguishes between "instituted" and "mental" models:

> Instituted models are the external or public aspect of culture and
> represent common source domains by which individuals schema-
> tize conventional mental models. Games and other cultural per-
> formances are especially useful for demonstrating the complex
> relations between the external structures of rules and norms and
> the personal experiences that make these possible. The movement
> between instituted and mental models goes in both directions.
> Instituted models are made by people and are the objectification
> over time of someone's inner experiences. The internalization of
> instituted models and the externalization of mental models usu-
> ally occur on quite different time scales, but taken together they
> comprise the basic dialectic of cultural life (1996:312).

Mental models can be either personal (such as the distinction I made earlier between my wife's mental maps and my own) or conventional, widely
shared cultural models that we have internalized as personal.

Concluding on the topic of cultural models, Shore (1996:313) writes,

> Though cultural knowledge is, by definition, shared, the nature
> of this sharing is a complex matter. Cultural knowledge is best
> thought of as a distributed system of models. Cultural models are
> socially distributed in that not all members will share all models
> or will have the same variant of a model. An adequate description
> of cultural models necessarily includes an account of which, or
> whose, perspective is being modeled. A player's model of baseball
> is not that of a spectator, and viewing a game through a television
> tube will engage yet another model of the game. These models

would all be expected to share important properties, however—
properties motivated by the framework of the constitutive rules
and strategies that underlie all play.

Shore's contribution has enhanced our understanding of the complex
process of meaning making, both personal and cultural. He has further elucidated many of the characteristics of cultural models that had remained,
to this point, quite "vague" among many anthropologists. He has provided
a fuller understanding of the psychological and cultural processes involved
in both personal and cultural meaning construction via schemata. Shore's
adaptation serves as an amalgam uniting the usually mutually exclusive
theories of psychology (the psychic unity of mankind principle) and of anthropology (relativism) into one grand theory. His work is an important
contribution to the study of how people make meaning.

4.3.5 Other types of schemata

Besides the kinds of schemata elucidated above, other scholars have proposed
additional types of schemata that warrant at least a brief mention during
this discussion on schemata. Because the main interest of this research is
cultural models however, this will only be a cursory look. Fiske and Taylor
(1984), social psychologists, propose four kinds of "social schemata" that
are also involved in helping individuals navigate through their social worlds.
The emphasis for Fiske and Taylor (as social psychologists) is more on the
individual's cognition (yet as a member of a group), while the cognitive
anthropologist's primary interest is in the cultural part of cognition. Fiske
and Taylor (1984:149) suggest that it is through the application of prior
built knowledge (in the form of schemata) that we are able to "function
in a social world that otherwise would be of paralyzing complexity." The
application of social schemata is a simplification process that helps us make
sense of others as well as ourselves. Fiske and Taylor propose four kinds of
"social schemata." These are (1) person schemata, (2) self schemata, (3)
role schemata, and (4) event schemata.

For instance, person schemata is knowledge (structured through the schema process)
we have "about the traits and goals that shape other people's behavior"
(Fiske and Taylor 1984:149). Fiske and Taylor define person schemata as
"Peoples' understanding of the psychology of typical or specific individuals, composed of traits and goals [that] helps them to categorize others and
remember schema relevant behavior" (Fiske and Taylor 1984:149).

For instance, we build a schema for what the typical "introvert" is like.
We bundle traits or characteristics that we consider to be typical of introverts (under an introvert prototype) and "understand" introverts through
this person schema. Fiske and Taylor conclude that although schemata use
is not always an accurate assessment of a person, it is efficient:

> Person schemata of all sorts shape the processes of perception, memory, and inference to conform to our general assumptions about other people. The effects of schemata upon perception, memory, and inference are not necessarily well suited to accuracy in identifying individual instances. Schemata are used by the mind to manage such processes economically, if not always accurately. (1984:154)

The second type of schemata mentioned by Fiske and Taylor are self schemata. They comment that "general information about one's own psychology makes up a complex, easily accessible verbal concept that guides information processing about the self" (1984:155). Fiske and Taylor term this a "self schema." This includes all of the characteristics (and their constituent meanings) that you would mention if you were to have to describe yourself to someone else.

The third type of schemata is role schemata. Each of us plays roles in the society. We all have an understanding (i.e., schemata) about the characteristics and behavior associated with people who fill certain roles. For instance, we might undress at the request of our doctor because that behavior is acceptable given his/her role, but we would probably not disrobe in front of our grocery store clerk even if requested. Role schemata are usually based on broad social categories such as age, occupation, gender, race, etc.

The final type of schemata mentioned by Fiske and Taylor is event schemata. This is the shared understanding of what happens at events such as birthday parties or at places such as restaurants. This is the same as event schemata mentioned above. Fiske and Taylor's observations focus more on how individuals (who are part of larger social groups) go about making meaning of themselves and others. Fiske and Taylor's observations have added greatly to an understanding of the role of schemata upon perception, memory and inference.

Alan Fiske (1991) takes another interesting approach to the examination of schemata. He proposes that there are four (and only four) irreducible schemata (which act as prototypes) that organize and construct all human social relationships[8]. These are (1) communal sharing, (2) authority ranking, (3) equity matching, and (4) market pricing. Every human society is organized (on a kind of sliding scale from high to low) around these four schemata[9]. These four, when combined in different ways, produce different societies. In American society, for instance, we would be low on communal sharing, mid on authority ranking (where the higher ranked person gets

---

[8] This is not to imply that Fiske does not recognize other schema. Rather, these four are considered meta-schemas under which all other schemata (such as those described above) would be applied (due to the embedded nature of schemata spoken of earlier).

[9] These would seem like "foundational schemata" to use Brad Shore's (1996) terminology.

more and has more choice), mid on equity matching (where all get the same regardless of need, desire, or usefulness), and high on market pricing. The former Soviet Union, however, would be high on communal sharing, high on authority ranking, high on equity matching, but very low on market pricing. Each society has a set of unarticulated rules (what he calls implementation rules), revolving around these four schemata, that people follow in order to organize social relationships. Fiske points out, however, that each culture gives different weight to the four forms and that there are certain contexts within each society where the four forms can be organized differently. It is the different combination of these four principles (a product of different implementation rules) that creates cultural similarities and differences between societies.

Although Fiske's proposal is provocative, various authors have been critical of his conclusions accusing him of cognitive reductionism (Stolte 1992; Lambert 1993). Lambert makes the point that he and many others (and even Fiske himself) have suggested that there are many other forms (besides the four) of human relations.

Recent discoveries in the field of neuroscience would seemingly support the schema concept. Researchers at the Max Plannck Institute of Cognitive Neuroscience have been interested in how language and music (both types of proposed schema) are processed by the brain. They have recently demonstrated that unfamiliar musical chords are processed by the area of the brain known as Broca's area and its right-hemisphere homologue (Maess, Koelsch, Gunter and Friederici 2001). In the experiment, when a conventional musical chord sequence was played to subjects, no unusual brain activity was noted. When a new chord (strange to the hearer) was inserted into the sequence, however, an unusual amount of brain activity was noted in the area of the brain known as Broca's area and its right-hemisphere homologue. These findings also supported earlier linguistic studies that discovered that syntax violation in spoken language also elicits strong brain activity in this same area. The conclusion of the studies is that it is the same "devices" that are the processors of both language and music. Although the authors of this paper don't identify these "devices" by name as schemata, the findings would support the schema concept. This study would suggest that new information is processed in the Broka's area and corresponding right hemisphere homologue of the brain and then incorporated schematically into the stored schema and the schema then becomes modified. Additional studies in neuroscience could further our understanding of how schemata are formed and function.

4.4 Cultural models of illness and HIV and AIDS

D'Andrade (1995) has demonstrated that schemata generally underlie beliefs about illness. In the American case, much of the schema (which he terms the "germ schema") is a "simplified version of the findings of scientific medicine" (1995:129). Some of our beliefs regarding illness, however, such as, cold weather causes colds, or that chicken soup cures colds, derive from the application of more traditional folk schemata of illness. D'Andrade considers illness schemata—because they are "culturally shared mental constructs"—to be cultural models. D'Andrade (1995:130) comments on the development of a cultural model, based on his data collected among Americans:

> Respondents have complex schemas about the function of the heart, the circulation of blood and the formation of blood clots and stroke. They also have complex schemas about the way cancer spreads, the effects of aging on the joints and muscles of the body, and some relatively loose conceptions about the way in which emotion and genetics interact with disease processes. Further, besides schema based knowledge, respondents also have a relatively large amount of particular knowledge about specific diseases; for example, that syphilis and gonorrhea are transmitted by sexual intercourse, that mumps is a children's disease, etc. Particular knowledge about specific diseases is then integrated with more schematic kinds of knowledge to make up a general folk theory of illness which gives informants the ability to answer a great number of questions about diseases and their properties. To understand folk beliefs about illness, more is required than just an analysis of the properties of illness. Knowledge of relevant cultural schemas is also needed.

So, according to D'Andrade, knowledge of a certain disease is integrated with cultural models (II) (schemata) to create cultural models (I) (general folk theories of illness).

Price (1987) has demonstrated that Ecuadorians use various cultural models in order to interpret and talk about illness. According to Price (1987:333), Ecuadorians "draw on cultural models of the family and of extrafamilial support, a cultural model of social hierarchy (with associated schemas of biomedical institutions), and a set of interrelated notions about illness causation."

Using narratives from fourteen individuals, Price traced the various cultural models individuals used to make sense of illness. This study is a good example of how narratives can be used to arrive at cultural models (I) and to understand the underlying schemata (cultural models II) associated with illness.

Paul Farmer (1994), using a synchronic approach, has traced the development of a cultural model (I) of HIV and AIDS in Haiti. Farmer discovered, as did Price (1987), that "illness stories contain numerous traces of cognitive models that bear on the interpretation of illness" (1994:801). The findings demonstrate that it is possible to document the elaboration over time of a widely shared representation of HIV and AIDS (1994:801). This study also demonstrates various interesting aspects of the development of the cultural model (I) of HIV and AIDS in Haiti. First of all, Farmer illustrates how the understandings of the cause of the disease shifted from a blame on "microbes" to a blame placed upon the government for bad conditions which has led to the epidemic; a sort of political economy discourse. When asked about the cause in the early years there was little consensus, but he claims that over time "the narratives became increasingly tinged with a new political sensibility" (Farmer 1994:803).

Farmer also demonstrates how old paradigms (schemata) were soon being applied to make sense of the new disorder. HIV and AIDS was associated with TB (because it was perceived to always come together with AIDS), and the traditional schemata explaining causation for TB (that it is caused by sorcery) was soon being applied to understand HIV and AIDS as well. Sorcery came to be understood as one of the causes of HIV and AIDS. We will see some of these same processes at work in the development of a cultural model of HIV and AIDS in Nepal in the coming chapters.

4.5 The limitations of the cultural model concept

Cultural models are shared understandings about the way that the world works. Cultural models are made up of various biologically and culturally formed schemata that structure the meaning we associate with any experience. The application of culturally formed cognitive schemata produces a shared understanding of an event or phenomenon. As Shore has demonstrated, however, the problem with the "cultural model" idea is that it can produce an over-reified view of culture. The early anthropological view of cultural models (as purely a psychological process) was reductionist in nature and it could not account for the noted differences between various personal models of individuals within the same culture. Further, this view could not account for the role of cultural ideas (like what we traditionally call "world view") in the shaping of cultural models. For instance, ideas about religion do not fit nicely into the model. How are such features of culture accounted for by the "strong constructivists?" Perhaps their position regarding cultural models is vulnerable to the same criticism levied against French structuralism—arranging the data to fit the model—or reducing the emotive elements of culture such as love and religion to purely psychological processes? And certainly the strong constructivists are guilty of ignoring the role of history and personal agency in the development of cultural models.

Having said this, it will not be my goal through the remainder of this book to organize (or reduce) the whole Nepali society into large irreducible overriding schemata. What I will try to do, however, is to elicit various Nepali cultural models (I) of HIV and AIDS searching for saliency among models which might suggest overriding foundational schemata (cultural models II), which are being used in meaning construction of the newly emerging disease known as "*AIDS rog.*"

Culture is indeed contested. Various cultural models of HIV and AIDS are currently being developed in Nepal and each is vying for primacy. The main negotiation seems to be between the western biomedical model of HIV and AIDS being presented by the major NGOs leading the fight against AIDS, and the more traditional cultural models of illness. The western model is a cultural model itself, built from underlying schemata, while the more traditional model is formed by applying traditional schemata to new diseases once they are classified as being similar. I will examine the interplay between these two models in part three when I discuss the construction of a unique cultural model (I) of HIV and AIDS in Nepal. Next, I discuss the different cognitive methodologies employed in the research projects.

4.6 Cognitive methodologies

For anthropology, methodology has been defined operationally as "a series of transformational rules and processes (including definitions of key concepts) that guide data gathering and relate the resulting data systematically to the hypotheses and other conceptual models in terms of which research results are expressed" (Pelto and Pelto 1996:297).

Underlying all social science methodologies is a set of taken-for-granted assumptions concerning the way the world works. The methodology utilized by cognitive anthropology is no exception to this. As mentioned previously, cognitive anthropology (and all cognitive science) employs a "mentalist" definition of culture that assumes that culture is (1) learned, (2) represented individually, and yet (3) shared by individuals of a group. It is also hypothesized from this paradigm that underlying cognitive structures (schemata) produce the shared nature (i.e., cultural models [I]) visible among a group. Further, culture, viewed from the cognitive paradigm, is considered to be a symbolic system with clear parallels to language (Doughtery1985:3), and as such, it is assumed to be amicable to linguistic analysis as well. For example, by studying how people talk about illness we can understand how people think about illness. We can study whether there are shared conceptions about illness (cultural models) and we can, in turn, uncover the underlying cognitive structures (schemata) used to produce these shared meanings.

4.6.1 "Systematic" data collection methods

Cognitive anthropology, based on the above assumptions, initially developed research methods or techniques designed to study cultural domains. This resulted in the ethnoscience type procedures such as those presented by Spradley (1972) and Tyler (1969) that were discussed earlier. A major limitation to these methods is that, although they demonstrate cultural domains, they often tell us nothing about the cognitive distance between categories or about the relationships between members of a class. With this criticism in mind, later scholars have refined these cognitive methods, adding various techniques designed to rectify the shortcomings. Weller and Romney (1988) have proposed "systematic" data collection methods that allow for cognitive mapping of cultural domains. They propose that these empirical methods used for hypothesis testing within structured domains have proven effective at illuminating shared conceptions regarding illnesses. For instance, Trotter (1981) used the free-listing technique to study illness beliefs among Mexican-Americans. Informants were asked to list all the home remedies they were aware of and they were also asked to list the illnesses for which these remedies were used. The data revealed shared perceptions among Mexican-Americans regarding illness and home remedies. Frame elicitation methods (another of the methods proposed by Weller and Romney) have been used to study the distribution of various beliefs regarding the causes of illness and cures for them (Bernard 1995:243). Regarding frame analysis, Bernard (1995:244) has suggested that this technique has also been instrumental in our understanding of the role of intercultural variation:

> Sankoff's[10] analysis was an important milestone in our understanding of the measurable differences between individual culture versus shared culture. It supported Goodenough's notion (1965) that cognitive models are based on shared assumptions, but that ultimately they are best construed as properties of individuals. (1995:244)

Both free-listing and frame analysis are precursors to other cognitive methods, such as cluster analysis and multidimensional scaling, which have been useful at further refining our understanding of the shared nature of illness beliefs. For instance, Weller (1983) used multidimensional scaling, following free-listing and pile sorting procedures, in order to demonstrate how her informants collectively perceived the various illnesses elicited. Several of these methods, such as free listing and pile sorting, were used during the rural phase of this research in order to understand how rural Nepalis categorize and understand illness (including HIV and AIDS). The various cognitive data collection methods employed throughout the rural research will be discussed in greater depth in the next chapter.

One limitation to the use of the cognitive techniques mentioned above is that interviews with informants generally produce a personal mental model rather than illuminate the instituted (cultural) model. This highlights the

---

[10] Gillian Sankoff (1971) employed frame analysis to study land tenure and kinship among the Buang people of Papua New Guinea.

importance of using larger numbers of informants in cognitive research. Garro (1986) used twenty informants and was able to demonstrate that 78 percent of the personal mental models collected reflected a shared cultural model. Likewise, Young and Garro (Young 1981) used data collected from 509 Mexican households to discover cultural consensus on illness beliefs. From the data collected, Young and Garro were able to derive a cultural model of illness that is employed in decision making, particularly for illness episodes. In my research, many informants were used (in a focus group format) during the rural study, and a questionnaire was developed and distributed more widely in order to test the validity of these findings. The exact procedures followed will be explained in the next chapter.

Although the cognitive methods developed have been very useful for investigating how various peoples divide up their illness universes, there are limitations to this approach as well. Mark Nichter (1994) distinguishes between what he calls the denotative features and connotative aspects of an illness. For Nichter, the denotative features are referential. These are the shared aspects of illness, such as physical signs and symptoms, severity, treatments, etc. (e.g., Kleinman's explanatory model), while the connotative aspects are multidimensional and less clear-cut. For Nichter, the connotative aspects of illness "emerge as a cluster of loosely associated image schema and feelings about an illness experience, bringing to mind personal experiences and indexing cultural meanings linked to illness" (Nichter 1989:116).

While cognitive approaches (which he characterizes as being used mainly in "disease-focused behavioral research") have been useful for identifying denotative features of illness (e.g., local illness taxonomies), they are much less effective at getting at the connotative aspects of illness. Nichter claims that they "identify schemata subject to negotiation and underestimate ambiguity" (1989:148). According to Nichter, the connotative dimension of illness is "evocative, episodic and contextual, flowing from what Good (1977) has described as a semantic illness network: a pool of illness related associations embedded in culture, enriched through personal experience and condensed around core cultural concerns" (Nichter 1989:116).

For Nichter, the connotative dimensions of illness are more likely to emerge from methods such as discourse analysis of illness histories, than they are from these traditional cognitive methods. Nichter (1994:229) suggests that traditional cognitive methods are useful "as a starting place" (i.e., they get at the denotative features of illness), but he pushes us to seek answers for the connotative aspects as well, which can only be derived using a different type of data.

4.6.2 Narrative analysis

Recently, within the cognitive anthropology paradigm, there has been a growing interest in the use of the narrative analysis method (Mattingly and

Garro 1994:771). Narrative analysis, one specific type of linguistic discourse analysis, has been proposed as a means for understanding illness experience and is a popular technique these days among medical anthropologists working within the cognitive framework. Mattingly and Garro (1994:771) demonstrate how various medical anthropologists, mainly intent on understanding cultural models, have discovered narrative analysis to be a good tool for illuminating shared cultural models of illness.

The underlying assumption (theory) behind narrative analysis is that narratives are vehicles through which meaning is made. Mattingly and Garro suggest that the sequence of events presented in relation to time in a narrative helps one understand life:

> Narrative offers what is perhaps our most fundamental way to understand life in time. Through narrative we try to make sense of how things have come to pass and how our actions and the actions of others have helped shape our history; we try to understand who we are becoming by reference to where we have been. (1994:771)

For Mattingly and Garro (1994:771), narrative also "offers a way to think about illness," as well as "a logic for explaining illness,...provides metaphors for understanding the experience of illness,..." and "provides a powerful means for communicating and giving meaning to experience." Narratives are not simply a telling of the past, but are also "used to express one's present understandings of a disorder, and may anticipate the future as well" (Garro and Mattingly 1994:771).

Holland and Quinn (1987:16) have also suggested that cognitive methods (e.g., the systematic data collection methods described earlier) be used to supplement other approaches, such as discourse analysis. Cognitive methods, because they allow for a large quantity of data to be gathered and reduced, can effectively be used to "sketch in a map of the territory and orient it relative to other domains, while different methods provide the higher resolution needed to explore a given terrain closely." To this, Holland and Quinn add, "Reconstructing the organization of this cultural knowledge, however, requires kinds of linguistic data richer in such clues than the data provided by naming and sorting tasks, and it requires eclectic exploitation of all possible sources of such data (1987:16).

The type of research methodology they advocate for this purpose is the analysis of natural discourse. Holland and Quinn (1987:16) suggest that narratives are a productive new data source for cognitive anthropologists intent on the reconstruction of cultural models. They also illustrate how natural discourse has been used by cognitive anthropologists to reveal cultural schemata (1987:16).

Laurie Price (1984) has also provided an illustration of how discourse analysis can be used to arrive at cultural models of illness. Using a narrative analysis methodology, she traced various cultural models underlying individual illness stories from Ecuador. Models of various relationships (friends, family and neighbors) and of social hierarchy emerged from the analysis. Likewise, Viney has used the narrative analysis method to examine the narratives of "AIDS-affected people" in Australia. The Australian study, since it focused on AIDS, was principally used as a model for the research conducted during the urban phase of my dissertation data collection. The details of this model will be discussed at greater length in the narrative analysis chapter (chapter six).

4.6.3 Narratives and schemata

There is also a strong relationship between narrative and schemata. Schemata underlie narratives. Narratives employ schemata in their construction (i.e., the activation of schemata produces narratives). Narratives are the visible byproduct of the schematization process (i.e., events are made sense of and remembered through this process and then are retold as narratives). Narratives, therefore, might be best understood as a story told by an individual, verbal or written, that contains the expression of various schemata. Laurie Price (1987:316) has commented that "illness stories contain numerous 'traces' of cognitive models that bear on interpretation of illness." Narratives, therefore, as the theory goes, are a good source to study in searching for cognitive models and their underlying schemata.

Narratives can expose personal cognitive models but they can also reveal cultural models. Narratives are the property of individuals, and yet in them "the presentation and interpretation of experience is guided and shaped by shared cultural understandings" (Mattingly and Garro 1994:772). According to these same authors, "individual reconstructions are situated or contrasted within shared cultural models of illness" and "narratives provide a vehicle for confronting the contradictions between an individual's experience and expectations based on shared cultural models" (1994:771). Various other authors (Farmer 1994; Garro 1994; Mathews, Lannin and Mitchell 1994; Price 1987) have focused on the relationship between narrative and shared cultural understandings.

Regarding these studies Mattingly and Garro write, "While grounding their studies in the illness experience of individual sufferers, these authors transcend the particular histories and life circumstances to representations of cultural models" (1994:771).

So, it seems clear that while narrative analysis can be productive at deriving the personal cognitive models (the connotative aspects of the illness experience) of individuals (thus revealing the individual and contested meanings associated with personal illness experiences of various individuals), it can also be productive for deriving shared understandings of illness (cultural models). It would seem, therefore, that narrative analysis is sensitive to the earlier criticisms of Nichter.

4.6.4 A combined methodology

The point has been made that various systematic cognitive methods, such as free-listing and pile sorting, have proven effective at illuminating shared conceptions (denotative features) regarding illnesses among different groups. It has also been demonstrated that these same techniques are unable to effectively examine the connotative aspects of illness beliefs. Furthermore, it has been suggested that discourse analysis approaches, such as narrative analysis, have been successful at revealing both contested personal models as well as widely shared cultural models. For this reason various authors have advocated for a methodology that combines these various methods.

This research is built on the assumptions (methodology) of cognitive anthropology and employs various methods (techniques) designed to elicit both the connotative and denotative aspects of understandings about HIV and AIDS in Nepal. The village phase (employing "systematic" cognitive methods) is intended to demonstrate shared beliefs about HIV and AIDS in rural Nepal. The city phase (using a narrative analysis approach) is also designed to elicit shared cognitive models (cultural models) of HIV and AIDS (albeit among Nepalis with HIV and AIDS), but the type of research conducted should also demonstrate the individual connotative aspects involved in the negotiation of a cultural model. Both aspects are useful. Used in tandem these methods should produce data that will reveal both shared conceptions (cultural models) about HIV and AIDS, as well as illustrate the slightly different personal meanings associated with the illness by different individuals. As previously noted, various authors have advocated the use of multiple methods in order to increase validity. The findings of this book are based on two different studies using these two different approaches. Each of the methods has its own strengths and weaknesses. It is proposed, however, that the combination of methods will provide a more thorough perspective regarding cultural models of HIV and AIDS in Nepal. The specific methods employed in each study will be introduced in the coming chapters. Next, we turn our attention to the projects that were conducted to investigate the various cultural models of HIV and AIDS.

Part Two

The Projects

5

Saano Dumre Revisited: Changing Models of Illness and Cultural Models of HIV and AIDS in a Rural Village of Central Nepal

This chapter presents the findings of an ethnomedical study conducted in rural Nepal in the late 1990s. Although locked in the "ethnographic present" of that time period, many of the conclusions of this research are still presently visible in the contemporary cultural model of HIV and AIDS in Nepal, as will be evident in subsequent chapters. Likely things will have changed a bit in the ensuing years, but many things will have also remained the same (thus, the continuity seen with today's cultural model). Although the study was designed principally to examine illness beliefs and practices, it was also a major goal of the study to determine whether a salient cultural model of HIV and AIDS yet exists among the people of a rural Nepali village. The study, carried out using primarily a systematic cognitive approach, was conducted throughout the village of Saano Dumre in rural Gorkha District.

In section 5.1, I introduce the village of Saano Dumre and the methodology followed during the research. Besides illuminating beliefs and practices in regard to illness (including HIV and AIDS) among rural Nepalis, this study examines the changes that have taken place in health beliefs over the past twenty-five years. Using the methods of cognitive anthropology, I have explored several health-related topics. The topics covered in section 5.2 include categories of illness, treatment seeking order, causes of illness and factors that make one more susceptible to illness, ideas about transmission of illness, villagers' perceptions about what has changed over the past twenty-five years, and ideas regarding the efficacy of traditional and western medicines. In section 5.3, I look at people's understanding of HIV and AIDS in particular, proposing an emerging cultural model of HIV and AIDS in Saano Dumre.

111

5.1 Background and methodology

5.1.1 Background

Situated in the shadow of Lig Lig Mountain[1] in the western mid-hills of Nepal is the village of Saano Dumre. The village consists of 150 houses spread across an entire hillside, with some homes resting on the ridge at four thousand feet and others situated along the banks of the Chepe Kola River some 2,500 feet below. The village, which covers all of ward two of Palantar Village Development Committee,[2] is made up of several *gaauns* (mostly caste-based neighborhoods or hamlets). The total population of the village is listed as 705 and is made up of Bhramin-Chetri (51 homes), Sarki/Kami/Damai (49 houses), Giri (30 houses), and Muslim (20 houses) caste divisions. Most people in Saano Dumre are agriculturists (603 persons) and about half of the population is reported as literate.[3] It was also estimated that nearly 200 of the village's 360 males are working abroad in either the Middle East, India, or Kathmandu.[4] This would suggest that Saano Dumre now has much contact with the wider world, a theme that became apparent over the course of the research.

Saano Dumre was first put on the map of South Asian anthropology by anthropologist Harvey Blustain in 1976. Blustain (1976), basing his conclusions on data gathered over an eighteen month period from 1974 to 1976, described health beliefs and practices among the local villagers of Saano Dumre. This well-cited article, part of a special issue of Contributions to Nepalese Studies published by The Center for Nepal Asian Studies at Tribhuvan University, quickly became a landmark piece in the medical anthropology of Nepal.[5] The article has since continued to serve as a basis for understanding health beliefs throughout various other parts of Nepal as well (e.g., Beine 2001, Streefland 1985, Stone 1983, Stone 1989).

Opportunity arose during my research to visit Saano Dumre, the site of Blustain's initial research, to conduct interviews with villagers regarding their current beliefs and practices concerning illness. I felt this research,

---

[1]Lig Lig Mountain is famous in Nepal. It is from the fort atop this mountain that the great King Prithvi Narayan Shah, who unified Nepal, is said to have come.

[2]Wards are the smallest unit of political organization and are encompassed within Village Development Committees (formerly Village Panchayats), the next largest level of political organization.

[3]These statistics are from the HMG 2053 census (96–97) and were provided by the Palatar VDC Chairman.

[4]This estimate was provided by the ward chairman (Ward 2) who lives in Saano Dumre.

[5]This special issue on anthropology, health and development included five articles, which featured beliefs and practices regarding sickness of peoples from various parts of Nepal.

besides offering a look at rural conceptions of HIV and AIDS, might also provide a valuable opportunity for a comparative look at the changes in belief and practices about illness that have taken place in the village in the twenty-five years following Blustain's influential publication. Such a diachronic view might provide some insight into the culture change (or resilience) in light of great efforts toward the development of Western-style health care in rural Nepal over the last quarter century.

There are a few notable differences between Blustain's findings and mine. This is perhaps best explained by a difference of time and focus. Although Blustain attempted to describe villagers' beliefs regarding illness, the focus of his investigation quickly became the beliefs of the traditional healers (referred to as "*baidhyas*" by Blustain) who were his main inform-ants. Although I also interviewed the same traditional healers as Blustain, the local villager's beliefs, rather than that of the traditional healers, was the focus of my research.[6]

Not all of the differences can be simply attributed to a difference in fo-cus, however. Beliefs and practices have changed significantly in the years since Blustain conducted his field research in Saano Dumre. Perhaps it is a combination of both focus and the time factor that best accounts for the dif-ference of conclusions drawn between Blustain and myself. Having claimed such "great change," however, I must point out that *jhaankri kaam* 'shaman work' is still alive and well in Saano Dumre, but has undergone substantial modification as will be illustrated later.

This chapter also introduces indigenous ideas about sickness and catego-ries of illness not formerly identified by Blustain. Again, I imagine this is perhaps best explained by difference of time and focus as well as a result of using different tools (e.g., cognitive anthropological methods) to elicit information. I have also drawn upon the ideas of other South Asian medical anthropologists in order to confirm ideas in Saano Dumre that seem preva-lent throughout other parts of South Asia as well.

5.1.2 Methodology

The goal of the research conducted during the rural phase was ultimately to determine whether a cultural model of HIV and AIDS yet existed in the rural areas. Various cognitive methods such as free-listing, pile sorting, and

---

[6]I use the generic term "traditional healer" to describe the *dhaami-jhaankris* (Hindu shaman) and the *baidhyas* (Muslim shaman) of Saano Dumre. Both prac-tice "blowing," but only the Hindus "shake." The Muslims, although their practices are very similar to the Hindus (minus the shaking), prefer the term *baidhya*. For a further discussion of the distinctions see Blustain (1976). The beliefs and practices of the traditional healers of Saano Dumre also seem quite similar to those of other shaman in the inner-Siberian tradition, as outlined in the work of David Watters (1975), Casper Miller (1979), and Gregory Maskarinec (1995).

development of flow charts were employed to gain a better understanding of the general thinking and behavior of people regarding health and illness. These methods were incorporated into a structured interview schedule that was designed to further probe health-related topics among focus groups. Each part of the interview schedule was discussed in depth and developed in consultation with my Nepali research assistant. Focus group interviews were conducted in Nepali and the proceedings were tape recorded and transcribed for later analysis.

Visits were made to each of the ten major hamlets of Saano Dumre and in-depth interviews were conducted among focus groups made up of members of each hamlet. The interview schedule followed by these groups can be found in appendix A. Focus groups were generally made up of eight to twelve participants who had volunteered to talk about the questions. Nepal is a relational society where almost nothing is done alone so I felt the focus group format was more considerate of the culture than other types of research formats. Consensus in Nepal also is usually negotiated through extended family group discussions so the focus group format seemed a natural one to use. When we arrived at a hamlet (generally ten to twelve houses) we usually found one household where various neighbors (who were usually related) were gathered. We introduced ourselves and sought out volunteer participation in our study. We explained that we needed a group to discuss the questions and the villagers then gathered people who were available and willing. Although this was not a random sample and although the members knew each other,[7] I felt that this was more natural to the Nepali context and that answers flowed more freely than they would if I had attempted individual interviews. In the end, the groups worked well together and were usually mixed in gender and age.

These interviews (conducted in Nepali) commenced with an open-ended discussion about what the participants do when they don't feel well. This discussion culminated with the construction of a treatment-seeking flow chart based on the information given. Next, an elicitation (free-listing) of all of the various kinds of illnesses they could think of was conducted and a pile sorting exercise culminated in the construction of illness categories. Free-listing and pile sorting are both cognitive anthropological methods designed to elicit natural categories and discovery saliency among and between members of these categories.[8] Following these exercises, the remainder of the questionnaire was administered to the focus groups in order to further assess the nature of these categories, beliefs about the causes of illness

---

[7] Bernard (1995:225) suggests that, in general, focus group members should not know one another. In village Nepal, however, everyone knows everyone else. And most households in each caste hamlet are related in some way.

[8] For a further explanation of the rationale behind these methods, the reader is encouraged to consult Bernard (1995).

(including HIV and AIDS), ideas about susceptibility and transmission of illness, perceptions of symptoms and treatment of illness, ideas about separation of sick persons, notions of the efficacy of Western and local medicines, and thoughts on how things have changed in the ensuing years.

From the findings of the ten focus groups (based on responses to scheduled interview in appendix A), a survey questionnaire was constructed and distributed to eighty-five percent[9] of households in the village (n = 128)[10] in order to verify whether or not the findings of the focus groups were representative of the beliefs and practices of the wider village.[11] Of these questionnaires, eighty-five (67%) were returned.[12] The questionnaires were then collected, and the data was entered into a computer database and analyzed using the Statistical Package for the Social Sciences (Norusis 1991), a computer program designed for social research. The conclusions of this chapter are drawn both from the in-depth interviews as well as from the follow-up community-wide survey. The findings are discussed below.

5.2 Ideas about illness

5.2.1 Categories of illness

5.2.1.1 Thulo *'big' and* saano *'small' rogs*

Perhaps the most natural categories that emerged from the research were those of *thulo rog* 'big sickness' or 'great sickness' and *saano rog* 'small sickness' or 'disease'. There was much agreement in what villagers considered as

---

[9] All percentages presented in this chapter have been rounded either up or down to the nearest whole number.

[10] "n=" is taken from statistics, and represents the number of subjects, things, or whatever is in a sample. In this case, the sample size is 128 households.

[11] Questionnaires were explained to a literate member in each household. The directions asked for the literate person to read the question to the household and note the various responses on the questionnaire. Survey questionnaires were given to 128 of 150 households in Saano Dumre. Twenty-two households were either vacant (the occupants were living and working abroad) or the occupants were away during the days of our visitation.

[12] According to social science research methodology (see Bernard 1995), this is actually a fairly large return rate for this type of self-administered questionnaire. The higher than expected return rate is probably due to the fact that I regularly walked the village, encouraging people to complete the survey. And even though I had asked for the surveys to be delivered to a local shop, I collected over thirty surveys directly from the respondents who had completed the survey, but had forgotten to return them. Most were rolled up and stuck under a beam just below the thatch in the ceiling.

thulo and *saano* (or *saadharaan*[13]) illness. These are listed in table 5.1 at the end of this chapter. The free-listing exercise also revealed this distinction between *thulo* and *saano rogs* to be quite a natural and salient category in the minds of villagers. When asked to make a list of all illnesses that can be found in Nepal, nearly all began the lists with those they would later also classify (in the pile sorting exercise) as *thulo rogs*. These, of course, were then followed by those they considered *saano*, or 'less serious'.

An interesting feature, which also emerged from the pile sorting exercise, is that the most common "floating" (meaning some listed them as *thulo* others as *saano*) diseases were leprosy and tuberculosis. When asked about this, people attributed it to the fact that there is now treatment available for both of these once greatly feared and stigmatized diseases. One respondent said "TB and leprosy have become *saano rogs* because you can now get treatment for them." It seems clear, therefore, that a major characteristic of the category *thulo* is perceived efficacy of treatment.

There is, apparently, a cognitive shift underway in how Nepalis understand and think about TB and leprosy. As effective treatment has become available for these diseases, people have begun to incorporate this new knowledge into their individual cognitive models regarding illness. And as a result, the community's collective ideas (cultural model) regarding these diseases will slowly shift as well. As more learn of the treatment availability and as older individuals die off, these once highly stigmatized diseases will complete the shift from one cognitive category (*thulo*) to another (*saano*).

This process of cognitive shift (for TB and leprosy) is underway but not yet complete. In answer to a later question about which diseases require the practice of *chhichhi durdur*[14] 'separation' or 'seclusion', tuberculosis and leprosy were still the most often mentioned diseases that require separation from the community and social ostricization.

The other frequently listed "floating" illnesses were things such as headache, joint pain, stomach ache, cough, and worms. It seems, however, that when considered a chronic problem these were listed as *thulo*, and when considered of short duration (non-chronic) they were considered *saano*. Hence, I have categorized them as *thulo* or *saano* according to chronicity.

Another interesting feature that emerged during the free-listing exercise was a further unexpected categorization of illnesses. Nepali has many words for the semantic category of 'illness' (e.g., *dukhcha, bisancho, asancho, bimaari, birami, byathaa,* and *rog*). Various authors have attempted to define the meanings of these various terms (Allen 1976, Johnson & Johnson-Caroll

---

[13]The term *saadhaaran* 'simple' was often used synonymously with *saano*. Both terms connote a "minor" illness or sickness.

[14]*Chi* literally means 'disgusting' and *dur* (in Sanskrit) means 'far'. *Chhichhi durdur* is the phrase used to describe the practice of ostracizing a person with disease from the community. It is usually practiced for those diseases categorized as being both *thulo* and *saruwa* 'transferable'.

1994, Kristivik 1993, Nichter 1989, Peters 1979, Pigg 1992, Stone 1976).
Initially I had tried (with very little success) to understand how the terms
were being used and understood in Saano Dumre. I wanted simply to know
what all the terms for illness were and how they were distinguished. This
became problematic, however, and I gave up after the second interview, as
it seemed that I wasn't being well understood. The widely distributed questionnaire, however, asked for a list of all of the *bimaariharu, byathaaharu*
and *rogharu*[15] (three well-known terms used to cover the semantic domain
of sickness in all its related nuances). Most simply free-listed using the criteria above (i.e., *thulo* followed by *saano*). Several respondents, however,
actually divided the space into the three categories; *bimaariharu, byathaaharu* and *rogharu*. Simple things like 'headache', 'fevers', and 'cough', were
listed as *bimaari';* while 'craziness' *baulaaune* and 'shaking' *kaamne*—both
thought to be the result of spirits—were listed as *byathaa;* and diseases such
as AIDS, cancer, TB, leprosy, and asthma (all categorized as *thulo* as well),
were listed as kinds of *rog*. One informant described the distinction to me
as follows: "If I don't feel well but am still able to walk and work, then I am
birami.[16] If I am bed-ridden or have a chronic problem, then it is *rog*. And if
it is spiritually caused, then it is *byathaa*."

5.2.1.2 Sardi *'cold'* and garmi *'hot'* rogs

Another category, which emerged quite naturally from the interviews, was
the separation of illness into categories that require the eating of 'cold'
sardi or 'hot' *garmi* foods for therapy. Blustain also originally identified this
categorization as a major feature of disease classification throughout Saano
Dumre. It has been identified as an important concept throughout other
parts of Asia as well. The main concept underlying categorization of illness
as either hot or cold is the concept of balance. It is necessary to maintain
one's inner balance because an imbalance between hot and cold can cause
sickness. Certain illnesses are believed to be caused by a loss of balance
(mainly through mixing of "non-matching" foods). Therefore, illnesses are
classified as either hot or cold, and health must be restored by bringing the
body back into balance by eating hot foods for cold illnesses or cold foods
for hot illnesses.

   An interesting feature, which emerged during the elicitation of this category, was that there was much disagreement (within and between focus
groups) about which illnesses require hot foods and which require cold
foods. From the free-listing exercise, cards with the names of the diseases
were placed on the ground and participants were asked to make piles of
which diseases require hot and which require cold. There was usually much

---

[15]*-haru* is the Nepali suffix used to signify 'plurality'.

[16]*Birami* and *bimari* are alternate forms of the same word.

discussion (and disagreement) about which should go where, but table 5.2 displays a small list of illnesses that were consistently categorized by all of the focus groups as either hot or cold. Another interesting feature is that all groups created a third category of "it doesn't matter what foods are eaten for this illness." All groups (see table 5.2) consistently placed AIDS, cancer, paralysis and sprains or broken bones in this category. Three of the groups also constructed a fourth "in between" category saying that these illnesses required eating food that was "neither too hot nor too cold."

One of the focus groups explained why people disagree on whether an illness is hot or cold. The spokesman of this group, after much discussion, said that they decide if an illness is hot or cold through experimentation. Therefore, some have had success (meaning they have gotten well) after eating hot foods for certain illnesses while others have gotten well after eating cold foods for the same type of illness. Thus, disagreement exists over the classification of these illnesses.

5.2.1.3 Saruwa *'transferable'* rogs

Another seemingly natural cognitive category seemed to be the idea of *saruwa* 'transferable' illnesses. Thirteen different illnesses were listed as *saruwa* by the different focus groups. These are listed in table 5.3. Every group mentioned TB and cold and cough as being transferable and several groups mentioned AIDS, leprosy, malaria, chicken pox, diarrhea, and fever as also being transferable.

In response to how *saruwa rogs* are transferred it seems that there is much cognitive overlap. Because people classify these diseases as members of the same category, they seem to extend the idea of mode of transmission from one member of the category to all other members as well. Therefore, the most common ways that were listed for *saruwa* illnesses to spread were through (1) eating *jutho* (the "left-over" food which is considered ritually polluted) of the ill person, (2) sleeping in the same bed, (3) wearing the sick person's clothing, (4) and breathing the same air. It is natural, therefore, that people should stay away from (and practice *chhichhi durdur*) a person with a *saruwa* disease. The concepts of *saruwa* and *chhichhi durdur* will be discussed at greater length later in this book.

5.2.1.4 Baahira *'outside'* and bhitra *'inside'* rogs

I also asked groups to pile cards as "inside" or "outside" diseases as this concept has been identified as a significant concept in other parts of Nepal (Kristvik 1993). Although all were able to form inside and outside piles at my request, this was not without great difficulty and discussion. One of the more educated interviewees in one of the groups even asked me what I meant by "inside" and "outside" so that he would "know how to go about piling the cards." Thus, the concept of inside and outside illness is not as cognitively salient as those of the other categories mentioned above. Zvosec (1996) found the same to be true in the eastern part of Nepal as well.

Having said this, however, it was interesting how people ultimately did form grouping of inside and outside illnesses. If the illness was something obvious to the eye like a skin rash, scabies, or leprosy, then it was classified as "outside," and if it was not outwardly observable (like cancer or gastric problems), then it was classified as "inside."

Although this categorization seemed more of a forced category than a natural cognitive category of illness for the villagers of Saano Dumre, people did consider inside diseases generally to be of a more serious nature than outside ones. A few informants also suggested that certain outside diseases (e.g., a wound) could "go inside" and become a serious disease, such as cancer. This will be discussed at greater length in the section on transmission of illness.

5.2.2 Health-related ideas

5.2.2.1 Treatment-seeking order: A symptom-based approach

Interviews conducted throughout the village demonstrate a variety of treatment-seeking behaviors that are in practice in Saano Dumre. These ranged from that originally described by Blustain (i.e., extensive use of traditional healers for all medical advice) to the exclusive use of western practitioners. The main feature which all of these variations had in common, however, is that the treatments sought were all determined by the symptoms exhibited. Thus, the villagers of Saano Dumre seem to exhibit a symptom-based strategy for seeking treatment. This focus on symptoms rather than other aspects of illness is a well-documented feature in other areas of Nepal as well (Pigg 1992).

The follow-up survey demonstrates the use of multiple strategies for treatment seeking. Eighty-nine percent (n = 71) of respondents to the wider survey reported that they or a family member had been to a medical hall, health post or the hospital in the last year. Fifty-one percent (n = 71) also report having been to the traditional healer during that same time. A current trend throughout Saano Dumre for treatment seeking seems to be the combination of new "western-appearing"[17] elements along with elements of the

---

[17]I use the term "western-appearing" because, although it may appear "western" on the surface (e.g., many "western" medicines are used as home remedies or brought from the nearby medical shops, and a majority of villagers frequent the nearby "western" hospital), one can still clearly see "traditional" elements being modified and combined with the western methods rather than discarded altogether.

more traditional structure, to form a new sort of hybrid health belief model. Although it may appear to some that the "traditional" model is simply being replaced by the "western" model[18] (and the move away from exclusive use of traditional healers and traditional methods toward the use of a more "western-appearing" system would certainly support this contention), it seems to me that something deeper is going on here. There appears to be a complex process of hybridization underlying treatment-seeking strategies rather than simply a replacement of one model for another. For instance, in one domain (home remedies), products of western development are being applied in an ingeniously indigenous fashion, while in another domain (spiritually perceived sickness) the traditional healer's practices are being modified to incorporate new beliefs in the efficacy of western medicine. And in another instance the use of traditional healers is being modified to exclusive use in one domain only ("shaking" illness). These cases will be discussed at length later in this chapter.

This hybridization process is less of a dichotomous replacement of one system (traditional) with another (western), and more of a means for maximizing possible treatment seeking options, by combining traditional ideas with new "western" methods into one constantly changing hybrid system. Such a new hybrid medical system developing in Saano Dumre is based on the same pluralistic tendencies identified throughout other parts of South Asia. The characteristics of this hybrid system, in reference to treatment-seeking behavior, will be discussed below.

The survey began with a question: "What do you do when you don't feel well?" The answers were elicited from the focus groups and developed into a general flow chart of health-seeking behavior. In each of the focus groups there was some variation expressed among members regarding treatment-seeking behavior. Most suggested that they go to traditional healers for shaking and to the doctor for other illnesses; some suggested that they go to the doctor for everything; and a few still exclusively used the traditional healers as described by Blustain (1976).[19] The follow-up survey revealed a stronger use of the hospital than of the traditional healers, but it is clear that the traditional healers are still used by many.

The general pattern (meaning that supported by the majority of responses from the follow-up survey) of treatment seeking is displayed in table 5.4 and various modifications of these patterns will be discussed below.[20]

---

[18]A desire for replacement of the "traditional" with *bikaas* 'developed' has been identified as a major theme in development discourse in Nepal (Pigg 1995).

[19]Some still use the traditional healer as the first stop for medical problems and some no longer believe in their power at all. This will be discussed further in the section on "changes." The vast majority, however, use the system presented in figure 5.4.

[20]The categories listed, such as *thulo* 'big' and *saano* 'small', will also be defined in the next section.

Although it is clear that there has been much modification of the system first described by Blustain, in two of the ten hamlets there was still consensus confirming the use of traditional healers in a way much more consistent with Blustain's original findings.

Interestingly, all focus groups initially responded to this first question in exactly the same way: "We take the sick person to the hospital." Upon further inquiry, however, different patterns began to emerge. It seems that the respondents were, at first, anxious to tell me what they thought I would want to hear since they perceived me to be an agent of the hospital.[21] However, when this was followed up with a second question about whether they first tried to treat illness in the home, a list of various *gharko ausadhi* 'home medicines' emerged. These various home remedies will be discussed further in the section on home remedies below.

The main pattern of treatment seeking in Saano Dumre is symptom based and goes something like this: If it is a *saano rog* 'small illness', then they self-treat with various home remedies for generally three to five days. (The specific remedy used seemed to be much more a matter of personal choice—or as Blustain pointed out, perhaps contextually determined.) If there is no improvement, then they take the sick person to the hospital. In the follow-up survey 88 percent reported that if home remedies didn't work, they would take the patient to the hospital while only twelve percent reported that they would call the traditional healer (n = 78). For *thulo rogs,* they go straight to the hospital. If hospital treatment fails then many will seek referral to a Kathmandu hospital or somewhere further abroad. One man even mentioned seeking further treatment from a hospital in Bangalore, India. If he is *kaamne rog* 'shaking', then he goes to the traditional healer for advice as this symptom is readily identified as spiritual and this domain of illness is his specialty. This focus on patients' symptoms in order to determine treatment strategies was consistent throughout all of the interviews.

There were some variations on the flow chart presented in table 5.4, although the contrasts were minor and were still symptom based. Some classified *jworo* 'fever' and *baanta* 'vomiting' individually as *saano rogs,* while others said that when they are combined *(jworo-baanta),* they are considered *thulo* and the patient is taken to the hospital within two hours if it doesn't stop. One respondent replied, "We wait only for two hours to see if the diarrhea and vomiting stops; if not we immediately take the person to the hospital." Others replied that they would take a person to the hospital

---

[21]During my research I lived in a home owned by the Gorkha Project of the United Mission to Nepal, which also administrates the Amp Pipal Hospital. My wife, a medical doctor, also volunteered her services part-time at the hospital. It was interesting, however, that when asked where I had come from, the answer "Amp Pipal" automatically associated me with the hospital. Most certainly this is because all foreigners they have seen here have been associated with the Gorkha project. I was even assumed by most to be a medical doctor at first for the same reason.

for fever alone and others for vomiting alone, if the fever or vomiting did not cease after two or three hours. All agreed, however, that they would first try various home remedies before seeking further help in the case of other *saano rogs.*

In regard to the use of traditional healers, there was some disagreement. While a few disavowed belief in the traditional healers altogether and just as few claim they consult these shaman for all illnesses, most reserve their use only for symptoms they define as *kaamne rog* 'shaking'. One man said, "First we go to the *dhaami-jhaankris,*[22] and if the shaking is caused by gods then we will be healed. If they cannot cure it, then we go to the hospital." One respondent also had an interesting approach in the case of diarrhea. She said, "First we take the person to the hospital and they will be cured of diarrhea. But if it reoccurs, then we will take them to the *dhaami-jhaankri* (if terribly sick) or astrologer (if only mild), but if it doesn't stop we will take them back to the hospital."

The follow-up survey supports the claim that the traditional healers are still in use. (Fifty-one percent report having been to a traditional healer in the last year.) Most (76%), however, report less use of the traditional healers than during the twenty previous years.

When asked which traditional healers villagers seek out, a common response was that selection seems to be more a matter of access and personal choice than specialty. For instance one man stated, "Whoever we meet first along the trail, that one we will seek help from."

5.2.2.2 Home remedies

Although the responses of the various focus groups (concerning health-seeking behavior) were varied, they did reveal some common themes. First of all, each of the groups agreed that the use of home remedies was common before seeking advice from either the doctor or the traditional healer. This was confirmed by the wider survey in which sixty-eight percent (n = 71)[23] reported using home remedies before going to the hospital and sixty-eight percent (n = 66) tried home remedies before going to the traditional healer.

A few of the different types of remedies tried are illustrated in table 6.5. Perhaps the most interesting feature is the variety of medicines used as home remedies. These varied from products of western development (such as VICKS or rifle oil), to ayurvedic medicines, to locally available products and plants. This list displays an interesting pluralistic incorporation of very different types of medicines into the wider overriding system.

---

[22]This is the most common term used generically to describe both the Muslim *baidhyas* and the Hindu *jhaankris*, meaning 'traditional healers'.

[23]Here "n=" is the sample size of respondents (households) to a particular question.

Some of the specific home remedies reportedly used were very interesting. Rifle oil, for instance was mentioned as a good cure for body ache. Actually, mustard oil massaged into the hurting body part seems to be a traditional treatment, but several people told me that if one had access to rifle oil, "it is much more powerful." It is interesting that western products of development have replaced traditional items and are thought to be more "powerful." Again, this demonstrates the power that the mantra of *bikaas* 'development' has had on Nepal (see Pigg 1992). This idea of more power inherent in western medicines was also repeated later in the survey. It is also interesting that these western products of development are not necessarily being used as intended or prescribed by their makers, rather they are being applied in a truly indigenous way. The same was true for VICKS cough drops. Several people told me that these are dropped into boiled (but cooled) water and drunk like the traditional cures for cold and cough, rather than sucked in the mouth, as we would expect. They are also sometimes combined with *besi pani* 'turmeric water' and drunk as a mixed concoction.

5.2.3 Influences on health: Causes of illness

There were several factors that were identified by the focus groups as possible causes of illness. Among these were germs, spoiled planets, bad *karma*, spirits, and body weakness. As Blustain pointed out in his original article, beliefs about the causes of illness in Saano Dumre are contested. Although the various factors above were cited as causes of illness, the findings of the follow-up survey demonstrate that certain beliefs regarding the influence of certain agents in disease causation are more widely held than others. In this section I examine the various influences identified by the respondents of both the focus groups and the wider survey.[24]

5.2.3.1 Kira 'germs'

The most popular answer to the question, "What is the major factor contributing to illness?," was *kira*[25] 'bugs'. When asked if *kira* can cause sickness the answer by all focus groups was "yes." When asked what kinds of illnesses come from *kira*, the most common answer was "stomachache."

---

[24]Although it is clear from these findings that the majority of respondents attribute the greatest cause of illness to germs, the question discussed among focus groups also demonstrated the understanding of the possibility of multiple causes for illness in the minds of many of the villagers of Saano Dumre. One respondent replied "some diseases are caused by spirits (like heavy body and shaking), some from doing hard work, and some from eating an imbalanced diet."

[25]Although the Nepali language distinguishes between bugs (*kira*) and germs (*kitaanu*), the people of Saano Dumre use the word *kira* to mean both 'bugs' (when referring to insects one can see) and 'germs' (e.g., "bugs" in the water one cannot see).

The most common mode of transmission was thought to be through drinking the water in which *kira* are living.

The follow-up survey confirmed these findings. The possible answers (spirits, bad *karma*, germs, spoiled planets and weak body) were all derived from the focus group interviews given previously. Then the questionnaire was distributed to the wider group, and survey results revealed that sixty-four percent (n = 75) considered germs to be the biggest factor contributing to sickness (fig. 5.1). This certainly demonstrates that an education concerning germ theory has taken place and the belief in germs as the primary cause of sickness is now widespread throughout Saano Dumre. This may be a result of the nearby hospital, the health education given in local schools, or a combination of both.

5.2.3.2 Graha bigriyo 'spoiled planets'

The second most common answer to the question "What is the biggest factor contributing to illness?," was "*graha bigriyo* 'spoiled planets'." This answer was reported by twenty-four percent of the respondents (n = 75). Although a minority opinion, it is clear that many still hold to this traditional belief that if a person's planets are spoiled, then harm, in the way of sickness, can result. When asked which illnesses can be caused by *graha bigriyo* one respondent replied, "All diseases; unless you have *graha bigriyo* you won't be entangled in any illness. If you are sick it is a sign that your planets are spoiled." Another responded, "If our planets are spoiled then we may fall on the trail, or a witch can attack us."

This belief is similar to how we might view the process of an immunodeficiency disease. When asked why an immunodepressed person fell sick, we might mention a certain virus, but we would consider the person's immunodepressed status as the main cause of their higher susceptibility, which in turn facilitated the particular illness episode. So, because of spoiled planets people can more easily succumb to diseases that are caused by *kira* 'germs', they can be vulnerable to a witch and therefore become sick, or they can have terrible luck, which can lead to an injury like falling from a tree. Germs, witches and bad luck are all contributing factors, but graha bigriyo is perceived as the main cause, which makes people most susceptible to other factors.

5.2.3.3 Karaab karma 'bad deeds'

There are very few people who still hold to the traditional idea that certain diseases are the result of *karaab karma* 'bad karma'. Only sixteen percent (n = 69) reported bad *karma* as a contributing factor in illness. Of those who still hold this belief, tuberculosis and leprosy were the two most commonly mentioned diseases believed to result from bad *karma*. One man said, "Most diseases have a physical cause, but in the case of leprosy and TB, our traditional belief is that these are the result of bad *karma*." Traditionally, negative consequences or illnesses are considered the result of 'bad works' *karrab karma*, or sins in one's previous life. One focus group referred to TB and leprosy as *paapko rog* 'sin diseases'.

Another focus group offered a different interpretation of *karma*. With respect to AIDS, they said, "It is not a result of the sin of past lives [but] rather the *karaab karma* 'bad actions' in this life." One man added, "Bad actions are the result of a corrupt mind."

5.2.3.4 Spirits

There is still a fairly strong belief that spirits can cause illness. It seems, however, that this idea has lost some influence (given way to germ theory) over the past quarter century. Only forty percent (n = 70) attributed cause for sickness to spirits and only three percent (n = 75) considered spirits the biggest factor in disease causation. This would appear to be a big change from twenty-five years ago.

Among those who still attribute sickness to spirits there seemed to be a good ability to list the various gods who are reported to cause illness, list which symptoms are associated with each god, and which treatments are required for the illness associated with each god. For example, *aakaash devi, naag, masaan, dev* and *pichas* (various local gods) are all malevolent spirits believed to be able to cause illness. The symptoms associated with *aakaash devi* are fever, loss of appetite and tiredness. Although the *dhaami-jhaankri* or the *baidhya* may give diagnoses, treatment must be sought from an astrologer who will identify the exact time in which you must go to a high, clean place and offer worship through sacrifice. The god *naag*, on the other hand, will cause one to be bedridden with headache and fever. This condition must be diagnosed by the astrologer who will then prescribe *naag pujaa* 'snake worship' at either a 'dry place' *paakhaa naag* or 'wet place' *jaamaa naag* dependent on his astrology based assessment. The services of the *dhaami-jhaankri* or *baidhya* are then employed to offer the proper *pujaa* 'worship', for example, offering cow's milk to a snake. Or other gods (e.g., *masaan*) may require a black cock to be sacrificed on the banks of the Chepi River in order to appease him and relieve the symptoms associated with this deity. Unlike what Blustain described, the members of each focus group seemed quite knowledgeable concerning the particulars of each spirit caused illness[26]

---

[26]Blustain (1976:87) suggested that the *baidhyas* and *dhaami-jhaankris* were the "repositories of local medical knowledge" while the average villager was more or less impervious to these details.

5.2.4 Influences upon health: Greater susceptibility toward illness

Besides the causes (agents) of illness there were also factors identified that would make one more susceptible to illness. These are discussed below.

5.2.4.1 Kamjor 'body weakness'

Although only eight percent (n = 75) identified *kamjor* 'body weakness' as the main cause of illness, 97 percent did agree that being *kamjor* increased ones susceptibility to illness (n = 70). The main cause of weakness seemed to be diet related. One respondent commented that lack of food w-ill make one *kamjor*. If we are *kamjor* then we will be more susceptible to sickness. If we don't have a balanced diet and lack food then we will *kamjor* and then illness can come.

Another common association with weakness was "weak blood." One respondent answered, "If a person has weak blood then s/he is more susceptible to illness. For instance, if a person has weak blood then s/he can get AIDS. Also, if you have weak blood then *kira* can take advantage and make you sick."

5.2.4.2 Laaparwaahi 'negligence'

When asked if sickness can be the result of 'negligence' *laaparwaahi,* 100 percent of the survey respondents (n = 72) marked the affirmative. Discussion in focus groups illuminated that negligence most often resulted in behavior that led to sickness. For some, negligence focused on the issue of diet while for others it had more to do with bad actions and morality. For instance, one man said, "Many people do stupid things like drink liquor. When you drink liquor you become negligent and forget to eat, or mix the wrong foods and you will get sick. This is how negligence leads to sickness. When one is *laaparwaahi* 'negligent', they do stupid things."

Another respondent suggested, "If one drinks too much, they may become negligent and climb a tree and fall from it creating a bad injury. Or they may build their house incorrectly causing it to fall down during the rainy season, which may hurt someone."

And another respondent, tying negligence more directly to morality, commented, "AIDS is the result of negligence. A *randi* 'sexually promiscuous' person will be negligent in her/his sexual practices and AIDS will result." I will talk more about the popular concept of *randi/o* later in the section on AIDS. This concept is a major element of one of the cultural models of HIV and AIDS that is emerging in Saano Dumre.

5.2.4.3 Fear or worry

There is also a minority opinion that having fear can make one more susceptible to illness. Thirty-one percent of the follow-up survey respondents agreed with this contention (n = 71). One focus group member commented that "there is much greater possibility of us becoming sick if we are afraid. Fear makes one very susceptible to illness." Another respondent commented, "Fear or worry facilitates AIDS." She added, "If persons worry about their disease, they will lose their appetite, become thin (*dublo*) and this will lead to their quick demise."

5.2.4.4 Imbalanced diet

A large majority (88%) of the surveyed sample confirmed the finding in the focus groups that imbalanced diet can contribute to susceptibility to illness (n = 77). What was meant by an "imbalanced diet" was (1) not having enough food, (2) improper mixing of hot and cold foods, and (3) not eating on time.[27] Diet was also associated with several of the other factors influencing illness. For instance, I was told that if one is *kamjor,* then he will not be able to eat, which would make him susceptible to sickness. Also, if the climate is too hot, then one will not feel like eating and will become weak and sickness will result.

The emphasis on a balanced diet ran throughout many of the focus group interviews. This is not a surprise given the emphasis on food and eating in Nepali culture (Stone 1989). It seems clear that food (and the concept of eating) is an important schemata in Nepali culture that may also be used in meaning-making in wider domains. This idea will be revisited in the coming chapters.

5.2.4.5 Low places and hot climates

In the focus group interviews, low places and hot climates were most often associated with greater susceptibility to sickness. This belief was also confirmed in the wider survey. Eighty-two percent (n = 73) of survey respondents replied that living in a low place would increase one's susceptibility to illness. Thirteen percent (n = 76) felt that all places were equal for susceptibility and only three respondents (4%) felt that one is more susceptible in high places. Likewise, 92 percent (n = 76) felt that one is more likely to fall sick in the hot season than any other season. Two respondents (2.5%) felt that the cold season was the worst for susceptibility, two (2.5%) felt that the time between seasons was the worst and two (2.5%)

---

[27]I was told that it is very important to eat at approximately the same time every day otherwise a stomach disorder will develop.

said that one is susceptible to the same degree in all seasons. It seems clear from the data that low places and hot climates are believed to be the places where one would be most susceptible to illness.

A few focus group members suggested that the reason that people get sicker in the hot season and low places is food related. One respondent replied, "People lose their appetite in hot places and so, therefore, do not eat enough food. Also, the heat makes it extremely difficult to digest their food, which brings illness."

5.2.5 Transmission of illness

The list of those diseases considered *saruwa* is displayed in table 5.3. The follow-up survey confirmed the findings of the focus group and demonstrated the strength of the wider beliefs concerning the various ways people believe that *saruwa* illnesses can be transmitted from one person to another. The most common responses were through sharing blood (70%), by eating another's *jutho*[28] (66%), by breathing the same air (52%), by being sneezed on by a person with a *saruwa* illness (50%), by using the same utensils (29%), by sleeping in the same bed (28%), or by sharing clothing with someone with a *saruwa* illness (25%) (n = 76). It seems, however, that certain diseases spread more naturally through various methods. For instance, several informants told me that only skin diseases could spread through wearing clothing of a sick person, while all *saruwa* illnesses can be spread through sharing utensils or eating the *jutho* of another. Various other *saruwa* illnesses, such as cough and cold, TB, malaria, AIDS, and chicken pox,[29] can be spread through all of the above modes. One woman even expressed the belief that jaundice was airborne. She commented, "There is a house above, and there one person got jaundice. And here also (because of that) one person got jaundice—so this must be because of the air flowing from there to here."

Another interesting feature of illness that emerged was the *sarnu* 'shifting' nature of illness itself. For instance, it was often commented that an illness might start as a cold, then change to a fever and finally change to pneumonia or typhoid. On the surface this would appear close to our idea that one illness episode, for example, the common cold, might contain several stages that progress to a lung infection and finally, pneumonia. It seems, however, that rather than viewing certain symptoms as stages in a certain illness, one disease can actually *sarnu* to another completely different disease. For

---

[28]The sacred/profane dichotomy is very important in Nepal. One can become ritually impure by touching 'unclean' *jutho* things that are associated with either ritually impure people (such as a lower caste) or impure items such as the food of another person (since they may be unclean). Again, an importance upon food is noted.

[29]I was told that chicken pox can only transfer to children this way, not to adults.

instance, some suggested that a wound or ulcer, if not treated properly, can turn into cancer, others suggested that cancer can become AIDS and still others suggested that colds and coughs or boils can turn into AIDS. This idea that one disease can turn into another is a unique feature that warrants further investigation.

5.2.6 Changes over the last quarter century

Focus groups were asked what have been the biggest changes they have observed in medical care since the time that Harvey Blustain visited Saano Dumre.[30] They were also asked what influence the nearby hospital has had upon their treatment-seeking behavior. There were a number of interesting observations. In reply to the question one man responded:

> Things have changed greatly in Saano Dumre since the time Harvey was here. At that time the hospital had just been built but there were not sufficient numbers of doctors, so people didn't go to the hospitals. They went only to the *dhaami-jhaankris*. The *dhaami-jhaankris* were the only doctors. We had no choice but to go to them for our sickness. Today, everyone goes to the hospital. Today, perhaps, only five percent of the *dhaami-jhaankri's* time is spent in *jhaankri* work. Before, perhaps 50 percent of their time was spent in that work. Today no more *baidhyas* work here professionally, just part time. Most of the *baidhyas* are dead now and the younger generation has little interest in learning the trade.

The contention that people are using the *dhaami-jhaankri* less now than twenty-five years ago was also borne out in the wider survey. Seventy-six percent of the survey respondents reported using the *dhaami-jhaankri* less now than twenty-five years previously, 13 percent reported going as often these days as before, and 10 percent reported using the services of the *dhaami-jhaankri* more these days than previously.

On the surface it would appear that the belief in the efficacy of the traditional medical practitioners (TMPs) is declining. One man told the following story:

> Fifteen years ago my younger brother went to work in India. After a few years we no longer received letters from him. We wondered what had happened to him, so we sent another family member to search for him. They were unable to track him down. We waited for news but heard nothing. We hoped and hoped, but still we heard nothing from our younger brother. After a few more years, I

---

[30]Everyone I spoke with remembered "Harbyji." He left a very positive impression upon the villagers, which made it very easy for me to conduct my interviews as a fellow anthropologist.

consulted the *dhaami-jhaankri* to see if he could tell me what had become of my brother. He told me that my brother was dead in India. I was distraught. He told me that I must conduct the final rights for my brother. He told me I must take a black goat to the banks of the Chepi River and sacrifice it there and give him the meat. We mourned for our brother, but after the appropriate time, we let him go and got back to our lives. Two years later, my brother appeared alive with a suitcase under his arm. He was home from India! From that very day I did not believe in the power of the *dhaami-jhaankris.*

Another echoed this same sentiment stating that "only the stupid and uneducated still go to the *baidhyas.*"

Despite this contention, however, it seems clear that many people still seek the services of *dhaami-jhaankris* and *baidhyas.* This fact was borne out in the survey. Just a little over half of the respondents (51%) reported visiting a *dhaami-jhaankri* or *baidhya* in the past year (n = 71). This also proved true in my personal experience. In one instance, while interviewing a popular Muslim *baidhya,* four Hindu women sought his services during the twenty minutes I was interviewing him. I also observed each of the other TMPs treating patients during my visits. Further, despite the contention that only the uneducated visit the TMPs, one well-educated young man admitted taking his mother first to the *dhaami-jhaankri* for her symptoms of shaking. He commented that "we took her to the *jhaankri* for her own peace of mind since we (he and his siblings) don't believe in that."

It seems clear that many still use traditional healers in Saano Dumre, but in a much different way than previously noted. Their use has been retained in the case of symptoms of shaking (believed to be mainly spiritually caused), while for most *saano rogs,* villagers attempt self-treatment, and for *thulo rogs* they consult doctors at the hospital. The villagers of Saano Dumre are combining traditional beliefs and ideas about the power of western medicine in certain domains into a complex hybrid medical treatment-seeking system.

There has also been an apparent change in the behavior of the *dhaami-jhaankris* in terms of their acceptance of western medicines and referrals to the hospital. I was able to interview each of the *dhaami-jhaankris* who had previously been interviewed by Blustain and I found there to be quite an acceptance of the efficacy of western medicine. For example, as I approached the house of one shaman, now an old man, he came out and greeted me asking if I had brought any medicine from the hospital, which would heal his deafness. In another case, the medicine-giving *baidhya* consulted me to know which medicine would be best for acid reflux. And in another case, the shaman told me that he enters a trance and consults the gods and that many times they tell him to refer the patient to the hospital. Most of the traditional healers themselves claim that they only attempt to treat *saano rogs* while *thulo rogs* are referred to the hospital. It seems that *laago* 'spirit caused' diseases are usually *saano*, which is a big change from earlier years.

As an interesting aside, one Muslim *baidhya* told me that most come to him only with *saano rogs*, but now and then a really poor person with a *thulo rog* will come to him in hopes that he will be able to treat them, thus sparing them the expense of the hospital visit.[31] This is in vain, however, as he tells me that he always refers *thulo rogs* to the hospital.

The belief in the stronger nature of western medicine was also reflected in the wider survey. Seventy-nine percent of the sample reports the belief that hospital medicine is stronger than *gaaunko ausadhi* 'village medicine', nineteen percent report the belief that village medicine is stronger than hospital medicine, and one percent report that both are equally effective (n = 68). Likewise, 77 percent report the belief that after taking hospital medicine, village medicine will no longer be effective (n = 71).

As has been noted, there has been a change in villagers' use of the traditional healers of Saano Dumre. The help of TMPs is still sought, but in a much more limited domain (mainly for *kaamne rog*) than before. And what will happen to this age-old trade? Currently, none of the Hindu *dhaami-jhaankris* are teaching their children their trade and there are also no young Muslims training to replace the aging *baidhyas*. One Hindu *dhaami-jhaankri* told me that he hopes to teach his sons, but that the oldest two are in Calcutta and are drinkers (apparently not allowed in this work) and that his youngest "also wants to depart for some foreign place." Likewise, the sons of the leading *baidhya* are working abroad and their father considers it unlikely they will return to take up *baidhya* work.

It seems clear that culture, at least in the domain of treatment seeking, has changed during the ensuing years since the publication of Blustain's study. Treatment seeking seems much more contested these days than at that time, and it seems the trend has now shifted away from the exclusive use of traditional healers.[32] And, even the practices of the *dhaami-jhaankris* seem to differ significantly from those described by Blustain.

Far from replacing one medical system (traditional) with another (western), however, the majority of the villagers of Saano Dumre employ a hybrid medical system that maximizes the use of all available resources. This hybrid system seems to combine elements of the traditional and western systems in a way that they feel maximizes efficacy. Traditional home remedies are best for *saano rogs,* the treatment of the TMPs for symptoms of shaking and western medicine for *thulo rogs,* especially those perceived to be 'foreign' *bidesh* such as HIV and AIDS.

---

[31]This practice matches the pattern observed in Eastern Nepal (in reference to T.B.) as well (see Zvosec 1996:201).

[32] As mentioned previously, perhaps this is due to a difference in the time of our studies, a difference in the focus of our studies, or a combination of both.

5.2.6.1 Reasons for change

Perhaps the biggest precipitator of change was the building of a western mission hospital thirty years ago that is within walking distance from Saano Dumre. The previously noted preference given to anything *bikaas* 'developed' has also contributed to the changes. During the interviews a number of respondents replied to my questioning, "Why are you asking us these questions? You are educated—you are developed."

Education has certainly contributed to a growth in the understanding of germ theory. Most families have at least one child studying in a local school, and the national curriculum now includes a health class in the eighth grade that uses a comprehensive health reader. I also was shocked to see that because of education, many parents are even giving deference to the opinions of their educated children. This is a big cultural change. In one instance I was interviewing a family about their understanding of HIV and AIDS. The oldest daughter who was studying in college in Kathmandu was home for the holidays. As I asked questions, the father would begin to answer, but then was interrupted and corrected by his daughter. After about the third question, the man said, "What do I know about these things? These are educated topics. Ask my daughter; she is educated."

Major demographic changes have also had an impact. Most families have at least one member working abroad in order to provide a subsistence living. There is a much larger awareness of an outside world than previously. In regard to treatment seeking, there is much more awareness of alternatives. One man responded, "When we get sick, we go to Amp Pipal. If we don't get well there, they will refer us to Patan hospital in Kathmandu. If we still don't get better we can go to teaching Hospital in Kathmandu. And if we cannot get good treatment there, we can go to Bangalore [in India]. There is a good hospital there as well."

The wider Nepali attitude toward the mantra of *bikaas* has also had a negative impact upon the occupation of the TMPs. It is now illegal to practice medicine in Nepal without a license. So, many of the TMPs are "practicing medicine" illegally. One of the TMPs we interviewed was hesitant to speak with us at first. He first reported that he no longer did that kind of work (*jhaankri kaam*). Later, we saw him treating people and he told us that when he first saw us, he thought we were there to arrest him for doing *jhaankri* work and throw him in jail. He had a court case against him by the government for practicing without a license. Such an attitude will certainly influence the eventual demise of the tradition.

The village of Saano Dumre is no longer "untouched" by the outside world; two of the three sons of one shaman are in Calcutta, the girl spoken of above is studying in Kathmandu, and one of the baidhya's sons works in Qatar. From these places they are bringing in new ideas. And these new ideas are being accepted because they are *bikaas*.

5.3 Perceptions about HIV and AIDS

The second half of the focus group interview centered on HIV and AIDS. Many of the same questions were asked about HIV and AIDS that had been asked about all illnesses in general in the first half (see appendix A). The findings are summarized below.

5.3.1 Knowledge of HIV and AIDS

As figure 5.2 demonstrates, a majority (86%) of the survey respondents reported having heard about HIV and AIDS (n = 72). This number was higher than expected, given many of the reports about the lack of knowledge about HIV and AIDS in the rural areas. One focus group reported, however, that although they had heard about HIV and AIDS, at first they thought AIDS was a brand of beer since advertisements about AIDS had begun to be aired in the place of beer advertisements that had formerly followed the nightly newscast on Radio Nepal. A minority (12.5%) reported having never heard of HIV and AIDS while one percent of the sample marked more than one answer, inferring that some in the household had heard of AIDS while others had not.

The marking of multiple answers on the questionnaire was an interesting phenomenon. There were a few questions that inspired multiple answers on several of the returned questionnaires. The survey was distributed to homes and participants were asked to (1) select a reader, (2) read the questions, (3) discuss the questions, and (4) mark the appropriate answer (or answers if members of the home didn't reach a consensus). For the most part, only one answer was marked. On three questions, however, several families marked multiple answers. This demonstrates that although Nepali culture generally appears to be one of societal consensus building, personal differences of opinion can exist and this type of research can, indeed, allow for differences of opinion to be expressed. This displays that meaning, even in this homogeneous society, is negotiated and can still be contested.

In response to the question about where they had heard about HIV and AIDS, the majority (72%) reported the "radio" as the main source of information, followed by the hospital, doctor or health post (46%), informational pamphlet (34%), poster (26%), school and TV (both 25%). One respondent reported hearing about HIV and AIDS from the *dhaami-jhaankri* and one reported hearing from other villagers (n = 76). Figure 5.3 illustrates the responses to this question.

5.3.2 Ideas about HIV and AIDS

In response to the question about whether HIV and AIDS requires hot or cold food for treatment, there was no consensus (fig. 5.4). The majority

(76%) claimed that they didn't know, sixteen percent felt that it required the eating of hot foods to restore balance and, nine percent felt it required cold food (n = 77).

5.3.2.1 AIDS as thulo rog

One of the strongest consensuses noted about HIV and AIDS was in response to the question of whether HIV and AIDS was a *saano* 'small' or *thulo* 'big' illness (fig. 5.5). Eighty-seven percent of the respondents felt that it was a big disease while only three percent felt it was small and one family gave multiple answers (again reflecting the ability to demonstrate a contested answer in response to a question in the survey) (n = 71).

5.3.2.2 AIDS as saruwa rog

Community consensus was also clear on the question of whether AIDS was a *saruwa* 'transmissible' illness (fig. 5.6). Over eighty-seven percent (87.5%) responded "yes" while only three percent said "no" and ten percent said they didn't know (n = 72).

5.3.2.3 AIDS as a fatal disease: 'Final' antim and 'finished' khattam

Another clear consensus is seen in response to the question of whether or not AIDS was a 'final' *antim* disease (fig. 5.7). Again over eighty-seven percent responded affirmatively, four percent said no, and just over eight percent (8.5%) claimed that they didn't know. In a related question 82 percent said that they would consider one with HIV and AIDS 'finished' *khattam*, while six percent said they wouldn't, and twelve and a half percent (12.5%) didn't know (fig. 5.8).

5.3.2.4 Perceived causes of AIDS

In regard to perceived causes of HIV and AIDS there was great consensus that HIV and AIDS is not a result of the traditional factors spoken of earlier. AIDS is generally not perceived to be caused by spirits (fig. 5.9), bad *karma* (fig. 5.10), spoiled planets (fig. 5.11) or bad luck (fig. 5.12). The community was divided almost equally about whether AIDS is the result of germs (fig. 5.13). What did seem very clear, however, is that the villagers of Saano Dumre make a strong association (87%) between AIDS and prostitutes (fig. 5.14).[33] This strong association between AIDS and prostitutes is most likely

---

[33]Two families returned surveys with multiple answers marked to the questions regarding spoiled planets, bad luck and prostitutes. Again, this displays differences of opinion on these issues.

a result of the various prevention campaigns developed in the city and disseminated to the rural areas of Nepal.

During the course of focus group interviews the traditional concept of *randi* or *rando* 'promiscuity' was often mentioned in reference to HIV and AIDS. In Nepali society a person who is known to be sexually promiscuous is considered as *"randi"* (if female) or *"rando"* (if male).[34] According to traditional custom, this person would be considered as a person of bad character and s/he must be 'despised' *ghrinaa* because of her/his bad actions, and *chhichhi durdur* 'social ostricization' would be practiced against her/him as a sort of social sanction. When I asked during the focus groups, who is at highest risk for contracting AIDS, the answer was usually "prostitutes and others who are *randi.*" In reference to the question about negligence, one informant responded, "Yes, getting AIDS is caused by negligence. You know, going here and there being *randi.*" And in regard to whether or not a person with AIDS should be 'despised' *ghrinaa,* another informant replied, "The type of persons who get it are *randi,* therefore it is our responsibility to disapprove of that kind of behavior and despise them." Because of the strong association of HIV and AIDS with sex and prostitutes, the traditional concept of *randi* is being employed as a major component of the emerging cultural model of HIV and AIDS here in the rural area.

In response to the question about the other ways AIDS can be transmitted, there were four popular answers among the eleven possibilities condensed from the focus group interviews. These most common answers were: having sex with someone who has AIDS (85%), having sex with many partners (79%), sharing needles with an infected person (67%), and using razor blades or scissors (used in shaving or hair cutting) of people with AIDS (53%). Various other answers did receive some attention as figure 5.15 illustrates.

5.3.2.5 Beliefs about susceptibility to HIV and AIDS

The traditional ideas identified earlier regarding susceptibility to illness do not generally carry over strongly to beliefs about the susceptibility to HIV and AIDS. *Kamjor* 'body weakness', weak blood, and fear are not felt strongly to contribute to one's susceptibility to HIV and AIDS as figures 5.16–5.19 demonstrate. Likewise, the majority does not know in which season one

---

[34]It is interesting to me that although the *randi* or *rando* concept can be applied to males or females, I only heard it applied using the feminine form. It seems that, like in our society, a woman is considered a "slut" if she is sexually promiscuous while there is no negative equivalent to describe a male who practices the same behavior. "Playboy" is probably the closest and it does not carry the negative connotations that "slut" does. It seems that in Nepal, the main burden for promiscuity falls on the female and she will be labeled as *"randi"* 'a woman of bad character'.

would be more likely to get AIDS. It is interesting, however, that of those who hazarded a guess about which season, 30 percent of the overall sample chose "hot" while only 14 percent said "cold." Again, perhaps there is some association with moral geography, as will be discussed shortly. There were also three questionnaires returned with multiple answers to this question of seasonal susceptibility to AIDS (fig. 5.19), and one questionnaire was returned with multiple answers for the question regarding a weak body (fig. 5.16).

There is also little consensus about whether females or males are more susceptible (fig. 5.20) to AIDS, although among those who felt that one group was more susceptible, 32 percent felt women were more susceptible compared with only nine percent who felt that men were. Diet is also perceived to have little effect on one's susceptibility to HIV and AIDS (fig. 5.22).

5.3.2.6 Moral geography of HIV and AIDS

When asked in which place one is more likely to contract AIDS, 46 percent of the sample answered "in a low place," 31 percent felt that one was at equal risk in either low or high places, and 23.5 percent claimed that they didn't know (fig. 5.21). Interestingly, not one person responded that AIDS was more likely contracted in a high place. Attitudes about HIV and AIDS mirror the association between low places and susceptibility to illness mentioned earlier.

Although several cited diet as the connection between geography and illness (as mentioned before), the villagers of Saano Dumre also practice a kind of moral geography in which they are more apt to attribute immoral behavior to people from lower regions than to people from their own location and higher places. When asked in the questionnaire why one is more susceptible to AIDS in lower places, several focus groups offered suggestions that implied more of a moral geography. Besides the relationship to food, the villagers of Saano Dumre also seem to associate a kind of low morality with the lower region of Nepal known as the Terai, which they view as a place of low moral values. As to whether one is more likely to contract AIDS in a low place or high place one informant replied, "A person is more likely to get AIDS in the Terai. This is because there are more "bad" people there than here, so you are more likely to get it there." Another respondent replied, "In the Terai and cities people are so rampant. But in the mountains people are not so much this way. That is why there is less fear of getting AIDS here in the mountains."

Clarke (1980) has demonstrated that the Helambu Sherpa people of Nepal also demonstrate a kind of moral geography in which they ascribe higher morality to their own group and other groups found up higher.

According to Hepburn (1994:450), "Clarke points out that the upper and middle-dwelling peoples ascribe morality according to a combination of 'lamaness', wealth, and altitude, such that morality usually resides in your group and all of the people residing higher than you do."

Likewise, Hepburn has demonstrated (using the case of a missing trekker) that other Nepalis also exhibit this same kind of pattern. She comments, "What is striking—and not surprising—is that morality is shifting, and is relative to who is speaking and how they situate themselves with respect to others in the local moral geography. It is also not surprising that the epicenter of morality always seems to be just where the storyteller, ethnically speaking, is standing (Hepburn 1994:449)."

Other authors have also made note of this "social geography." In noting differences between various groups of Tamang, Campbell (1997) identifies this phenomenon as well. He comments

> Overlaying the east-west cultural axis is that of north-south. This reveals a stronger correlation between ecological adaptation and social estimation, in that people living higher 'up' the valley than oneself *(turpa)* are considered somehow better than those further down *(murpa,* or the derogatory *chyoba). Tur* meaning 'up' connotes respect. An honored guest is invited to sit up by the window of the house, or in a feast up would be among the elder men *(kyekpama* or *memema).* Conversely *mur* meaning 'down' has lowly, inferior connotations: 'by the door', 'among the children'. At the *ghewaa* the image of the deceased is eventually taken above the village on the path to the north. Images of harmful spirits, after exorcism are taken, by contrast, below the village to be shown the path to the south.[35]

In discussing the topic of nationalism and ethnicity in Nepal, Whelpton (1997:47) also makes the point that, despite the popular image of Nepal as a "unified" kingdom[36], there has long been a strong north-south division in Nepal and that an historical prejudice exists on the part of the people of the

---

[35]Besides illuminating the distinction between north and south, this also demonstrates that "up" and "down" may in fact be wider cultural schemata which are at play in the formation of illness beliefs.

[36]Gellner (1997:6) writes that "for the last 40 years it has been a cliché of Nepalese politics and tourist brochures that the many different castes, religions, languages, and 'races' of Nepal live together in tolerant harmony, without the violent conflict which has blighted the other countries of South Asia. The harmony may have been exaggerated—Bhattachan (1995:125) condemns it as a "'blatantly manufactured myth." Whelpton (1997) makes the point that the propagation of the dominant *prabati* culture (Hinduization) has been a hegemonic process that has been perpetuated historically by the Nepali school system (via the national history curriculum) and the media.

parbatiyaa 'mountains' toward the *madeshi* 'plains dwellers'. It seems that there has long been a derogatory association by higher people toward lower people in Nepal. Anyone who spends any time in Nepal is keenly aware of that fact.

5.3.2.7 Treatment of people with AIDS

People were generally divided over the issue of how people with HIV and AIDS should be treated. Over 40 percent felt that *chhichhi durdur* 'separation' should be practiced against those with AIDS while almost an equal number (43.5%) felt that it should not be (fig. 5.23). About half the sample (49%) felt that 'disdain' *ghrinaa* should be shown toward those with AIDS, while 43.5 percent said it should not be (fig. 5.24). Only a small group (4%) claimed no knowledge of such things and 3 percent of the sample supplied multiple responses to the question (fig. 5.24). Over half the respondents (51.5%) also felt that people with AIDS should be excluded from community participation (fig. 5.25). Another 32 percent felt that persons with AIDS could be included in community activities while 4 percent claim no knowledge of such things, and 3 percent returned multiple answers (fig. 5.25).

It appears that the traditional *rando/i* concept is being applied toward those with HIV and AIDS by about half the group and that the traditional ideas of practicing *ghrinaa* (a form of social control) and the practice of *chhichhi durdur* (to protect the group) are still in force with about half the group. It mirrors the earlier findings regarding *saruwa* illnesses.

5.3.2.8 AIDS as a foreign disease

When asked whose medicine is most appropriate for treating AIDS, the large majority (87.3%) answered that the medicine of the doctor or hospital would be more powerful (fig. 5.26). Five respondents (8%) responded with multiple answers, one respondent (1.5%) claimed the *baidhya's* medicine to be the most powerful, and five respondents (8%) added a "don't know" box and checked that instead (fig. 5.26). The findings here would seem to mirror the earlier findings about the perceived efficacy of hospital medicines over village medicine. During the course of the research I heard many references to AIDS as a foreign (*bideshi*) disease. This is no surprise since early information disseminated from Kathmandu identified it as a foreign disease.[37]

---

[37]When AIDS was first discussed among the medical community in Nepal it was approached as a foreign disease and some even advocated testing of entering foreigners. Also, the government education campaigns have focused heavily upon prostitution in India. It is no wonder that AIDS is perceived as a foreign disease. The strong association with America and other European countries that is

5.4 Conclusion

In this chapter I have presented the findings of an ethnomedical study designed to examine health beliefs and practices of the people of Saano Dumre as well as the changes that have taken place in treatment seeking over the past twenty-five years. It was also a major goal to examine beliefs and practices regarding HIV and AIDS in order to determine whether any cultural models of this newly emerging disease yet exist in the minds of rural Nepalis. The data indicate that there are, indeed, at least two main cultural models (I) of HIV and AIDS emerging among the villagers of Saano Dumre. (See 4.4 for previous discussion of cultural models I and II.) The first model (held by about half the population) is fairly close to the quasi-western model being disseminated from the capital while the second (held by the other half) is more of a hybrid model that combines elements of the quasi-western model with traditional ideas about illness. Cultural schemata (cultural models II) also seem to underlie this model. The emerging cultural models of HIV and AIDS and the underlying schemata will be discussed in this section.

5.4.1 Two major cultural models (I) of HIV and AIDS

In response to various questions regarding ideas about HIV and AIDS, villagers demonstrated a strong consensus, which would imply a cultural model of HIV and AIDS. The majority have heard of AIDS (fig. 5.2) and view it as a 'major' *thulo,* 'infectious' *saruwa,* 'fatal' *antim* and *khattam,* and 'foreign' *bideshi* disease that is mainly associated with prostitutes. Much of this cultural model has developed from the information people receive from Radio Nepal, their main source of information. The government agency commissioned to lead the way in the fight against HIV and AIDS in Nepal has widely disseminated this model, having been heavily influenced by a western model of HIV and AIDS. This is also, therefore, the popular model being disseminated by the wider media.

The second model incorporates elements of the first model, but then modifies it by applying traditional ideas in the meaning-making process in order to make sense of this new disease. For example, because AIDS is so strongly associated with prostitution, people extend the traditional idea of *randi* to AIDS. Therefore, one with AIDS is generally considered *randi.* And since they are *randi,* the practices that are expected to be applied to all who are categorized as *randi* are practiced against people with AIDS as well. They are to be 'disdained' *ghrinaa* as a form of social ostricization, 'put out of the community' *chhichhi durdur* and kept from social interaction.

---

presented by most Nepali informational guides (e.g.,"AIDS was first recognized in the USA" (Suvedi 1994) has solidified it as a *bideshi* disease in the minds of many. This will be discussed further in chapter 7.

The treatment of people with AIDS in this fashion is also supported by other traditional ideas concerning other *thulo saruwa* 'big' and 'transmittable' diseases. These diseases (e.g., TB and leprosy) were traditionally considered sicknesses associated with bad actions in one's past life. Therefore, they warranted the practices of *ghrinaa* and of *chhichhi durdur* against those who contracted it. Given AIDS' association with prostitution and its classification as a *thulo saruwa* illness, it is no wonder that these traditional practices have been incorporated as major elements of a rural cultural model of HIV and AIDS.

In regard to HIV and AIDS as a *saruwa* illness, there seems to be a conflict between the traditional category of *saruwa* and knowledge about the way AIDS is perceived to spread. Almost all (87.5%) understand AIDS as *saruwa* (a traditional cognitive category), while only about half display an accurate understanding of how HIV and AIDS can spread. For the first half of the group, it seems that the new information concerning the way AIDS can be contracted has been successfully incorporated into their cognitive schema (about the way *saruwa* illnesses can transfer). And the schema has been modified to reflect this new knowledge. For the other half, however, the inclusion of AIDS as a *saruwa* illness has led them to apply only their traditional understandings of such illnesses, leading to incorrect conclusions about how HIV and AIDS can be spread. Perhaps in time, the new information (through education) will be incorporated and modify the *saruwa* schema of the larger group leading to a better understanding of HIV and AIDS (and perhaps a more compassionate treatment of those with HIV and AIDS). In the meantime, it would be very interesting to study whether it is lack of adequate information or some other factor which best accounts for the fact that some have modified their *saruwa* schema through the incorporation of new information while others have not.

Traditional ideas concerning a moral geography are also being applied to the cultural models of HIV and AIDS in the rural area as has been demonstrated. The people of Saano Dumre view the Terai as a place of low moral values where one is more susceptible to contracting AIDS among those "rampant people."

Interestingly, the young educated girl spoken of earlier exhibited a cultural model similar to others observed in Kathmandu. This is not surprising since she was studying at college in Kathmandu. She was the eldest daughter in the home and was home on holiday. I heard answers like hers from no other villager. The reason I introduce her ideas here is that certain elements were identical to one of the city cultural models, which illustrates a clear distinction between city and rural models. Like many city folk, she seemed quite knowledgeable about HIV and AIDS (in terms of the western biomedical model). She also shared ideas about the need for HIV positive persons to keep a positive attitude and that although AIDS is fatal, people will not die instantly, which gives them time to do "good works." These are two major elements of the city model, as we will see in the next chapter.

Another reason that this girl's answers are so significant is due to the changing nature of cultural models. The cultural model of AIDS developing in the village is being modified by people such as her, the educated children of the village. And, as I have already demonstrated, parents are deferring to their children's knowledge because they are "educated," while parents consider themselves "villagey," "backwards," and "ignorant." The mantra of *bikaas* 'development' as "good" and tradition as "bad" (Pigg 1995) will further influence deference being given to the cultural model of those considered *bikaas*. As we will see in the next chapter, there are many negative aspects to the cultural model developing in the city that, if they spread to the rural areas as well, will further facilitate the spread of HIV and AIDS in Nepal.

5.4.2 Proposed schemata

There are a few lower level schemata (cultural models II) that are influential in the construction of a rural cultural model of HIV and AIDS. These are (1) the *randi* 'promiscuity' concept, (2) the idea of food, and (3) the concept of "up" and "down."

As previously noted, the *randi* schema was applied quite naturally once it was determined that HIV and AIDS was associated with sex. This is a traditional Nepali schema that is well known and applies principally to women. It is this cultural schema that accounts for, in part, the taboo nature of the subject of sex, especially for women. As we will see in later chapters, this has repercussions for AIDS education campaigns in Nepal.

An even more fundamental schema in Nepali society is food. The village study indicates that food is an important schema running through the various topics: A person becomes weak by not eating properly. A person who is negligent will not eat properly and will therefore become sick. One who has fear will not focus on a proper diet. By going to a lower place, one will lose her/his appetite because of the heat or will not be able to properly digest food. Sickness spreads through eating the *jutho* 'pollution' of another, etc. This theme will be elaborated on further in chapter seven.

The moral geography concept illustrated the "up" and "down" schema. This orientation schema is used to associate morality with "up" and immorality with "down." This appears to be a popular orientation or image schema used by many Nepalis, as has been demonstrated, and is applicable to the domain of illness as well.

The cultural models and underlying schemata proposed for the rural area will be elaborated on further in chapter seven. Next, we turn to the city to examine cultural models of AIDS among HIV positive persons.

Table 5.1. *Thulo* and *saano rogs*

Thulo rogs	Floating	*Saano rogs*
Aids	Tuberculosis	Cold/cough
Cancer	Leprosy	Stomachache
Chicken Pox	Malaria	Fever
Vomiting/Diarrhea	Gastric	Diarrhea
Chronic headache	Tonsillitis	Headache
Chronic stomachache	Ulcer	Body ache
Chronic joint pain	Bloody stool	Sprain
Chronic cough	Asthma	Wound (minor)
Jaundice		Joint pain
Fast breathing		Worms
Paralysis		
Blood clot		
Gangrene		
Typhoid		
Polio		
Worms (chronic)		
Pneumonia		
Broken bones		

Table 5.2. Hot and cold diseases

Hot foods required	Cold foods required	"In between"	Disputed	Can eat anything
Cold/cough	Tuberculosis	Gastric	Headache	AIDS
Joint pain	Fast breathing	Chronic cough	Stomachache	Cancer
	Jaundice		AIDS	Paralysis
	Bloody stool		Cancer	Sprain
	Diarrhea		Cough	Broken bones

Table 5.3. *Saruwa* illnesses

Those mentioned by all	Those mentioned by many	Others
Cold Tuberculosis	AIDS Chicken pox Leprosy Malaria Fever Diarrhea	Jaundice Chronic cough Bloody stool Boils

Table 5.4. Treatment-seeking flow chart (general)

If thulo rog > hospital > if better > yes > home > no > Kathmandu hospital If saano rog > try home remedies > if better > yes > no further treatment > no > hospital > if better > yes >home > no > Kathmandu hospital If kamne rog > Dhadmi-Jhaankri > 1) treats > if better > yes > home > no > hospital 2) refers directly to hospital

Table 5.5. Home remedies

Western	Ayurvedic	Traditional

Cetamol
    (paracetamol)
Vicks
Rifle tel (rifle oil)
Esprin (aspirin)
Jiwan jel
	Maha jarankus
	Chandra shekar
	Nunilu paranisor
	Ananda bairva
	Kana sundari
	Nawras
	Sringaput
	Seto palaadhi
	Jesta palaadhi
	Agni khumar
	Batisa
		Besa pani (turmeric water)
		Nun pani (salt water)
		Beri nun (red [from Tibet] salt water)
		Phet-kiri (alum dissolved in water)
		Ghortabre (bitter leaf of small plant)
		Chini pani (sugar water)
		Todi tel (mustard oil)
		Nun panile sekne (hot salt compress)
		Saj bark lotion for cuts (from a tree)
		Sajiwan liquid for cuts (from plant)
		Tulsikopaat pani (marigold leaf
		    water)

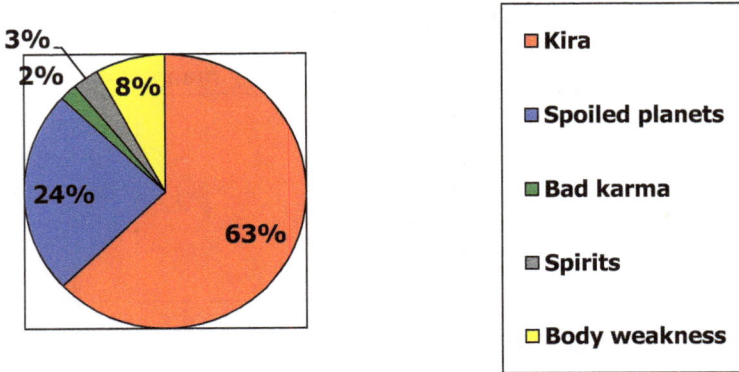

Figure 5.1. Biggest factor influencing illness.

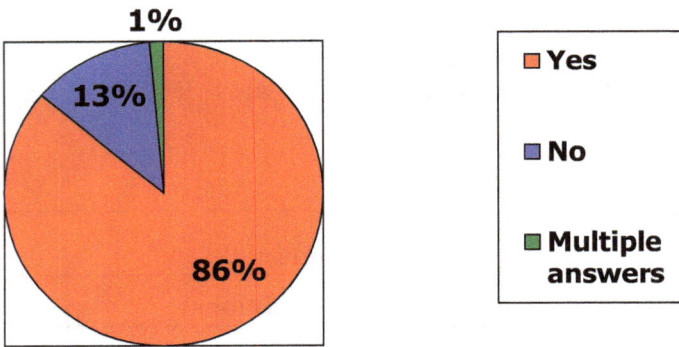

Figure 5.2. Have you heard about AIDS?

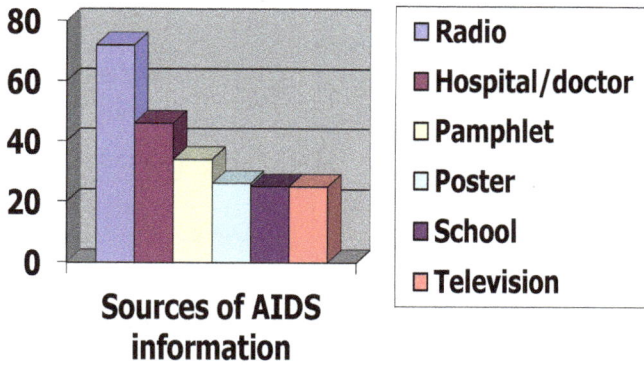

Figure 5.3. From where have you heard about AIDS?

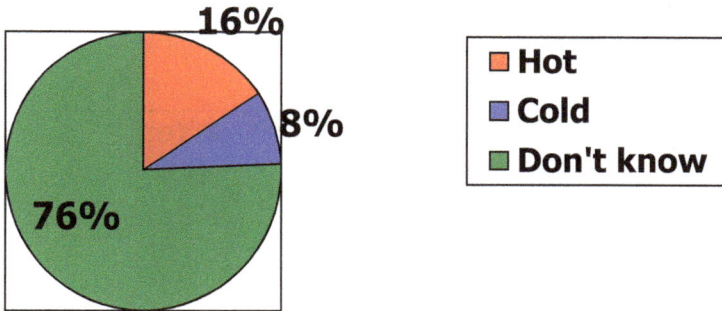

Figure 5.4. Does AIDS require eating hot or cold foods?

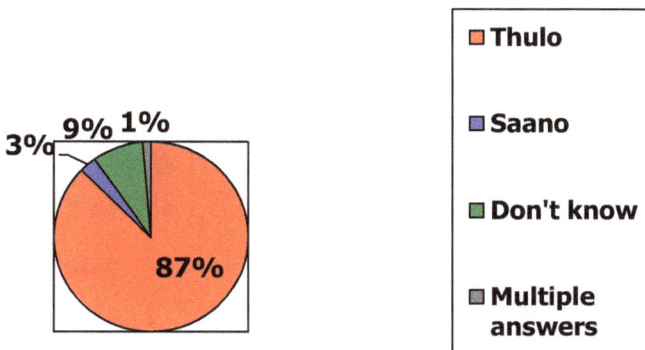

Figure 5.5. Is AIDS a *thulo* 'big' or *saano rog* 'small sickness'?

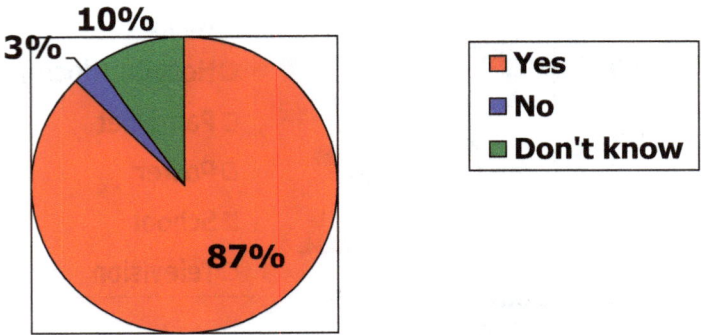

Figure 5.6. Is AIDS a *saruwa rog* 'transferable illness'?

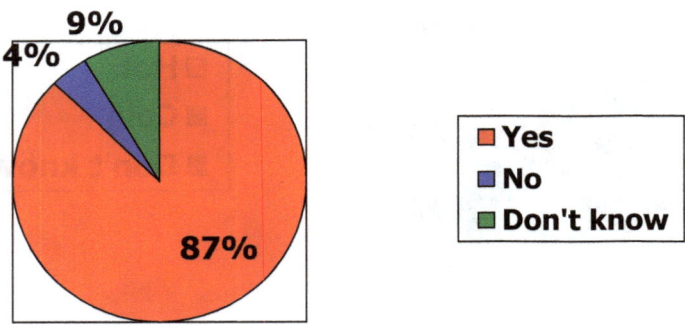

Figure 5.7. Is AIDS an *antim rog* 'fatal illness'?

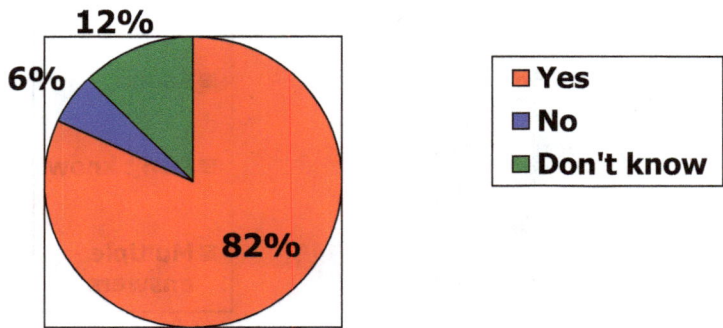

Figure 5.8. If you have AIDS are you considered *khattam* 'finished'?

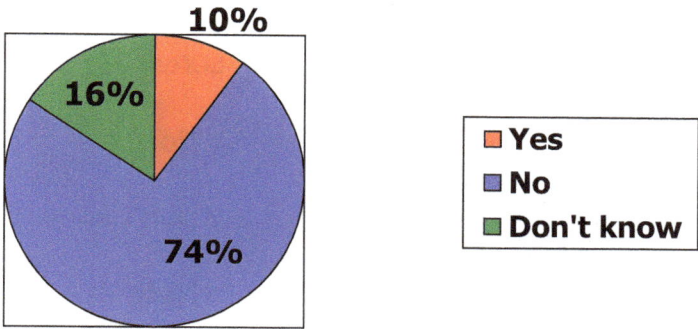

Figure 5.9. Can spirits cause AIDS?

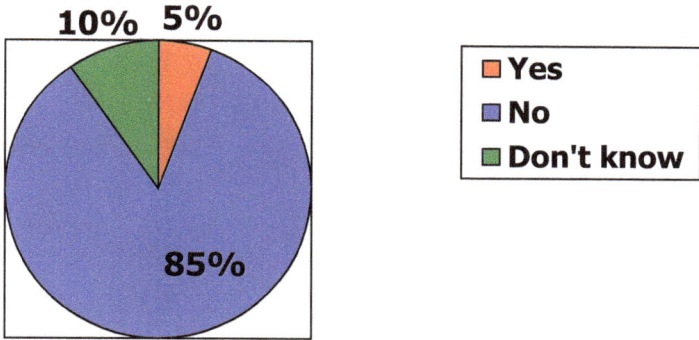

Figure 5.10. Is AIDS the result of bad karma?

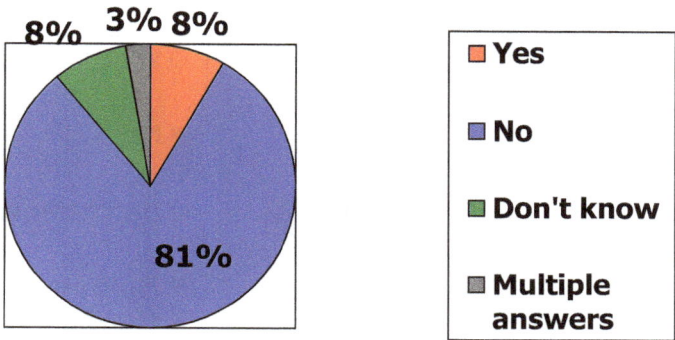

Figure 5.11. Is AIDS the result of spoiled planets?

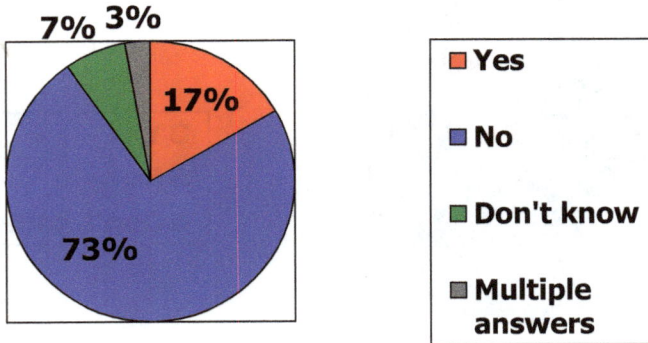

Figure 5.12. Is AIDS the result of bad luck?

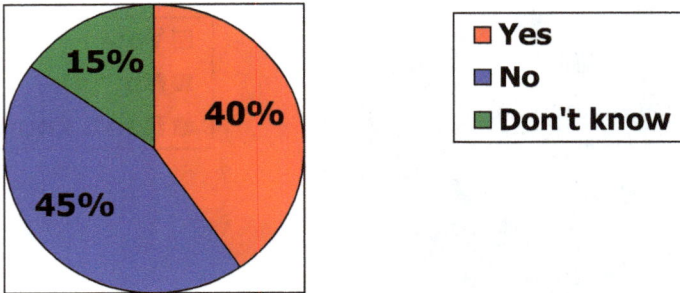

Figure 5.13. Is AIDS the result of germs?

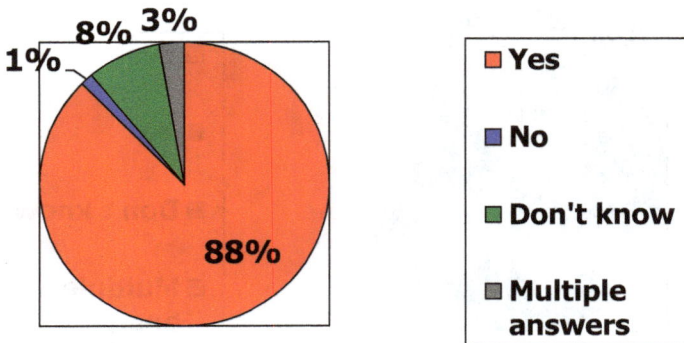

Figure 5.14. Does AIDS come from prostitutes?

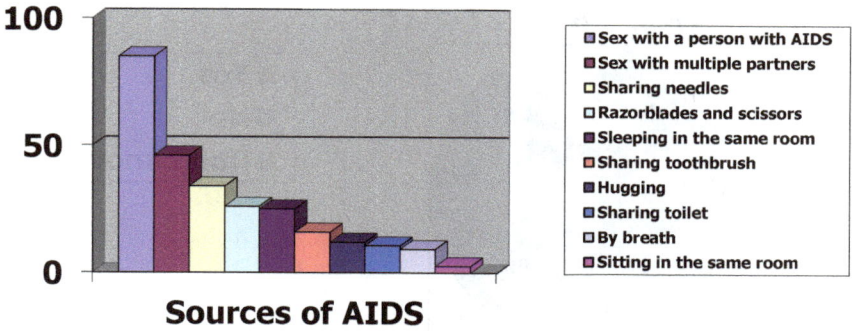

Sources of AIDS

Legend:
- Sex with a person with AIDS
- Sex with multiple partners
- Sharing needles
- Razorblades and scissors
- Sleeping in the same room
- Sharing toothbrush
- Hugging
- Sharing toilet
- By breath
- Sitting in the same room

Figure 5.15 What other ways can you get AIDS?

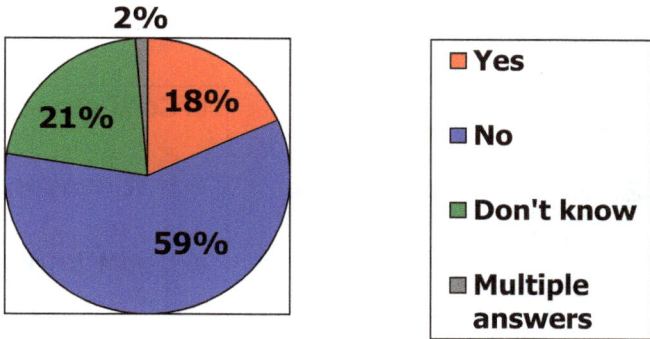

Legend:
- Yes
- No
- Don't know
- Multiple answers

Figure 5.16. If *kamjor* 'weak in body', are you more susceptible to AIDS?

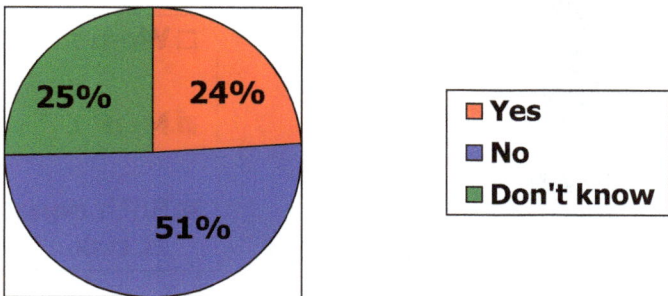

Legend:
- Yes
- No
- Don't know

Figure 5.17. Will weak blood make you more susceptible to AIDS?

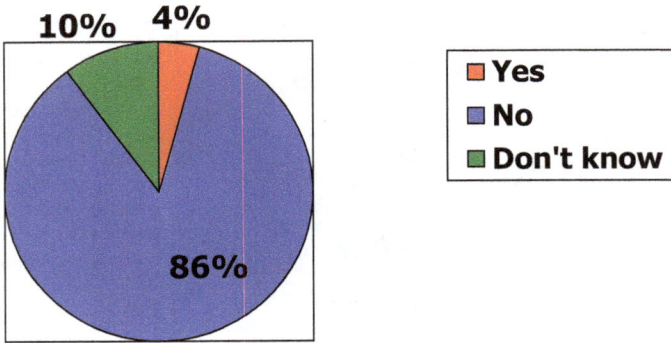

Figure 5.18. Will fear make you more susceptible to AIDS?

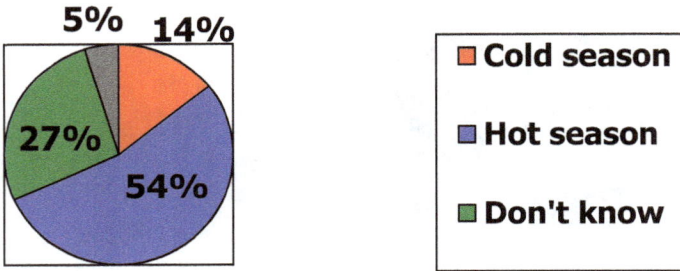

Figure 5.19. In which season would you be more susceptible to AIDS?

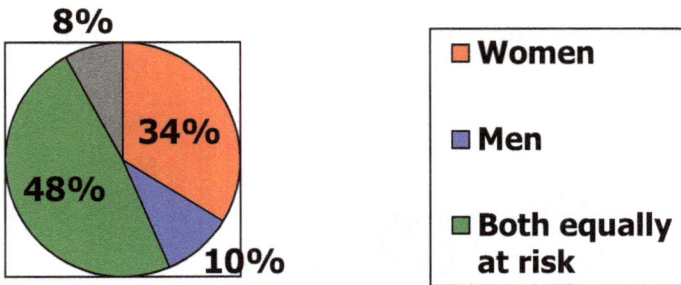

Figure 5.20. Who is at greatest risk for AIDS?

0%

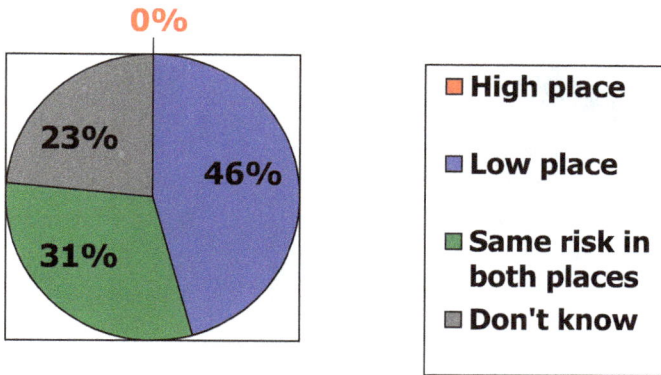

| High place |
| Low place |
| Same risk in both places |
| Don't know |

Figure 5.21. In which place would AIDS be more likely contracted?

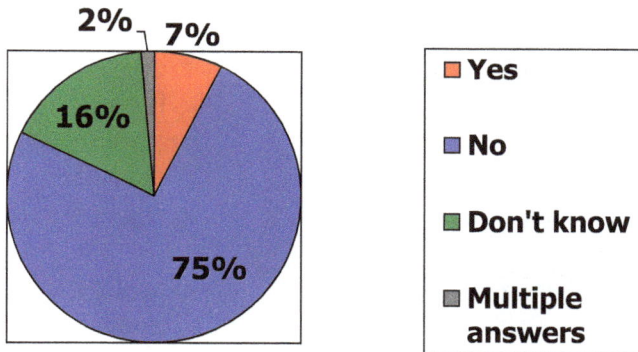

| Yes |
| No |
| Don't know |
| Multiple answers |

Figure 5.22. Will an unbalanced diet make you more susceptible to AIDS?

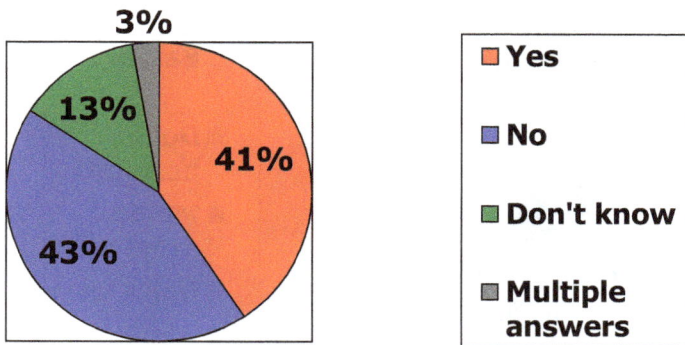

| Yes |
| No |
| Don't know |
| Multiple answers |

Figure 5.23. Should *chichi durdur* 'ostracism' be practiced towards a person with AIDS?

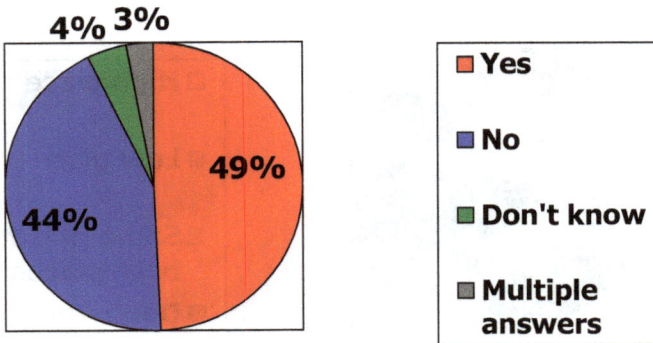

Figure 5.24. Should *ghrina* 'societal hate as a form of social control' be practiced towards a person with AIDS?

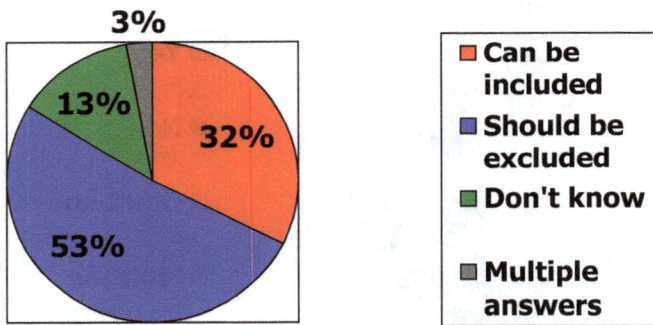

Figure 5.25. Should a person with AIDS be included in community activities?

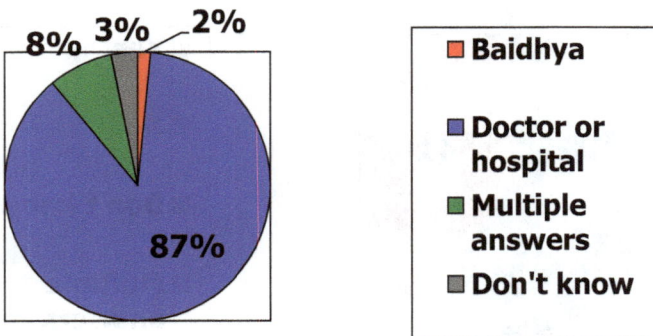

Figure 5.26. Whose medicine is best for AIDS?

6

HIV and Me—A Discourse Analysis of HIV and AIDS Narratives

This chapter introduces the findings of a narrative study conducted among HIV positive persons in Nepal. The two different locales for this study were (1) in the capital city, Kathmandu; and (2) in the rural setting of Gorkha District. I carried out this research with those who have HIV and AIDS in order to determine how they understand their illness. The scientific significance of this approach is multifarious. First of all, since AIDS is a relatively new phenomenon in Nepal, we have a chance to see a cultural model develop before our eyes. This affords us the opportunity to study the development process of a cultural model, and then cross-culturally compare and contrast it with the growth of HIV and AIDS cultural models in Haiti (Farmer 1994), France (Herzlich 1989), Australia (Viney and Bousfield 1991), and America (chapter 1). Secondly, the narrative analysis model is currently under critique (Good 1994) and has only been applied to limited data, providing tentative results (Viney and Bousfield 1991). Using this approach will allow us to test the validity of this new model for studying agency using a larger sample. Finally, this model has not been tested cross-linguistically. This research will apply narrative analysis methods to narratives of mother tongue Nepali speakers in order to assess the value of using this method cross-linguistically to understand how people create meaning.

In addition to the theoretical significance mentioned above, the study also provides insight into how HIV positive persons in Nepal think about their disease. There are, indeed, widely held meanings associated with HIV and AIDS among those infected. As mentioned previously, stigma, blame, and hate (partially a result of the various governmental prevention campaigns) are all elements of the dominant HIV and AIDS discourse in Nepal, and as we will see, these same elements are embedded in the narratives of HIV positive persons living in Nepal.

Although elements of the dominant cultural model can clearly be seen in the narratives of HIV-positive persons in Nepal, this analysis also reveals other common themes within this group that are not generally shared by members of the wider culture. Besides the thematic commonality of HIV positive sufferers, the narratives also reveal slight differences of meaning attributed to HIV and AIDS by rural and urban dwellers and between urban males and females. The narratives will also allow us to explore the various illness schemata that underlie these HIV and AIDS stories. These findings will be discussed further in this chapter.

While these narratives are set in the "ethnographic present" of 2001–2002, at the end of the chapter I include summary analysis from narratives collected in 2012 for comparative purposes; they illustrate that many elements of the former cultural model are still strong in Nepal, while new elements—reflective of the current wider discourse on HIV and AIDS in Nepal (e.g., living with HIV vs. dying of AIDS)—are also being woven in to the ever-changing cultural model. For the sake of brevity I have not included these recent narratives in chapter 10, but these texts will be included in full in a forthcoming publication.

6.1 Methodology

A relatively new strategy of understanding the meanings associated with illness is a narrative analysis approach (Cortazzi 1993; Riessman 1993). One of the strengths of this approach is that it presents the voices of the research participants, which are rarely heard in more traditional ethnography. The socially shared meaning of AIDS, like other culturally constructed meanings, is likely to express the multivocality commonly understood to be part of all cultural representations (Herrell 1991). Social scientists studying illness, however, have tended to neglect agency (the voices of the patients), presenting findings which often imply a single cultural meaning attributed to disease by all members of the society under study (Viney and Bousfield 1991) and research participants have often felt misrepresented in the findings. For this reason, we have been encouraged to use methods that are more considerate of the voices of our research participants (Viney 1988). The narrative analysis approach may be a good way of investigating the multivocalic nature of cultural models of illness. Researchers (Viney and Bousfield 1991) have successfully applied narrative analysis to AIDS research in Australia and their work has been used as a model for this study.

6.1.1 Data collection

A total of thirty Nepali texts were collected for the narrative study. This included twelve texts that I collected personally. Fifteen texts came from a book titled *Ajhai Dherai Banchnu Chha* 'Still Much Time Remains for Rescue', recently published by Panos South Asia (1999).[1] The final three texts were taken from a book titled *Maiti Phakreka Cheliharu* 'Girl's Returning Home', published by ABC Nepal (1998).[2] The English translations of these texts can be found in the appendices of this book.

In collecting twelve of the twelve narrative texts, I first needed to identify HIV positive persons willing to tell me their stories. This proved somewhat problematic as the social stigma makes having HIV and AIDS something that many keep very private and are unwilling to talk about openly. I spoke with many doctors who were actively involved in treating HIV positive persons and asked if they could provide me with contacts. They told me that because of doctor-patient confidence they could not introduce me to their patients, but they could give their patients my card and ask them to contact me privately if they were willing. Although I assured them complete anonymity, I didn't receive a single call from any of these patients. This fact in itself confirmed my growing suspicion that AIDS is a highly stigmatized disease in Nepal.

Next, I began visiting several of the NGOs working with HIV and AIDS infected people in Nepal in order to build relationships with people with AIDS (PWAs). It is principally from three of these NGOs that I found willing participants to tell me their stories. The first NGO is Prerana,[3] a Nepali organization founded recently as a support group for those living with HIV and AIDS. The second NGO is the Freedom Center, a drug rehabilitation center. Both of these organizational names occur frequently throughout the narratives. The third NGO is a rehabilitation home for former prostitutes.

After obtaining permission for the interview, we moved to a private room where we proceeded with the interview. I found that the best way to get a natural narrative was to simply ask, *"Ke bhayo"* 'What happened'? As will be seen, this resulted in narratives of various lengths focusing on the participant's personal HIV experience. The interviewing format followed was basically that introduced by Bernard (1995).

After the completion of the story, I often followed up with questions designed to probe further for the meanings the interviewee associated with HIV and AIDS. This unstructured interview format (Bernard 1995) was based primarily on parts of the narrative that were of particular interest to me. I also then conducted a short, structured interview eliciting responses for Kleinman's (1980) explanatory model of illness. This included (1) the symptoms which characterize the illness, (2) what is believed to cause the illness,

---

[1]This book is a collection of stories from HIV positive people about their life experiences.

[2]This book is principally a collection of stories from women trafficked to India for prostitution. Three of these women were infected with AIDS and talk about their experience in the midst of their wider discourse.

[3]In Nepali *prerana* means 'inspiration.'

(3) the recommended treatment, (4) the way the illness is perceived to work (pathophysiology), and (5) the prognosis. All interviews were conducted in Nepali, although many urban participants interspersed English with Nepali in their stories. The interviews were tape recorded (with permission) and then transcribed into a computer database called Shoebox 4.0 (SIL 1998) for later data analysis. The names of all the villages and their participants were changed for the sake of the participants' privacy and their protection.

The basic justification for using narrative analysis to understand social meaning is that narratives are a linguistic device by which both speakers and listeners construct meaning (Ozgood 1952) and recapitulate experience (Labov 1972). Narratives can, therefore, be analyzed to derive the speaker's understanding of the concept of AIDS. The narratives can then be compared for salient features shared with other research participants in order to arrive at some common meanings (cultural models). For further elaboration on the narrative analysis technique, consult Cortazzi (1993), Riessman (1993), and Viney and Bousfield (1991).

As will be seen shortly, at Prerana, every narrative revolved around drugs, in one way or another, as the personal cause of AIDS. As would be expected, this was also the case at Freedom Center since it is a drug rehabilitation center. Many of the narratives collected from the other sources also revolve around this theme. The fact that I could only get people from populations already considered stigmatized by the society, and the fact that almost all storytellers associated the cause of AIDS more readily with drugs (less stigmatized in Nepal) than sex, further confirmed my suspicions about the cultural model of AIDS as a "bad persons" disease.

6.1.2 Data analysis

Data analysis of the narratives has been conducted using the model introduced by Mishler (1986) and outlined by Viney and Bousfield (1991). In this model, narratives share the following common structural features that must be identified in the text:

- orientation—the involved characters, the setting, and the context are all identified

- abstract—usually a brief summary of the narrative

- complicating action—an elaboration of the story that also includes secondary narratives (stories begun but not finished).

- evaluation—the emphasis or the main point of the story

- coda—something that brings the narrator and listeners back to the present

Once these features of the text have been identified, the text is then thoroughly read for themes and condensed into a "core" narrative. The core narrative is the "essential meaning of the story in terms of its informational content, its interpersonal impact and the language in which it has been told" (Viney and Bousfield 1991:759). For my purposes, the "essential meaning" of the texts is arrived at by identifying "major themes" as proposed by Spradley (1972). The text is read for repeating themes that occur over and over again (either in exact or slightly different forms). The core narrative can then be used to suggest a hypothesis concerning the personal meanings of AIDS given by the research participants. Comparing the "core idea units" of all research participants then allows us to discover the salient features that are shared by all of them.

This was the basic model followed in analysis of the various texts. Common themes did emerge as well as various personal themes. Again, the strength in this approach is that it allows us to get at both the denotative and connotative aspects of culture, the denotative being the shared, referential attributes associated with HIV and AIDS, and the connotative being the aspects unique to each individual's personal illness history.

6.1.3 The sites

The first ten narratives I collected were recorded in the Kathmandu valley. Kathmandu, the capital city of Nepal, is a large urban center with many problems common to other large developing-world cities. With a population of nearly one and a half million in the valley, pollution and overpopulation are major problems. Immigration, largely from the rural areas of people in search of employment, has stretched the already insufficient infrastructure. It should be noted that although these narratives were collected in Kathmandu, many of the storytellers identify themselves with their father's ancestral village somewhere else in rural Nepal. Most, however, have spent the better part of their lives in Kathmandu. Kathmandu also has a growing problem with drug use among the young in the middle and upper classes, as many of the narratives will reflect.

As mentioned previously, six of the stories that I collected in the city were gathered from an organization called Prerana. Prerana, located in the Dilli Bazar section of Kathmandu, provides a drop-in style atmosphere for those living with HIV and AIDS. Workshops about various AIDS related topics are held almost daily and Prerana also sponsors educational outreaches and an AIDS hotline. Three of the narratives were gathered at a drug rehabilitation center in the Lagenkhel section of Kathmandu, and the final narrative from Kathmandu was collected at a rehabilitation center, for FSWs, just outside the ring road that encircles the city.

The final two texts that I collected personally were given by HIV positive patients at Amp Pipal Hospital in Gorkha District. Amp Pipal Hospital is a fifty-bed hospital administered by the United Mission to Nepal. Amp Pipal is a small village, of about five hundred, situated at about five thousand feet in the shadow of the Himalaya mountains. This hospital is located eighty miles west of Kathmandu and is twelve miles from the nearest road. It serves a catchment population of five hundred thousand, from villages as far away as a ten-day walk. There are hundreds of small villages with populations around two hundred within a day's walk of Amp Pipal.

As mentioned previously, the remainder of the narratives were gathered from published literature. There is no way to know of the locality from which these storytellers originated.

6.2 The findings

6.2.1 The Nepali narrative structure

Although there were significant differences between the content of the narratives, there was a striking amount of similarity in the structure of the various narratives. This would imply a general Nepali narrative structure. Although the order in which narrators presented the different elements (noted below) differed from text to text, these basic structural elements were common to all:

Discussion of family background
AIDS Narrative
Family/societal response
Conclusion

Most storytellers began their narratives by describing their family backgrounds. It was this introduction that set the stage for a discussion of how they came to be HIV infected. It is no surprise, given the importance of family in Nepali society, that each story began by situating the narrator within the larger social context of the family.

Next, the story focused on how the person became HIV infected. Here there were notable differences between the narratives of men and women and between urban and rural dwellers. Various gender specific and geographically specific schemata seemed to emerge from this analysis. These differences will be addressed shortly.

Almost all storytellers spent a significant time talking about the response of their families, as well as the wider society, to their condition. Some families were supportive while most were not. The narratives express fear of hatred and contempt on the part of the wider society. This feature demonstrates that the elements of fear, blame and hate (major components of the wider cultural model spoken of earlier) are embedded elements in the cultural models of PWAs as well.

There was a notable difference between the lengths of the narratives of the city dwellers as compared to rural dwellers. City stories tended to be much longer. For instance, the narrative of a city girl with AIDS (Prabita) is ninety-three pages long while the narrative story of a village man (Hari) is only ten sentences long.[4] I often found that I could simply ask city dwellers, "What happened?," and it would most often result in several minutes of text, which I would then follow up with various questions that had come to mind during the telling of their story. Although the length of city dwellers' stories varied as well, they tended to generally be much longer than the rural dwellers. City dwellers seemed to have much more experience with this type of personal story telling. Rural dwellers, however, would usually summarize their story in less than two minutes requiring much elicitation of specifics following their story. It would be interesting to study further the main influences of this phenomenon.

Finally, an interesting feature of a majority of the stories is that narrators seemed to try to avoid mentioning AIDS directly, and preferred the use of euphemisms for other culturally taboo topics, such as sex and prostitution. Rather than mentioning the name "AIDS" directly, many talked about 'being made sick' (Maya), 'coming to this situation' (Rageena), 'being ensnared' (Hari), 'getting such type of disease' (Akash), 'getting this dreaded disease' (Sarina), or becoming 'positive' (Thuli).[5] Narrators also avoided talking directly about having sex with prostitutes. They spoke euphemistically of 'walking in mischievous deeds' (Hari) with the girls of Bombay, 'becoming ensnared in bad places' (Hari), 'walking with the girls' (Fulmaya), and 'walking in roughness' (Shoba). Prostitutes were often referred to as 'that sort of girl' (Rajan) and their occupation as 'that kind of work' (Sita).

As has been mentioned previously, it is not considered proper to discuss sexual issues in public in Nepal, therefore the preference for euphemistic language (as it refers to sex) is understandable. It is also noteworthy that drug use does not appear to have the same stigmatization as sex. This is not to say that euphemistic language was not used at all for drug use. Often people referred to "bad deeds" which seemed to be a category inclusive of both drug use, and sex outside of marriage. Much less euphemistic language was used to describe involvement with drugs than sex, however. There seems to be more stigmatization attached to sex outside of marriage than to drug use and more compassion shown toward drug users than to those branded as *randi*. This will be addressed further in this chapter.

---

[4]All names have been changed to protect the privacy of the narrators.

[5]It should be noted that those in the city used "AIDS" or "HIV" more often than those in the village. Usually, however, even among city dwellers, there was still a strong preference to use a euphemism instead. Several of the texts avoid using these terms altogether (Sarina, Maya, Rajina) and many used these terms sparingly, usually only after it was first mentioned by the interviewer. Even those who opened their conversations talking about "AIDS" used many euphemisms to describe the disease, sex, drug-use and prostitution throughout the rest of the text.

6.2.2 Common themes and cultural schemata

Various common themes emerged from the analysis of the narratives. Many of the general themes noted in the rural cognitive study were also obvious in the narratives. Besides these similarities, however, differences were also noted between the narratives of city folk and rural folk. And even within the city sub-grouping, there were differences between the narratives of men and women. This section examines the general themes and schemata evident in all narratives, and also investigates the differences in discourse that emerge from the narratives of city versus rural folk and urban men versus women.

6.2.3 The general cultural model

6.2.3.1 Hate, fear, and blame

Perhaps the most obvious themes emerging from the narratives (both city and rural) is the concept of HIV and AIDS as a fatal, infectious, sexually transmitted disease. A majority of the narratives (76%) contain direct evidence that suggest the narrator understands AIDS to be a fatal disease. Although there was no direct evidence that the storytellers of the remaining 24 percent of narratives understand AIDS to be fatal, there were often comments made that would imply such an understanding. Eighty-three percent of the texts contained direct remarks concerning the infectious nature of AIDS. And 76 percent of the texts contained some sort of reference to an understanding of AIDS as a sexually transmitted disease. These key elements, identified as elements of an emerging cultural model of HIV and AIDS in the village (chapter five), are important elements of the cultural models expressed in the narratives of PWAs as well.

Most narratives then focused on the response of the family and the wider society to PWAs. While some families showed compassion, most showed disdain and the narratives were clear that HIV and AIDS is a stigmatized disease in Nepal; it is one in which the sufferers are blamed for their own condition and hated. Blame and hate are two major elements of the wider cultural model of HIV and AIDS and they have been incorporated as major elements in the cultural models of PWAs as well. Seventy-six percent of the texts contained references regarding the hate shown (or that would be expected to be shown) toward those who have HIV and AIDS by either their own families and/or the wider society. Twenty-four percent of the text-givers had not told their own families about their disease due to fear of their reactions. And another 14 percent had not told other members of the wider society for the same reasons.

One narrator, Prabita, talked about her family's negative response:

> We (Prabita, her husband, and her son) have been thrown out of the home and greatly despised *(hela)*. We have to live in a small room. We live there hiding our bodies, we have even found it

difficult to find enough food... I have seen many who have HIV
that have double problems. If they remain quiet, not telling their
family that they have the disease, then they worry about transferring the disease to another member of the household. But if
they tell, they will be kicked out of their home with a vigorous
hatred at a time when they need a good diet,[6] counseling, love,
care, acceptance, and sympathy.

Another, Jyoti,[7] responded, "My family has pretty much disowned me. My
older brother who is now in America has said that he will not even look at my
face ever again. No one ever comes to see me, and why should they really?
After all, because of my reckless ways, I have brought shame to all of them."

Rajan, another narrator, gave the reason she feared telling her own family: "I have not told my family that I have AIDS and I don't think they know.
If they find out I have AIDS they will detest me even more."

One woman, Sarina, who had been tricked into prostitution, expressed
an expectation of societal hate. She said, "Don't put my name or picture in
the book. How will I live if the people who have never gone beyond the
imagination of only one wife and husband, knew that I have returned (from
India) lying daily with eight to ten men?"[8]

And another, Saritya, replied, "All of us were in fear of what others
would say—what the society would say. I too remained silent to protect
my parents...and since I am HIV positive I have to accept that I shall be
discriminated against and stigmatized until I die. The society does not care
about these infected people."

Likewise, one narrator, Sali, claimed that when the doctors discovered
she was positive, they even refused to dress her wounds. And another,
Rama, claimed that the doctors even refused to touch her when they learned
she had AIDS. It is not difficult to see that the concepts of hate and blame
run deep in the minds and in the narratives of PWAs in Nepal.

6.2.3.2 *Worry and health*

Another common theme emerging from both the city and the rural
narratives is the idea that worry can contribute to sickness. Thirty-eight

[6]This idea of a good diet (and the embedded food schema) will be discussed at
length later in this chapter.

[7]Interestingly, this girl feels a large sense of personal responsibility for her condition (and the shame it has brought to her family) even though she was duped by
her husband, a drug user. This schema of female responsibility and male irresponsibility will be addressed shortly.

[8]The Nepali magazine Janmanch had run a story (including name and picture)
of a Nepali woman with AIDS. She was, subsequently, treated horribly as is documented in Red Light Traffic (ABC Nepal 1996:56–63). This story became well
known among PWAs in Nepal.

percent of the narratives included this discourse. For instance, Jyoti, a city girl, commented, "I constantly think of my uncles, aunts and grandparents, brothers; and cry a lot, even though I've been told not to worry so much because I'll become weaker and sicker, so I try to hold myself together."

Likewise, Laxmi, another young city girl, claimed that her mother-in-law became "so anxious" over her son's condition (HIV positive) "that she herself became sick." Another young city man, Indra, responding to his condition replied, "The thing that should not have happened has already happened. Therefore, there is now no advantage to worrying about it. Worry will only harm rather than lead to health."

An older male PWA in the rural area, Hari, told me, "If you are doubtful in your heart (worry) then the disease can catch you. If you aren't doubtful, then it won't catch you. Sickness is a thing caused by psychological attitude; the same is the case with HIV as well."

6.2.3.3 Chhichhi durdur

Associated with an understanding of the fatal and transmissible nature of AIDS among some of the storytellers was an idea of separation of a PWA from other members of society. This concept was present in the narratives of both urban and village dwellers. Twenty-eight percent of the narratives acknowledge the practice of separation of those with AIDS, an idea akin to the concept of *chhichhi durdur* 'separation' introduced in chapter five. Again, in traditional society, because a disease is considered *saruwa* 'contagious', separation of the infected person is expected in order to prevent further spread.

6.2.3.4 Randi

Given the strong association between AIDS and sexual transmission (76%), and therefore, prostitution, it is not a surprise to see that many associate AIDS with one who is *randi* 'promiscuous'. Although not using the term verbatim, 30 percent associate AIDS with bad sexual practices. This concept was present in both the rural and urban narratives. Rajan told the story of meeting a girl, falling in love, having sex with her, and only later discovering that she was "that kind of girl" (retired prostitute from Bombay). And Rama, a young girl sexually abused and impregnated by her boss, commented, "Even though she (the boss's wife) was a woman, she found fault in me, a woman. I'm sure she knew that I wasn't that kind of girl (sexually promiscuous), but naturally she was not going to blame her own husband."

Likewise, Asha, a young girl kidnapped by a family friend and forced to become the wife of this former drug user, worked hard to assure us that although he took her away to his home; she wasn't involved with him sexually.

> One day he took me forcibly to his place. He didn't let me go home
> for two days so I had to stay with him; not that he did anything
> bad to me. When I finally managed to go home, my family thought
> I had eloped with him. My mother explained that it would now be
> better in fact if I remained with him since I was an unmarried girl
> and had spent two days with him already. I thought about it too
> and decided that it was the best situation and went back to him.
> But I did not get involved with him in any sexual way.

Asha worked hard to convince us that she is not "that kind of girl" even though it is clear that she believed (along with her family) that the society would brand her *randi* after the experience that she had. And since she was *randi*, she would most likely be *ghrinaa* 'disdained'. And a "ruined" wife (Prabita) tells of the "shame" that Nepalis feel in talking about condoms. She commented that "many people feel shame (*laj manne*) when they talk about condoms, the process of using one, and even when they just get sight of it."

Why is it that people feel shame in such situations? It seems clear that this "shame" is a product of the application of the *randi* schema. In Nepal, only one who is *randi* would dare talk openly of these things. And of course a *randi* person is to be despised, as Janaki suggested, "I heard that you could get it (AIDS) simply by wearing the clothes of an infected person. I used to believe that one should detest such people. And now I am like that. I wonder what evil things I did.

Janaki's narrative not only confirms the idea that anyone who is *randi* (due to association with AIDS) should be despised; it also demonstrates the application of schemas introduced in chapter five, of (1) *saruwa* 'disease spread by clothing' and (2) *karma* 'result of evil deeds in the last life'.

In each of the examples given above it seems that the *randi* schema is implied. As suggested in chapter five, one (usually a female) who is sexually promiscuous is considered *randi* and must be treated with contempt by the community as a type of social punishment for bad deeds.

6.2.4 City-specific narratives

Besides sharing elements of the general cultural model (described in section 6.2.3) with the rural narratives, the city narratives also demonstrated themes and schemata that set them apart from the rural narratives.

6.2.4.1 A drug-related disease

Not only was AIDS identified as a sexually transmitted disease by many, but also a large majority of the city narratives identify drugs as a possible mode of transmission. Seventy-eight percent of the texts identify drug use as a means of contracting AIDS. Most of the narratives of male city dwellers focused on this issue. As I have previously noted, I found the most receptivity to my research at the organization called Prerana (where the majority claim to have contracted AIDS via drug use) and at drug rehabilitation centers. Again, this reveals something about the stigmatized nature of HIV and AIDS in Nepal. Drug use seems to be a less stigmatized "sin" than extramarital sex.

6.2.4.2 *Karma*

Over half (67%) of the narratives expressed the concept of *karma* in one way or another. Consistent with the findings of the rural cognitive study, the concept of *karma* was either expressed as the "bad deeds" practiced in this life or as the "bad deeds" committed in the last life. And one city dweller provided an interesting dualistic explanation of how he contracted AIDS:

> According to our Buddhist religion, I got this disease because of my previous life (*pahile janam*). It is all because I might have committed some kind of sin (*paap sap*) that I don't know about. I'm not sure, this may be the cause. In order to have the drugs I had to use syringes. In my previous life I might have committed some bad act (*naramrai karma*) of sin and I think it is the consequence of the sins of the previous life that I am suffering now... I know it transmits by using injecting drugs and through sex... but infection (HIV) might also be the result of previous bad deeds. Therefore, having gotten this disease in this life, I must bear the consequences of the bad I did in the last life. In my previous life I must have done something and now I am bearing the consequences. I know, however, that it is really because of my injecting that I have become infected, but the other answer gives me peace of mind. I'm now infected, and there is no way out. Thinking that previously I might have done those bad kinds of things gives me self-satisfaction. (Gopal)

Seemingly related to the concept of *karma*, a large number (56%) of the city narratives focused much attention on doing good once one was diagnosed with AIDS. The major discourse went something like this: "I got AIDS by doing bad deeds, now with the time that is left, I should do good things for society." For instance one young man, Raju, made the following comment:

> I thought it over and decided that it would be better for me to spend the coming days doing good things rather than to remain a bad man (*naraamro maanche*) continuing to take drugs and ruining my own health... Whatever remains of my life I should spend working among those who take drugs advising them not to do so... In this way the coming generation may be saved from the disease.

It is this young man's conviction that doing good will equate to a 'good life' *raamro jiwan*. Others echoed these same sentiments. For instance, Sharad commented, "I had ambitions to go abroad, to make something of myself, but these plans have now been cancelled. But now, I hope to save the young generation, to counsel them, spread the word about AIDS, save others, this is my last aim."

Likewise, Bijay wanted to "do something constructive" and "spend the rest of (his) life as a clean and honest individual." He concluded, "I want to spend the rest of my life as virtuously as possible. I want my own people—my friends and family—as well as the society at large to say that even though he had been a bad person once, he did good work later."

And Sudha echoed a common sentiment:

> My brother has advised me to tell everyone slowly, but how can I do that? I now feel so sensitive that I only want to cry. I gather and hold on to my sons' toys and cry away. But now I think that it's time that I start doing social work to keep myself occupied. Surely there must be others like me out there. Probably in worse situations. I think I should try to help them so that I can help myself.

6.2.4.3 Positive attitude and a good diet

Closely related to the schema of worry and health mentioned earlier is the idea that maintaining good health requires a positive attitude and good diet. Ten of the city narratives (37%) included elements suggestive of this discourse. Many of the city texts discuss the importance of maintaining a positive attitude in order to preserve health. One young man, Gopal, states that the proper attitude and living happily in the present is the only treatment for AIDS available:

> The main treatment for it (AIDS) is to make one's heart happy, strong and have a positive attitude... One should not worry too much about the future, thinking "the disease has caught me, what will happen in my life, I will die soon," or so on. We should not worry about the future, rather we should live happily on this earth for as long as we have. Worrying about the future is not important, but what is important is for us to keep a positive attitude and live happily in the present. I think this is the only kind of treatment available. Because the more a person feels happy, they will get good things in this life. If a normal man also lives unhappily, he automatically gets disease.

One young HIV positive woman, Shoba, even told me, "There are many that have been finding their positive blood to be changed to negative after a long time. If one controls him or herself mentally (has a positive attitude) it can be so."

Combining the concepts of positive attitude and good diet, one young man commented,

> Thinking over my past, I now want to change tracks. I want to spend my life in a better way. I got married eight months ago. My family knows that I have HIV. When I myself found out, I did not panic. I have to accept this. It's not going to go away if I scream and shout. I will be better off if I maintain the proper mental attitude. I believe there will be a cure for it soon because this is a very old disease. I am convinced of this. And when the cure is found I will go to any spot in the world for treatment. This conviction has kept me alive so far. If a cure is not found soon, then I shall try to live as well as I can until my death. If I take care of myself and eat properly then I will probably live for another fifteen years or so. (Ashish)

And another young man, telling a similar story, highlighted the necessity of "eating well" when he stated,

> Well, I am told that there is no cure for AIDS, that no medicine exists, but the doctor told me that if I eat well, take care of my health, and stay free from drugs, then I may live for another fifteen or sixteen years. I am now 25 years old... The doctor showed me an athlete's photograph; he said that the man played football, even though he had been infected with AIDS eighteen years ago. But, you see, the athlete is a foreigner. He has money. But how long will I live? Maybe five or six years. You have seen my condition. I have no food. I live on the streets. (Ram)

As an interesting side note, there were a very few who talked about the possibility of a cure. Each that did, however, associated a cure with the West in one way or another: one with a foreign football player (mentioned above); one with the former American basketball great, Magic Johnson; and the third mentioned the expectation of a cure coming from elsewhere around the world. As noted in chapter five, AIDS in Nepal has been considered as a foreign disease, so these associations with the West are not surprising. It is also interesting to see the American cultural model of HIV and AIDS (e.g., AIDS as a chronic, manageable condition) beginning to have an influence upon the narratives of Nepali PWAs, and in the long run, perhaps upon the developing cultural model of HIV and AIDS in Nepal.

6.2.4.4 Gender specific cultural models

Perhaps the most interesting feature of the city narratives was the emphasis on different discourses that emerged between the narratives of males and females. It is very interesting that most city female discourses focused on the unfaithfulness of men while the male narratives focused on drugs. Among men there was a general desire to disassociate their contraction of the disease with sex. Even the discourses of those who admit uncertainty about whether they were infected through sex or drug use focused their attention on drug use. It seems there is less stigma (and more compassion) associated with drug use than sex.

Seventeen of the thirty narratives (57%) were given by females. These narratives, in one way or another, usually revolved around the woman having been deceived or mistreated by men. Of the female narratives, eight (47%) involved the story of unfaithful husbands but faithful wives, six stories (35%) revolved around a girl trafficking discourse, and three (18%) revolved around prostitution.

Within the "unfaithful men" grouping of texts, some interesting schemata emerged. The first of these is the Nepali expectation of (1) the unfaithfulness of men and (2) the faithfulness of women to their husbands (despite the men's unfaithfulness). After describing such unfaithful behavior among men, one woman, Rageena, adds that this type of a man is a coward:

> Our Hindu scriptures also don't talk much about a man's faithfulness to his wife while they speak much about the loyalty a woman is to show to her husband. Why do men always want to be like Krishna?[9] Why do men, seeking adventure and behaving as men, always dote on every young and beautiful girl every time their eyes see one, while at the same time they are unable to provide properly for their own wives and households? What an amazing tradition—using up a woman by having outraged her virginity and then leaving the useless part behind and seeking another. If they can't accept a woman for who she is (stay with one woman) for life then why can't they stop their burning passion? What a coward this type of man is. He can't introduce his wife to his own father, mother, friends or brothers, yet he can make an innocent girl, who desires to live a pure life, pregnant by giving her hollow promises. (Rageena)

The unfaithful husband schema was borne out in many of the female narratives. One woman comments on her husbands lamentable behavior:

> As for my husband, he had not changed his pampered ways. He made fun of me because I was from the village. He would say to me, "You are an ignorant country girl. Here, even in the alleys, you see lovely girls. There are lots of beautiful Nepali girls and they know how to make themselves attractive. And they fuss over me when I go to see them." Of course, that was when he had money to spend. When he didn't then he would come to me. Oh, what an ungrateful man he was. (Laxmi)

---

[9]The Hindu god Krishna is well known and admired (by men) for his sexual prowess and promiscuity.

Another spoke of a man's unfaithfulness to his own wife when she told of the man who seduced her and ultimately deceived her, selling her into prostitution:

> At that time I was sixteen years old. One day, he found me alone and said, "You are so beautiful, I want to marry you." At first I didn't believe him and I told him that I would not go with him because he was already married. So he took a vow (bit his finger) telling me not to worry about his wife. He said that he would rather die than to stay with her. He said, "I have divorced my wife, but don't tell Mahili (a mutual friend) about it." I promised him I would not tell anyone. Then, without telling Mahili, we went to Pokhara and he put sinder on my head (married me). (Sarina)

In a follow-up interview I asked one woman why Nepali women seemed to be so accepting of their husbands' infidelity. I was told, "What to do *(ke garne)?* That is just the way Nepali men are and it is our position in life to accept it."

There was much in the texts about the expectation of faithfulness of women (even when men are faithless). Even in the face of his unfaithfulness, one woman, Sudha, expressed her devotion to her husband. She said, "My husband got so sick that he had to be hospitalized. The blood test revealed that he had HIV. That was it! I was mad at him. I felt like divorcing him...of course, given my husband's illness, I couldn't leave him. After all, I have a woman's heart."

Laxmi, who knew that her husband "roamed around," "got drunk" and "gambled," spoke of receiving her mother's advice concerning her husband's behavior. "She (her mother) told me that woman is like the earth. She must bear every hardship, and that a husband is like a god. So, no matter how he treated me, I must respect him. Her words soothed me."

And one male PWA spoke of this "extreme devotion" of a Nepali wife toward her husband when he told of his wife's reaction to his condition:

> I'm on the right track these days. I feel trusted and loved. My wife has not had a blood test yet. I want to think that because she has not had a test that she is all right. We use condoms (when we have sex). Once or twice the condom has broken, so I don't know if my wife has been infected or not. On the other hand, my wife says that she too should contract AIDS. I have it and she doesn't. She tells me not to use a condom. I say, "No, just because I have it, you shouldn't get it." But she asks why should only she live? "You have it, I should too" she says... My wife has said "Infect me too. It's better if we both have it. If you die, what will I do all alone?" (Ashish)

Very closely related to these ideas of a man's unfaithfulness and a woman's faithfulness is the concept of "fate." Interestingly the concept of fate (outside of one brief mention of the idea by one male PWA) was limited to female narratives. Among the female narratives fate was a popular theme. Eight of the narrators (44%) devoted a significant amount of their narratives to the topic. For instance, Laxmi began her life story in terms of her fate:

> I was born in a small village in Syangia thirty-four years ago. Since I was born on the day of Aunsi (the 15th day of the Hindu lunar calendar), both of my parents were very sad. According to our Hindu tradition, it is very inauspicious to be born on Aunsi. And not just inauspicious, you know, but people say that a girl born on this day will also cause the early death of her husband. So people say that a girl born on Aunsi should marry a boy also born on this same day. My two brothers and one sister were born on normal days, but I, the youngest, was born on a very inauspicious day. So imagine how worried my parents must have been. And so I suppose that it has been my fate to have such a hard life.

Laxmi continued her story telling how her mother, commenting on Laxmi's unfaithful husband, suggested that it is a woman's fate to bear such hardships. She continued to explain how her husband left her to marry another, and how she was sent off to a foreign country to work and was enjoying it. But then she fell sick and discovered she was positive. She concluded, "Oh well, what can you do when you are not fated for happiness?" and "I suppose the evil committed by the husband has to be borne by the wife." Likewise, Jyoti, a promising athlete and scholar infected by her husband (who, unbeknownst to her, had been a drug addict before their marriage), concluded, "I attended class in Kathmandu and always did very well in school. I even won many essay contests and a quiz competition. I was also very good in sports and won several awards. But you know, all these achievements mean nothing if your fate dictates otherwise."

And Sarita, having just told her sad story of being married off to a drug user, thrown out of the house, and yelled at by her drug-using husband for requesting him to use a condom, concluded, "And so now too, I have been infected. I guess such is life. You never know where it will lead." So, it seems clear that two schemata are at play here—a Nepali man is expected to be faithless and a Nepali wife is expected to be faithful. And within the faithful Nepali wife schema is a sub-schema of fate.[10]

The narratives of city men focused mainly on drug use. Nine of the eleven (82%) AIDS discourses in the city male narratives revolved around telling

---

[10]These findings lead one to wonder if perhaps these same schemata underlie the traditional South Asian practice of Sathi (the custom of a widow burning herself to death on her husband's funeral pyre).

the story of having gotten AIDS through drug use.[11] Subsumed within this discourse was also the discourse of having first fallen under the influence of "bad people." All (100%) of the male drug related narratives include this sub-plot to their story. For instance, several of the men made the following claims:

> Because of the kind of people I met, I also started to smoke and drink, and this led me to try anything and everything...later, because of bad company I contracted AIDS. (Ram)

> I studied up to class nine in my village, but dropped out because I was hanging out with the wrong crowd. (Ashish)

> As to how or why one gets into drugs...you do not succumb to drugs right away, no, not quite so quickly and easily. What happens in the beginning, you see,...well, you are about sixteen or seventeen years old, and your behavior, attitude, has been steadily worsening. At home, you begin to lie; skip school. You cheat, you steal—and generally begin to act dishonestly. You also associate with a certain kind of people, the disreputable kind, that is. (Bijay)

Others mentioned "hanging out with the wrong crowd" (Sunil), being around "bad people" (Raju) and having "bad friends" (Gopal).

Another very interesting sub-plot to the drug-use narratives is that most of these men admit being sexually active, but they prefer to believe (or prefer us to believe) that they contracted AIDS through drug use:

> Turns out I had AIDS. My main guess is that I got it at the center (drug rehab center). It was not very strict there. We all lived there like a big family. We used to share blades to shave. We shared needles while injecting tidigesic (a type of drug). I have not had very many sexual relationships, but I did indulge in it occasionally. However, I don't think I was HIV positive before I entered the treatment center. (Ashish)

> I did not get AIDS from sexual contact because I had sex perhaps three or four times with one woman only. And she was not that kind of a girl *(randi)*. (Ram)

> I have not had many sexual relations. I had relations with two or three girlfriends when I was in school in India. When I came back to Kathmandu, I visited prostitutes three or four times. I used condoms. This happened about five or six years ago. And in those days,

---

[11]Only two of the male city narratives focus on the use of prostitutes as the main cause of their condition. And one of these (Rajan) still includes a large discourse on drug use in which it seems he tries to disassociate his condition with sex and focuses on drugs.

> I had never heard of HIV and AIDS. It wasn't publicized very much
> either. Since I was more into drugs than prostitutes, I suspect I got
> HIV because of drugs and not sex. One or two of those in my circle
> (drug sharing) have also contracted AIDS. (Bijay)

Because there is a preference to think one became infected via drugs
rather than extramarital sex, it is my contention that a greater stigma is
attached to extramarital sex in Nepal than to drug use. There is no doubt
that drug users are stigmatized, but more sympathy seems to be shown by
the society toward drug users than those who are branded as *randi*. Aschich,
who had been *randi*, communicated to his family that it was only through
drug use that he had AIDS:

> When my family found out I had HIV, they told me not to do
> drugs anymore but to take care of myself. They gave me a lot
> of love and care. I can't say the same of the environment out-
> side of my home. Those who do not understand drugs take a
> negative position, but those who are aware of the destruction
> caused by drugs tend to be more sympathetic. They are not so
> quick to judge.

Following up on this thought, I asked one Nepali friend why he feels
more sympathy is shown toward those who have contracted AIDS via drug
use versus those who have contracted it through sexual transmission. He
replied,

> It is very understandable. No one is willing to admit he has had sex
> with a hooker. It is about prestige in our society. If you say, "Okay,
> I had sex with a hooker and got AIDS," you will be looked down
> upon by the society. Even though drug users are also looked down
> upon in our society, more prestige is lost if you are caught having
> used hookers."

> It's like this, most people use drugs because of some kind of
> problem they have within the family. We would probably think,
> "Okay, that poor fellow has some kind of problem with their
> family. His parents might be the cause of his taking drugs." Most
> people would blame his parents saying, "Okay, because of you
> guys, he went down the wrong path and started using drugs." So
> we would show a bit of compassion toward that fellow. These
> days most people who don't have a good family or good parents
> are into drugs.

> But, for the one who went to a hooker and had sex with her has
> created his own problem. No sympathy is due here. It is their own
> fault. Nobody else made him do it.

> Also we don't talk about sex in public in Nepal. How could we talk
> about having sex with a hooker? It would be big trouble.[12] We fear
> talking about these things. We would be secluded from our society
> if we were discovered doing these things.

It should also be noted that one female also deferred to the drug use narrative. Sali, even though a self-professed prostitute, also disassociates her condition from sexual transmission, claiming that "I suppose that (drug use) is how I contracted AIDS."

6.2.5 Village-specific narratives

I was only able to collect two narratives of HIV positive persons from the village area.[13] Given this small number, any conclusions drawn from these narratives must be considered tentative. Having said this, however, conclusions regarding a rural cultural model can be checked against the findings of the cognitive study conducted in the rural area (chapter 5) and such a comparison should strengthen the support of any such conclusions. It was also impossible to contrast the narratives of men and women in the rural location, as both storytellers were male.

As has previously been noted, the narratives collected in the rural area were generally shorter than those collected in the city. The format of the interviews also differed as the rural storytellers did not seem as adept at providing long life histories as the urban dwellers had been. Therefore, much of the rural interviews were in question-answer format. The interviews did provide some useful data, however. Besides exhibiting many of the features of the general cultural model described above, the rural narratives also displayed characteristics unique to themselves.

---

[12]My informant told me that he has never heard anyone talk publicly about sex with a prostitute. He now lives in America so he was more open to discussing the topic with me. It was also interesting, however, that he insinuates that it is the conservative nature of Nepali society that causes men to use prostitutes. According to him, Nepali boys cannot have sex with their girlfriends because of the stigma for the girls if they do. For instance, if a girl has sex with her boyfriend and then they break up, she may never find a spouse because she has lost her virginity. As a result, boys are forced to go to prostitutes for sex. I got the sense that the blame (for men going to prostitutes) must fall on the girlfriends, who are abstaining due to the conservative nature of Nepali society. His opinion seems to reflect an attitude that I saw among many men in Nepal; sex is required for a young man. In response to my question as to how many of his close friends he would suspect have visited prostitutes, he suggested that 60% had.

[13]Although there were several new HIV positive diagnoses made during my stay in Amp Pipal, it was very difficult to find willing participants to tell me their stories. Again, I suggest that the strong stigma associated with HIV and AIDS in the urban areas is also a common feature in the rural areas as well.

6.2.5.1 AIDS via eating

Both of the village narratives display an idea similar to the urban men's attempt to disassociate themselves with AIDS through sexual transfer. In the village case, however, rather than defaulting to drug use, they default to the more traditional eating schema. For instance, although the first narrator (Hari) expresses understanding of how AIDS is transferred (through "mischievous deeds"[14]), and he has contracted AIDS, he claimed not to have been involved in such things. He explains, "I might have got it (AIDS) while I was eating, through sharing food with someone. I don't know for sure. People won't tell when they have it. Not telling, we eat together. So while we are eating together (sharing one plate), if they had blood coming from somewhere, perhaps it ultimately transferred to me."

And when asked why he didn't tell his family of his condition he said, "I plan to live alone by myself. I will prepare my food separately. I don't want to put my parents or brothers at risk." Likewise, although the second storyteller (Ramesh) readily admitted having visited brothels while living in India, in response to the question "How do you think you got AIDS?," he replied, "I used to drink and smoke." Cigarettes and liquor are both "eaten" in the Nepali language rather than smoked and drunk as in English. "Eating" is a popular schema for anything put in the mouth. Just prior to the interview this narrator also admitted to me that he believed that a PWA could spread AIDS through breathing the same air and sitting together while eating with others. These same beliefs were identified through the rural cognitive study (chapter 5).

6.2.5.2 The sarnu nature of AIDS and weak blood

The second village narrative, given by Ramesh, displays several ideas about the causes of AIDS that were also consistent with the findings of the rural cognitive study (see narrative in full in chapter 10). When asked if he believed his condition (AIDS) might have first begun as a smaller disease, he replied, "First I had fever so I went to the Malaria Control Center and took ('ate') medicine." And when asked if he thought, therefore, that his AIDS condition had first started as that malarial fever, he replied, "Yes, I do." This idea of a disease changing from one kind to another (*sarnu*) was noted among rural dwellers (chapter 5).

Likewise, the second rural narrator expressed a belief that his susceptibility to AIDS had increased because he perceived himself to have weak

---

[14]He also says of a woman who died of AIDS at the hospital that "it was rumored that she used to live in Bombay." The use of "Bombay" like this in the rural area was a euphemistic way of talking about prostitution. Again, he reiterated that he was not involved in "that sort of thing."

blood. He said, "This is all because of my own weakness of blood in my body. After the blood in a person's body becomes weak *(sarirko kun kamjor bhaepachhi),* the disease will ensnare[15] you. This is a fact." Again, this idea of *kamjor* being a major factor in disease susceptibility was identified in chapter five.

6.2.6 An explanatory model of AIDS

As mentioned in the introduction, questions designed to elicit an explanatory model (Kleinman 1980) were asked following each of the thirteen interviews that I conducted. The explanatory model seeks to understand basic elements that people associate with certain illnesses. The basic elements of this model are (1) the signs and symptoms by which a particular illness is distinguished, (2) the assumed causes of the illness, (3) recommended treatments, (4) how the illness is believed to work inside the body (pathophysiology), and (5) expected prognosis.

6.2.6.1 Signs and symptoms of AIDS

There was a set of three symptoms that were said to be characteristic of AIDS when they occur together. These were (1) swollen glands, (2) diarrhea for more than one month, and (3) fever for more than one month. These were the most common symptoms associated with AIDS according to all those interviewed in both the urban and rural areas.

6.2.6.2 Causes of AIDS

As has been noted, drug use and prostitution were the two most commonly given causes of AIDS. Again, however, we see individual variation throughout the narrative texts with some attributing cause to bad *karma,* sharing food, or other more traditionally accepted causes for illness.

6.2.6.3 Treatments for AIDS

Although it is clear from the narratives that AIDS is understood to be fatal, the following treatments are believed to help one survive longer: (1) do not worry (as worry can accelerate the progression of illness), (2) maintain a positive attitude, and (3) maintain a healthy diet. This is one element of the earlier cultural model that has shifted radically in recent years as will be illustrated at the end of this chapter.

---

[15]The title of this book was prompted by the Nepali word, phansu 'ensnare', used in this narrative.

6.2.6.4 *Pathophysiology of AIDS*

Self-reported knowledge of how AIDS is believed to affect the body showed great differences between rural and urban dwellers. The rural PWAs expressed very little knowledge concerning this issue while the urban PWAs gave descriptions very similar to the Western biomedical model. The great amount of knowledge expressed by city PWAs is probably due to the extensive education and counseling services provided by Prerana.

6.2.6.5 *Prognosis*

Most suggested that AIDS is a 'final' *antim* disease, meaning that it will end in death. It seemed to be well understood by all that one who had AIDS is *khattam* 'finished'. Three PWAs (all city dwellers), however, expressed hope, suggesting that no cure for AIDS currently exists but a cure may be just around the corner. And another (also a city dweller) suggested that some PWAs' conditions (their blood) had changed from HIV positive to HIV negative through positive thinking. Interestingly, three of these four cases seemed to tie a possible cure to a wider Nepali discourse of Western *bikaas* 'development'. Again, this is an element of the earlier cultural model that has undergone radical transformation due to the introduction of ART into Nepal as I will illustrate shortly.

6.2.7 Recent narratives

In 2012 I collected eight narratives of HIV positive persons (six female and two male) attending the Tansen Mission Hospital, Palpa District, in order to compare themes with the narratives collected ten years previously. My goal was to compare the cultural model expressed in 2002 to the newer cultural model, based on the experience of PLWAs in the ensuing decade. Also, I sat in on two pre-test counseling sessions (both female) that allowed me to assess current trends in HIV and AIDS. The findings of these narrative interviews are given below.

The first obvious feature is that the composition of the narratives reflects the wider epidemiological reality that wives of migrant laborers (particularly to India) now make up the biggest number of HIV sufferers; all six of the women giving narratives reported that their husbands had worked in India, as did one of the males. The second male didn't mention where he contracted HIV. One of the pre-test counseling seekers had also worked in India.

Three of the narratives explicitly confirm the belief (either on the part of the narrative giver prior to receiving counseling or on the part of their village neighbors) that HIV is fatal, while two other implicitly imply the same. One woman commented, "When I first got the disease I didn't think that there was any treatment and I thought that I would probably not live more than ten years. I felt sorrow, like I will surely die... Even today many of my villagers consider that AIDS is fatal and that there is no treatment available."

And mainly on this basis, five of the narrative givers spoke of their fear, or fear that others had when first learning of their positive status. One woman commented, "Of course I had fear. After getting this kind of disease who wouldn't fear? Because I lacked knowledge about treatment, when I first heard my test results, I had great fear of dying."

Likewise, five others mentioned the fear or the actual experience of being 'despised' *ghrinaa* or 'hated' *hela* by their family and neighbors (who retain the belief that AIDS is fatal). For example one women replied, "My own mother treated me with contempt (*hela*) when I first told her" and another said she "hid herself away" for twelve years in fear of what others would do or say. And one of the men mentioned, "When I told my family they feared greatly. They despised me and said, "Leave him in the forest to die." People believed that HIV positive persons should be killed.

Another responded that she expected villagers to react with "violence" and "hatred" if she told them of her status. And yet another would not tell her family because of fear of their expected response, stating that "if the family knew about it they would expel me from the house." For the same reason many others report that they did not disclose their status at first (and some have still not done so).

Seven of the eight narratives use language that confirms that the eating schema is still used strongly in association with HIV and AIDS. Most referred directly to "eating medicine" and the need to "eat good foods." Several confirmed the wider village narrative, of the belief that HIV is spread "by eating together." And one of the women combined the hatred and eating schemas when she commented, "I was despised by my family excessively. They wouldn't eat what I touched, they would not eat what I cooked and they wouldn't even let me wash the dishes."

Another combined the beliefs that AIDS is fatal and is transmitted by what one eats (elements of the old cultural model) with the new element of hope (which will be addressed shortly) when she proclaimed "If we don't eat [ART] we die." And in an interesting use of the eating schema one of the women getting pre-test counseling expressed shock at the thought of her husband potentially having been unfaithful (she knew that she hadn't been), commenting, "but he speaks so deliciously to me."[16]

All eight narratives confirm that many people still associate HIV with the traditional illness beliefs identified in chapter four, such as eating together,

---

[16]This idiom might serve well as a potential prevention slogan as will be discussed in the following chapter.

living together, the possibility of HIV being spread by mosquito or lice, HIV as the result of "spoiled planets," "ghosts," "spirits," "witchcraft," or "bad works," and the belief that a person with HIV should be separated from all others (i.e., "expelled from the house"). In regard to treatment, the wearing of amulets and the use of herbal medicines is mentioned by several, and all eight mentioned that treatment is still sought either from the astrologer or the shaman (*lama, dhaami,* and *jhaankri* were named by several), "requiring the killing of roosters or a goat." So, it is evident that many of the elements identified ten years prior are still part of the wider cultural model of HIV and AIDS in Nepal.

The separation schema also seems prominent (although less so than formerly). Three talked explicitly about the fear of being thrown out, kicked out, or removed from the home, and two others inferred the same. The traditional belief that HIV can be spread via "living together" (noted previously) implies that those with the disease should be separated. One woman mentioned that "the villagers feel it is better for us to live apart from them." Another woman speaks of voluntarily separating herself and one daughter (also HIV positive) from her second (non-HIV positive) daughter and the rest of the family, feeling that this action protected others. She even confesses to having two sets of nail clippers—one for herself and her positive daughter and the second for the other daughter, thus protecting her.

Probably the most noticeable change between the early narratives and these later narratives is the addition of hope associated with ART. The once fatal HIV is no longer viewed as such by all of these narrative givers. All eight speak of the future with hope. Hope for good health and a long future. One woman, now in her seventeenth year of ART states her belief that "I can now live confidently, pretty strongly, for twenty to twenty-five years." Another (the same one who felt she would die when she first got the news, or certainly not live beyond ten years) now expresses hope confessing, "Others believed that I would die from the disease, that there is no treatment or medicine, but I did not listen to them in this regard."

And another comments on her experience among an HIV support group, "Seeing all of these other people living I now feel as if I will live as well." Many mention the long-term hope of seeing their children grow, being married and holding their grandchildren. One of the male narrative givers is the first HIV positive person in Palpa District to get married and another "can imagine the day when the HIV positive children of Palpa will someday marry each other." They speak of being healthy and of being able to remain productive members of their society into the indefinite future. It seems that, at least for these HIV positive persons, their personal schema has shifted from dying of AIDS to living with HIV.

To one who has studied HIV and AIDS in Nepal for well over a decade, the transition that I am seeing take place between resident elements of the cultural model is shocking (and encouraging!). Although four of the participants tell directly of families and neighbors who still despise and hate them, two of the storytellers report facing no such discrimination in their own particular situations and two others tell of the change from "hatred" to "love" on the part of their families, friends, and neighbors since HIV and AIDS education has reached their villages and been applied. The one who spoke of once "hiding herself away for twelve years" because of her fear of neighbors at the time, confesses after living with HIV for nineteen years, "Now I can tell openly. I have only hope and courage." The same one who once thought HIV a sure death sentence now confides, "All have to die someday after being born; at the end, HIV-infected and non-infected both die." Another whose own mother once 'despised' *ghrinaa* her because of HIV, but who has since been educated along with the village, now proclaims, "At first everyone thought I would die from the disease (as did I), but now they even tell others I am healthy and can even work!" And the man whose family once 'hated' *hela* him for the disease and left him in the forest to die now lives in a village that loves him; a village that has been transformed. In this village an educated resident once expressed the belief that an HIV positive person should be killed; now this resident (a university professor and campus chief) gives love.

There are a couple more interesting elements of these narratives I should address before bringing this chapter to a close. The first is that HIV or AIDS was only mentioned by name by one of the ten persons interviewed (8 narratives and two pre-test counseling sessions). Often they mentioned getting "this" disease or of others being afraid of "that" disease, but only one (the one who now works for an NGO that focuses on HIV and AIDS) mentioned either HIV or AIDS by name; this even after the counselor or I used the terms many times throughout the interviews. There still seems to be a strong stigma associated with HIV and AIDS (much revolving around its association with sex), even among this group. And when one man was asked how he contracted HIV he responded that maybe he had made a "mistake." When asked to elaborate on "mistake" he avoided talking about his sexual activities, commenting only that "it might be so—it did not come from flying (i.e., it didn't come from nowhere)." Although it is lessening, stigma, especially as it is related to sex, still seems to play a strong part in the cultural model of HIV and AIDS in Nepal.

Turning to the pre-test counseling sessions now, there were two interesting observations. The first is that both contained much teaching about the "facts" of HIV and AIDS, but the explanatory model used was exclusively the western war schema. For example, while explaining to the first woman in the pre-test counseling session what HIV does in the body, the counselor describes the disease in terms of war:

There is a microbe called HIV, but normally our body has immunity power (he uses English here), that fights the disease and kills
it...our immunity power and the virus have a fight.... And if the
virus called HIV wins over our immunity it kills us.... Our body's
ability to fight against the disease is weakened.... On the one hand
our body continues to increase the ability to fight the disease, on
the other hand it goes on killing it...over time the ability of our
body to fight the disease becomes weaker and weaker...and then
the disease catches (*samaatnu*—more of a military term) us.... Now
in such a condition, when that disease catches us, after winning, it
becomes serious. Our body becomes tired.... AIDS is not a disease
itself, it is the condition of being caught by the disease (HIV).

And in describing the treatments available to the same woman, the counselor says, "Until now the medicine to completely kill the microbe has not
yet come. But there is a kind of medicine that increases the body's ability
to fight against the disease in our body, to control the microbe, to keep it
from growing."

There are only two other narratives that contain even a hint of the warfare schema. The first comes when, after completing the narrative, the
counselor asks the first woman if she knows what the disease does inside
the body, to which she answers, "It causes one's immunity power (she uses
the Sanskrit word *pratiraksha* which best translates as 'defense') to weaken."
In response he asks, "Do you mean that it causes the immune power that
fights the disease to weaken?," to which she answers in the affirmative.
I find it ironic that even the counselor has to ask for clarification on this
point because that schema is so infrequently used among villagers to talk
about illness. The only other occurrence of the warfare schema is found in
the second narrative, but here again the usage is initiated by the counselor
in the same context, educating the narrative giver about the disease post
narrative. Here he says, "HIV reduces the power of the body to fight against
the disease." It is clear that usage of the warfare schema is common among
HIV educators, but uncommon among rural HIV sufferers.

The second interesting feature was the form of education used. It followed the same patterns I have observed elsewhere; discussion of what
HIV is, what it does, followed by a list of how it is spread (e.g., sexual
contact, blood transfusion, injecting drug use and mother to child transmission). This mirrors the pattern (and the various materials) I have
observed across the country and around the world. What intrigues me
most is why the counselor, once he understood the specific context of
each narrative giver (the faithful housewife of a migrant laborer), which
was obvious through the interviews, often continued to talk about other non-relevant and stigma promoting vectors of transfer. And why he
chose to be so explicit with these obviously naïve women? For instance,

the first pre-test counseling patient was a shy young housewife.[17] It was obvious within a few minutes that we need not focus on anything but her sexual relationship with her husband (the only relevant vector for her—all others would be stigma enhancing), yet the counselor goes ahead, using the most direct and stigma-producing term for sexual contact *(yon sampark),* and tells her of the various ways sexual contact can happen (i.e., oral, anal, and vaginal, "men with men") and then moves on to talk about blood transfusion and injecting drug use; all of this in the context where the woman most likely has no ability to speak to her husband's sexual choices (e.g., demand he wear a condom) without having him brand her as *randi.* Transfer by blood transfusion is not an issue at this hospital (and no longer much of an issue elsewhere in Nepal) and she certainly didn't seem at risk for illicit injecting drug use. The only real concern for her, and within her control, is the possibility of mother to child transmission, which he addresses next. He then addresses the various misnomers about how HIV can spread, such as those already mentioned, and asks her if she understands; to which she sits silent, and he moves on to talk about HIV treatments. In the case of the second pre-test counseling session, another housewife, being told that "out of the husband comes semen and out of the wife comes a greasy substance," is advised that it is better to use a condom to protect against this and that the condom is "the best way to protect against this and other such diseases." Again, I am not anti-condom, but I doubt she really has much choice in the matter. And as I watched the interaction I could tell that she was visibly uncomfortable as the counselor talked directly and openly about these stigma-producing topics in her culture.

Besides the counselor, only four of the narrators (the two males, one female who works for an HIV and AIDS NGO, and one other woman) use the direct word for sex, while the others, if they talk about it at all, chose to use euphemistic language. It seems to me the prevention education needs a bit of cultural sensitivity adjustment in this area in order to be more effective.

And finally, perhaps one of the most personally interesting things that emerged from the collection of these new narratives, is that I heard a new folk-treatment mentioned, which I had never heard before. One woman mentioned that they had been told by their neighbors that "drinking an excessive amount of beer" would cure AIDS." In this case the HIV-positive husband "overdosed" and was hospitalized, but the reference to beer makes me wonder if this perceived "cure" might actually be a product of the phenomenon mentioned in chapters three and seven? Certainly speculation, but not without merit.

---

[17]This woman was sent for testing because she had a very small child (seven months) and if positive they wanted to protect her against potential mother to child transmission.

It is evident from the analysis of these new narratives that a shift in the cultural model is taking place. Many elements of the earlier model are still solidly embedded, but other key elements of the model are shifting. The most prominent change is that the idea of AIDS being fatal is slowly but steadily giving way to the inclusion of the newly embedded element of hope. This transition between models, while not likely yet universal across all of Nepal, is a strikingly positive adaptation for the individuals who are experiencing it. And certainly as the cultural model continues to shift further in this same encouraging direction with time, the element of fear (associated with fatality) that was so evident in the earlier model should lessen as well.

6.3 Chapter conclusions

In this chapter I first used thirty narratives of urban and rural-dwelling HIV positive persons to examine early emerging cultural models of HIV and AIDS among PWAs in Nepal. The results demonstrate that hate, fear and blame were (and still are) three major elements of a cultural model of HIV and AIDS among PWAs in Nepal. The narrative study also revealed a shared understanding of HIV and AIDS among PWAs as a fatal, infectious, and sexually transmitted disease. And a belief in the strong connection between worry and health was also a notable theme throughout the various PWA narratives.

Besides these shared elements of a cultural model among PWAs, however, we have noted differences between the narratives of urban males and females, and between urban and rural dwellers in the earliest emerging cultural model. For instance, city dwelling PWAs shared ideas among themselves that they didn't seem to share with rural PWAs. These ideas include injecting drug use being a major mode of transmission of AIDS, the necessity of building good *karma* once diagnosed as HIV positive, and the importance of maintaining a positive attitude and good diet once infected. Among urban male PWAs, there was an attempt to associate the cause of their illness with drug use and disassociate it with sexual transmission, while the narratives of female PWAs expressed common themes of unfaithful men and fate. Meantime, the narratives of rural PWAs exhibited common themes more closely akin to the findings of the cognitive rural study: ideas such as AIDS being transmitted through eating, the *sarnu* 'shifting' nature of illnesses, and the concept of weak blood.

An examination of the common themes running throughout the texts leads to a proposal that there are, in fact, various underlying schemata of various types and levels that produce the shared elements noted in the narratives in this earliest cultural model. For example, the lower-level eating schema is evident throughout the narratives. Other higher-level schemata (meaning that they are comprised of various lower-level schemata), such as the worry-will-make-one-sick, a-positive-attitude-will-keep-one-well, the faithful-wives-unfaithful-husbands, and *randi* schemata, have all been identified through narrative analysis, and these in turn, are embedded into even higher-level schemata and cultural models. The significance of these findings will be discussed further in the next chapter.

The findings of this chapter also afford cross-cultural comparison. It seems clear that the early emerging model of HIV and AIDS in Nepal shared some common features with the Haitian cultural model illuminated by Farmer (1994), with the early French model elucidated by Herzlich (1989), with the Australian model described by Viney and Bousfield (1991), and with the early American model (as introduced in chapter 1). In all of these cases, AIDS has been associated with a marginalized group, and blame and fear quickly emerged as key elements in the models. The similarity noted between the various models suggests that perhaps there are biologically based survival schemata that also underlie the cultural models demonstrated. This will be discussed further in the coming chapter.

The findings of this study also help to confirm the validity of the narrative analysis method as a form of discourse analysis. In the original study (Viney and Bousfield 1991) only twelve texts were analyzed providing only tentative conclusions. Such a small sample size limits the validity of any study. Viney's findings (concerning narrative analysis as a valid form of discourse analysis), however, were confirmed through the course of this research, and the increased sample size of thirty narratives (plus 8 more recent narratives) should add weight to the validity of the use of narrative analysis as a discourse analysis method.

As suggested earlier, narrative analysis has proven to be a useful tool for getting at both the denotative and connotative aspects of culture, the denotative being the shared, referential attributes associated with HIV and AIDS, and the connotative being the aspects unique to each individual's personal illness history. The stories bring to life the role of personal agents (people) in their own illness experiences, while at the same time illuminating shared understandings that exist among members within a cultural group. The results of this narrative analysis study confirm the findings of the cognitive study. Beyond this, however, this form of analysis provides a finer level of discrimination, illuminating differences between various sub-groups of PWAs as well as demonstrating individual variation between the various narratives. It seems, as suggested by Viney and Bousfield (1991), that narrative analysis is more sensitive to the issues of personal agency.

This study also confirms the validity of the use of the narrative analysis method cross-linguistically. To date, the method had not been employed extensively cross-linguistically and has not been used at all to study illness beliefs and practices in Nepal. The method seems to work well for analysis of Nepali texts. Although Nepali texts differ structurally from English texts, they still exhibit core narratives that are easily identified and analyzed using the narrative analysis method as described by Viney and Bousfield (1991). Narrative analysis is likely a good tool for cross-linguistic analysis designed to elicit cultural models.

Finally, I have added conclusions drawn from recent narratives, confirming that many of the earlier embedded schemata are still in use in Nepal today, but which also display a wider cultural model that has adopted the element of hope and is slowly displacing the key "fatal" element in the earlier model. And as this model continues to shift, I anticipate that fear and stigma associated with HIV in Nepal, if HIV education and prevention efforts are conducted with cultural intelligence, will lessen in time as well. The findings of this chapter imply that a wider cultural model of HIV and AIDS exists and is currently being modified in Nepal. This model, including its various constituent schemata, will be the focus of the next chapter.

Part Three

Wrapping it Up

7

Nepali Cultural Models of HIV and AIDS and Underlying Illness Schemata

In this chapter I examine the cultural models that have emerged from the findings of the cognitive ethnosemantic study (chapter 5) and the narrative analysis project (chapter 6). The two studies have demonstrated different cultural models, expressed by various communities in Nepal. Having said this, however, I would add that the various models also exhibit a great deal of similarity to one another. In this chapter I propose the emergence of a dominant cultural model of HIV and AIDS; a basic model that informs the various sub-group models. I will also examine the underlying illness schemata made evident through the findings of both studies. An understanding of the various cultural models (and their constituent schemata) is essential because it is these cultural models that people rely on to make sense of AIDS and it is these same cultural models that people use to determine appropriate behavior to exhibit toward those who have HIV and AIDS.

As a reminder, books are locked in the ethnographic present. Many of the conclusions of this chapter are based mainly on the earlier studies. While it is clear that these findings still have relevance today in the formation and promotion of a Nepali cultural model of HIV and AIDS, at the end of the chapter I will take a cursory glance at the implications of more recent research.

7.1 Nepali cultural models of HIV and AIDS

In the last chapter we used thirty narratives of urban-dwelling PWAs (persons with AIDS) to discover whether there were any shared understandings of HIV and AIDS in Nepal. The results of the narrative analysis study confirm the earlier findings of the rural cognitive study (chapter 5), that hate, fear, and blame are three major elements of an emerging cultural model (I) of HIV and AIDS in Nepal. Both studies also revealed widely shared understandings of HIV and AIDS as a fatal, infectious, and sexually transmitted disease. And both studies illuminated common themes regarding AIDS as a "bad person's" disease, AIDS as the result of bad *karma*, and the belief in a strong connection between worry and disease. Based on the data, I propose an overarching composite cultural model (I) of AIDS in Nepal that encompasses these features as major elements (fig. 7.1). As can be seen in figure 7.1, however, there are also slightly different cognitive models held by different sub-groups (e.g., rural versus city PWAs and urban female PWAs versus urban male PWAs). These sub-group models still encompass the major features of the wider model, but differ from one another in significant ways. For instance, the findings among rural PWAs confirm the findings of the rural cognitive study (among non-PWAs) in the beliefs that (1) AIDS can be transmitted through eating and (2) AIDS may first begin as a "smaller" disease (like malaria). These features were unique to a rural cultural model of AIDS. Likewise, urban female PWAs' discourses revolved around issues of unfaithfulness of men, faithfulness of women and ideas about fate, while urban male PWAs' discourses revolved around drug use (not sex) and the influence of bad people upon their lives. These features were unique to urban PWAs.

Each of the widely shared understandings (the elements of the composite model) regarding the meaning of HIV and AIDS carry with them a host of related cultural beliefs and social expectations that are closely attached to the meanings that have been attributed to the disease. For instance, since AIDS is 'fatal' *antim* and 'infectious' *saruwa*, which equates to *thulo* 'big', then 'separation' *chhichhi durdur* of infected persons is expected. And since AIDS has been associated with prostitution, traditional ideas concerning *randi* 'promiscuity' have been applied as well. When Nepalis apply certain schemata associated with HIV and AIDS to someone infected with AIDS, they are able to behave in a culturally appropriate manner toward that person, based on the elements of response that have developed within the current cultural model. The various schemata embedded within the cultural models are discussed below.

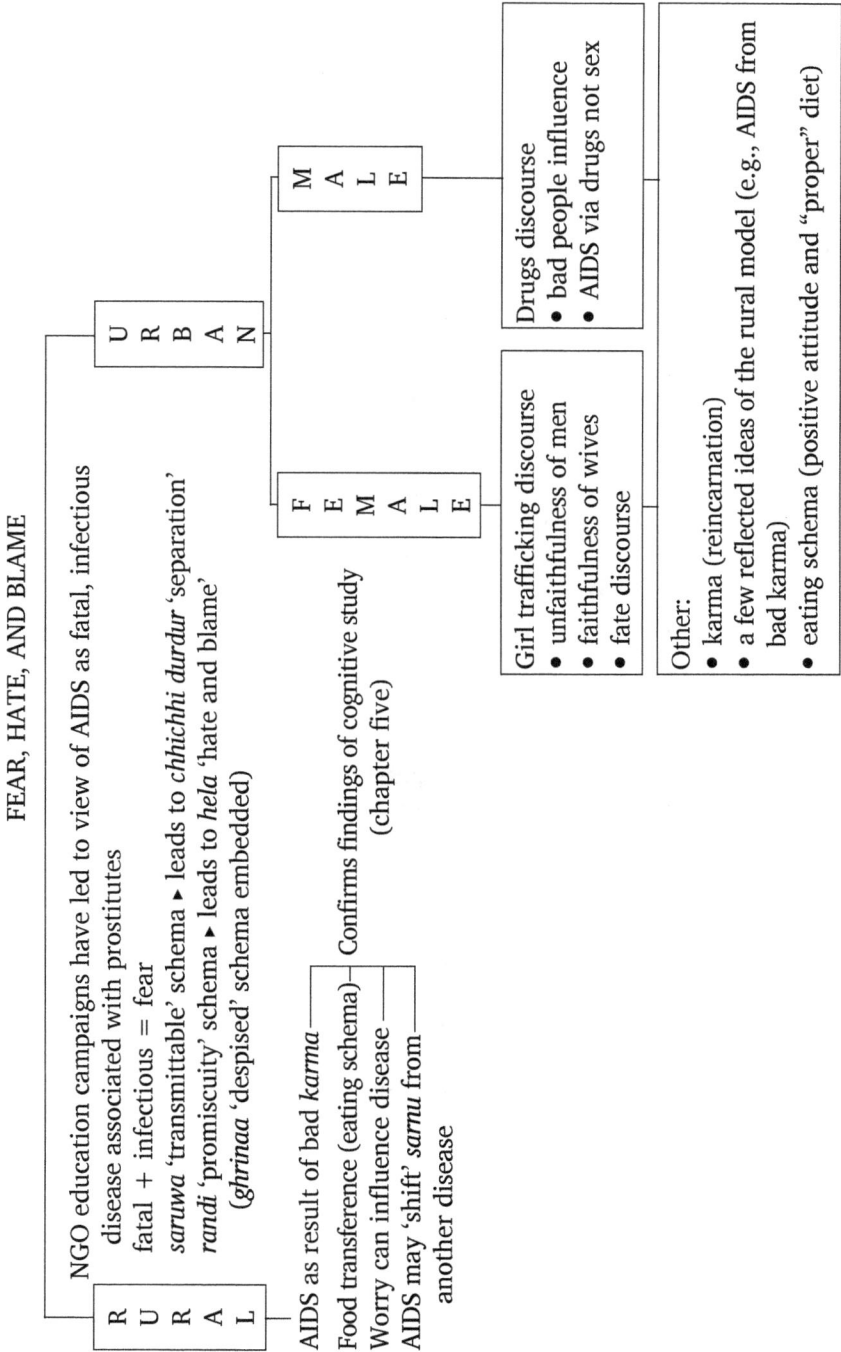

FEAR, HATE, AND BLAME

R
U
R
A
L

NGO education campaigns have led to view of AIDS as fatal, infectious
   disease associated with prostitutes
fatal + infectious = fear
saruwa 'transmittable' schema ▶ leads to *chhichhi durdur* 'separation'
randi 'promiscuity' schema ▶ leads to *hela* 'hate and blame'
   (*ghrinaa* 'despised' schema embedded)

AIDS as result of bad *karma*
Food transference (eating schema) —— Confirms findings of cognitive study
Worry can influence disease   (chapter five)
AIDS may 'shift' *sarnu* from
   another disease

U
R
B
A
N

F   M
E   A
M   L
A   E
L
E

Girl trafficking discourse
• unfaithfulness of men
• faithfulness of wives
• fate discourse

Drugs discourse
• bad people influence
• AIDS via drugs not sex

Other:
• karma (reincarnation)
• a few reflected ideas of the rural model (e.g., AIDS from
   bad karma)
• eating schema (positive attitude and "proper" diet)

Figure 7.1. Cultural Model of HIV and AIDS in Nepal, including embedded schemata.

7.2 Underlying illness schemata

An examination of the common themes running throughout the narratives leads to the proposal that there are, in fact, various underlying schemata (of various types and levels) that produce the shared elements noted in the cultural models. Many of these schemata have been identified in the previous chapters. Again, some of these schemata are present in the overarching cultural model (i.e., there is evidence of the application of those schemata in all the various sub-group models) and some are specific to certain sub-groups. For example, the lower-level eating schema is quite evident throughout both studies. As noted, the research (both cognitive and narrative) is full of examples that imply the application of this schema. Various other higher level schemata (meaning that they are comprised of various lower-level schemata), such as the a-positive-attitude-will-keep-one-well, the faithful-wives-unfaithful-husbands, and the AIDS-via-drugs-not-sex schemata, are embedded in the cultural models of specific sub-groups.

As discussed in chapter four, embeddedness is a characteristic of schemata. Schemata are embedded in other schemata, which are themselves embedded in even higher level schemata such as cultural models. For example, the eating and separation schemata are embedded as major elements in the *saruwa* 'transmittable' schema, resulting in the beliefs that *saruwa* diseases can be spread via food and people with *saruwa* diseases should be 'separated' *chhichhi durdur* from others. The *saruwa* schema, in turn, is embedded along with the *khattam* 'fatal' and *randi* schemata, in the wider cultural model of HIV and AIDS. Likewise, the *ghrinaa* 'societal-hate-as-a-form-of-social-control' schema encompasses the *randi* schema. The application of these various schemata within the cultural model results in the elements of fear, hate, and blame that is currently associated with HIV and AIDS in Nepal.

Within sub-groups, various other schemata are embedded in their specific cultural models. For example, the rural population includes the *sarnu* 'shifting' schema as an element of their cultural model of HIV and AIDS while the urban women include the expected-unfaithfulness-of-husbands and faithfulness-of-wives schemata (which encompasses the embedded fate schema) in their cultural model of HIV and AIDS. And urban men encompass the bad-people and the AIDS-via-drugs-not-sex schemata in their particular cultural model. And, of course, each of these schemata is embedded by other schemata. For instance, the AIDS-via–drugs-not-sex schema of urban males incorporates the *randi* schema along with a more-compassion-is-shown-toward-drug-users schema.

As has been noted, the eating schema was a prevalent theme throughout both studies.[1] At the lexical level, various narrators used the Nepali verb

---

[1]Interestingly, the root of the Nepali verb *khaanu* 'eat' is the Nepali word for food itself, *khaanaa*.

'eating' as an image schema to semantically fill the slot that would be filled by the English glosses 'smoke' (as in cigarettes), 'drink,' and 'take' (as in drugs).[2] "Eating" also appears to be used as an image schema extended to many illness ideas. For instance, the verbs *khattam* 'finished' and *bigriyo* 'spoiled', often associated in the texts with the idea of finality (e.g., AIDS is the final disease—meaning fatal), are terms normally associated with food in other contexts. For instance, when food spoils it is *bigriyo*, and when one is done eating, the food is *khattam* 'finished'. Concerning the association between *bigriyo* and illness, Zvosec (1996:150) writes, *"Bigriyo* may refer to food, either in terms of food that goes rancid, for example, or of spoiling that results from a person's failure to observe dietary restrictions. This is said to make a person more susceptible to illness, or even cause tuberculosis, according to one *dhaami* (traditional medical practitioner)."

At a higher conceptual level, many of the findings of both studies support the contention that eating is a major schema used in Nepal to inform higher level schemata and cultural models of illness. For instance, eating played an important part in illness and treatment in both studies. Diet was considered a major factor in illness causation (being 'eaten' by spirits, loss of appetite, not eating properly, not eating on time, mixing hot and cold foods, disease transferred through eating, 'eating drugs,' etc.) and illness treatment ('eating' home remedies, eating properly—including the right hot/cold foods, etc.). It seems that health, from the choice of the words used to talk about it (eating-image schema) to the things one must do to maintain it, depends in one way or another, on a relationship with food. It appears from the research, that eating is a major lower level schema that informs higher level illness schemata (including cultural models of HIV and AIDS) in Nepal.

Although it has never been identified explicitly as a schema, the relationship between eating and sickness is well documented in Nepal. For instance, Zvosec (1996:125) has written, "Dietary rules are among the most fundamental and influential concerns of health and daily life among rural Nepalis on individual, social and ritual levels." Likewise, Stone (1983:971) has noted "a cultural preoccupation with food and eating." Stone's research illustrates how conditions of food scarcity and harsh environment combine to pattern the nature of social relationships and ritual practices of high caste Hindu groups in Nepal. The ritual (and reciprocal) relationship between hungry spirits and humans is analogous to the relationship between hungry humans and the scarcity produced by living in a harsh environment. Stone demonstrates how, through the idiom of illness, hierarchical social systems (in which cooperation and care taking are constrained yet required) are reinforced. "Feeding the dead" is done through the ritualistic sacrifice of food to a hungry deity. Zvosec has also identified a preoccupation with diet within Tibetan and Ayurvedic medicine (1996:125).

---

[2]'Eating drugs' was even used as a generic cover term for injecting drug use.

I would argue that the eating schema is a fundamental element of a larger foundational schema of purity and pollution. Brad Shore (1996) has described foundational schemata as major schemata that inform many aspects of the culture throughout various domains. As such, foundational schemata are evident throughout multiple contexts in any given culture. For instance, Shore identifies the hub-and-spoke schemata as a foundational Western schema. This foundational schema organizes, for example, the layout of bus stations, train stations, and airports (via the influence of the hub-and-spoke schemata upon architectural design styles).

I propose that purity-and-pollution is a foundational schema in South Asia. It informs the caste system, which in turn informs various rules of social contact, eating, sexual contact, etc. The purity-and-pollution schema is also evident in rules about 'infectious' *saruwa* illnesses and ideas about moral geography, as well as in the ideas about 'separation' *chhichhi durdur* seen so clearly throughout this research. So many aspects of life in South Asia, including ideas about health and illness, revolve around the theme of keeping oneself pure. The purity-and-pollution schema is arguably a foundational schema in Nepal around which many aspects of Nepali culture, including cultural models of HIV and AIDS, are centered. The purity-and-pollution schema also encompasses various lower level schemata, such as the eating schema mentioned previously.

I have also noted a strong association in both studies between worry and disease. Worry is believed to make one more susceptible to sickness. This seems to be a schema that is embedded in the wider cultural model of HIV and AIDS in Nepal. It would be interesting to see if this same schema is applicable to all other categories of illness as well. Although this schema is a major element of the cultural model of HIV and AIDS, it may itself be, or may encompass, a biologically based schema. Much of the anthropological literature on stress suggests that various social and psychological factors can cause stress, and stress in turn can cause sickness (Dressler 1996). Although the definition of stress goes beyond the traditional idea of stress as a metaphor for psychological upset, worry, anxiety and frustration (Dressler 1996:255), the Nepali example would seem to fit this definition quite well. The Nepali schema posits that *chintaa*, usually translated as 'worry',[3] will increase a person's susceptibility to disease. So, stress may be the result of various social, historical, environmental, physical or psychological factors, but the reaction to it, namely sickness, appears to be a biologically based universal. Therefore, the worry-and-sickness schema, although it is a cultural schema and is not necessarily shared by all cultures around the world, does appear to have a biological basis. I will revisit the idea of biologically based schemata and their influence on cultural models in the next chapter.

---

[3]*Chinta* can also mean 'to be anxious, overwhelmed with cares, or saddened by circumstances'.

7.3 Implications of later research

Based on the most recently collected narratives (chapter 6), it is clear that a shift in the HIV and AIDS cultural model is underway. It is not so much that one cultural model is giving way to another, rather that key elements of the one are slowly being replaced as others are being introduced, resulting in the modification of the overall model. And it is likely that this transformation is not happening uniformly across the culture. Some segments of society are ahead of others in adapting this change. But it is clear that the overall trajectory is moving in a particular direction. So, while some of the later texts reveal a change for some PLWHAs toward an increased level of hope and away from fear, hate, and blame, these elements remain resident (but to a decreasing degree) for many other PLWHAs and in the wider Nepali cultural model of HIV and AIDS.

The key question in my mind is "What makes the difference in the Nepal context?" It would appear that where effective NGOs are working there has been dramatic change. The model of dying of AIDS is changing to living with HIV (the wider world cultural model) as a result of these organizations helping PLWHAs understand that there are now life-preserving treatments available. This has long-term implications on the directly associated elements of fear, hate, and blame. NGOs are providing moral and emotional support along with education; they are attempting to make ARV medications affordable and accessible to PLWHAs; and they are educating the wider population in the places PLWHAs live, reducing the societal stigma associated with HIV and AIDS. Where effective NGOs are working, I am encouraged by what I see. Their services are bringing a dramatic change for the individuals who are being reached. But it is clear by the responses of other PLWHAs that the wider societal model still needs to be addressed.

8

The Making of a Cultural Model

In the last chapter I examined the cultural models of HIV and AIDS that exist among different sub-groups in Nepal and examined the various schemata that inform these models. I also proposed a dominant model that influences these sub-group models. Three major components of this dominant model are fear, hate, and blame. In this chapter I examine the various factors involved in the creation and spread of this dominant model of HIV and AIDS. A complex combination of factors, both cultural and biological, seems to be the impetus for both the dominant model's creation and spread.

8.1 The role of NGOs

There are currently nearly one hundred non-governmental organizations (NGOs) working in the area of AIDS education and prevention in Nepal.[1] The education and prevention models employed by these organizations are drawn from the National Center for AIDS and STD Control (National Center), an organization charged with coordinating all AIDS education and prevention throughout the country. The education and prevention models promoted by the National Center are, as we saw in chapter two, borrowed from the West. The strategies employed and materials distributed focus primarily on the issues these Western organizations (based on the findings of Western KAP and KAB studies) have recommended. Western models dominate the AIDS discourse in Nepal. The result is an emphasis on awareness building

---

[1]This information comes from a list titled "Organizations Working on HIV/AIDS/STD Issues in Nepal" that I obtained from the HIV/AIDS Training Unit of the United Mission to Nepal.

that portrays AIDS (even using Western illness schemata[2]) as a highly communicable and fatal disease associated most directly with prostitution and drug use. The findings of both studies would suggest that the awareness building campaign led by the various NGOs, has been fairly successful at promoting these associations with AIDS across the country. The concepts of AIDS as fatal, infectious, and sexually transmitted, are, therefore, a direct result of the Western-style awareness building campaign.

In updating this chapter I have had to examine whether there has been significant change in the approaches used by NGOs since the first edition of this book was published over ten years ago. In chapter three, I made the point that some have recently begun to question the effectiveness of the "standard fare" prevention approaches and are beginning to advocate for more culturally sensitive approaches. And I have written about some of these innovative approaches being used elsewhere (Beine 2011). Many of the NGOs that are developing these innovative approaches are small organizations actually funded by very large INGOs who dedicate only a small amount to supporting such "innovative approaches," while the majority of their money (and effort) is still spent on projects that fit the earlier model.

In a recent example of this I sat with the head of a large International funding agency who told me that while she accepted my ideas and considered them "evidence-based" (a new criteria they require for funding), I would need to convince the implementer (a large INGO that is the recipient of these funds) to take up the innovative approach I was suggesting. Meantime I met with the supported INGO, who told me that I would have to convince the funder. I subsequently got the two together, asked the international funder if my research was considered "evidence-based" (in front of the funds recipient), and the funder assured me that it was. Then at this meeting, I mentioned that the funder told me I needed to convince the supported INGO, and that the supported INGO told me I needed to convince the funder. I was then able to share the ideas with the supported INGO, who enthusiastically embraced them and invited me to Kathmandu to share the idea. In a subsequent email, however, he communicated a disappointing decision:

> As a researcher and Program manager, I fully agree with you that the language we speak and IEC/BCC messages we direct to rural people are not always well understood and this varies across the ethnic domains... However, since we just started the program, many of the targeted interventions inclusive of the SBC (strategic behavior communication) materials are in the process of collection,

---

[2]The leading campaign slogan *Condom lagaaun AIDS bhagaaun* 'Lets wear condoms and chase away AIDS' employs a Western war schema (bhagaaun is what you do to enemies, thieves and dogs), a schema not usually associated with illness in Nepal.

compilation, collation and modification. Given this priority, we
will not be able to focus on translation work at this stage.

So, it seems despite the evidence, it is just easier to continue to support
the status quo. And while there is still an abundance of the same materials I saw ten years ago being promulgated by various government sources,
schools and NGOs, a few NGOs are now employing modern technology,
such as computers (e.g.,YouTube), mobile phones, music CDs and videos,
etc., in their HIV education efforts. One prominent INGO has produced a
series of Bollywood-style short films, music videos and full-length films (including comedies)[3] intended to promote HIV awareness. Unfortunately, in
most cases these various materials still primarily reinforce HIVs association
with the various stigma-reinforcing elements noted earlier. So, while the
"packaging" may have changed, the content (i.e., the focus and form of the
education) is, for all practical purposes, the same. It would appear that,
overall, the earlier noted focus still dominates the HIV prevention discourse
of NGOs in Nepal, and the international funding agencies and INGOs that
support the NGOs are still "beating the same drum."

In regard to the emerging "hope" theme, a music video entitled "Sayapatri:
Songs of Hope"[4] is a poignant example of the kinds of messages that are
being produced by INGOs and targeted for PLWHAs in order to convey
the message that there is life after becoming HIV positive. Again, however,
this video seems to reinforce HIVs association with injecting drug use and
sex (two of the stronger stigma-reinforcing elements). And it even seems
to glamorize life post HIV infection.[5] While certainly appropriate for those
with HIV (to give them hope for a future), I often found myself wondering
how a poor rural Nepali without HIV might interpret these messages? Might
it bring hope to their poverty as well to become HIV positive? I will speak
to this further in the next chapter.

And on a philosophical level, with the new demand certain funding agencies place on their local government and INGO partners to "produce results"

---

[3]In 2010 Family Health International's Asha Project, with funding from USAID,
released You are No Exception, eight short videos intended to promote HIV awareness and prevention. Likewise, a number of other DVD recordings, such as Left to
Right, Manish Sanga Manish Mile, Jiwanko Geet, Jeevanko Upahar, Tikeko tin
Mantra, Manko Awaaz, UNDP HIV and AIDS TV spots, Subha Yaatra, and a MTV
documentary entitled "Sold" were produced by the same project (with the same
funding) and shown on Nepal television and in Nepali theaters, and many of these
were uploaded to YouTube in August 2011.

[4]This music video CD of seven songs was produced by FHI with funding from
USAID and was uploaded to YouTube in 2011.

[5]While many PLWHAs I met with were alive and hopeful, they still faced regular
health problems and emotional difficulties that paint a "better than death," but a
far less than glamorous post HIV infection life than is suggested by this video.

or lose funding,[6] I often wondered if the encouraging numbers now being reported in Nepal (e.g., fig. 3.1) are an accurate reflection of what is really happening at the grassroots level, or if these numbers are simply produced by various government agencies and associated INGOs and NGOs to provide what they think (and what we have told them) we want to see? The WHO has commented on this problem as indicated earlier (i.e., structural weaknesses), and I think we need to keep the weaknesses of the various agencies noted at the forefront of our concern.

8.1.1 The influence of *bikaas* 'development'

I have already alluded to the deference shown by Nepalis toward anything *bikaasi* 'developed'. Implied in this is the assumption that traditional is bad (usually referred to as "backwardness") and *bikaas* 'development' is good, as demonstrated by Pigg (1992). Given this attitude toward Western development, it is no surprise that deference has also been displayed toward the ideas of Western experts in the domain of HIV and AIDS education and prevention. Deference toward Western models (even when their impact is questionable) is quite obvious. The Nepali director of the National Center recently agreed to continue the use of current Western approaches despite evidence that they may not be very effective. Karki (1998) displayed an understanding of the "KAP gap" problem when he acknowledged that "although awareness of sexually transmitted diseases (STDs) and HIV among female sex workers is generally high...there is a wide gap between knowledge and practice" and that "regardless of how much one knows, it is often not translated into action." Yet, "awareness building," the recommended strategy of the various NGOs involved, remains the major thrust of the prevention campaign. Although condoms are made available free to the population by the Nepali government, not many people use them. Karki (1998) freely admits, "It is irony that in spite of much effort to make condoms available to all sex workers and their clients, it is estimated that less than 50% of sex workers or clients use condoms." Even so, Karki (1998) concludes that "condom promotion and its use by a large number of clients should be the target for the future." Awareness building (stressing the fatal, infectious and sexually transmitted nature of AIDS) and condom promotion have been strongly promoted by Western organizations consulted by Nepali AIDS prevention planners. And despite an apparent understanding of the limitations of an emphasis on awareness building and condom distribution, deference has been displayed toward this Western (development) approach.

---

[6]USAID (2013) in establishing major reform requirements, is now "demanding a relentless focus on results," i.e., "evidence-based results" (http://www.usaid.gov/usaidforward).

Given the sexually conservative nature of Nepalese public life, I have been very surprised at the small amount of controversy that the emphasis on condoms in the public sphere has created. Although I have heard some criticism, there has generally been a wide acceptance of the saturation of the country with condom billboards. Again, this would seem to suggest that AIDS is understood as a Western disease, and the approaches to combat it (e.g., the media condom campaign) have been suggested by the West. Deference is given to the West, therefore, in the public display of sexuality, even when it violates cultural norms. Given the development in Nepal it is not a surprise that the evolving AIDS prevention campaign would be a product of Western development paradigms.

8.1.2 The development industry of AIDS in Nepal

Closely related to the idea of *bikaas* is the fact that Nepal, being a poorer country, has created a development industry. AIDS is no exception. Back in 1995 David Seddon expressed concern that the AIDS epidemic would attract those who were primarily interested in having access to the funds, which would soon be made available:

> There is a real danger that the prospect of an epidemic will attract organizations and individuals whose interest lie more in the resources that are now being made increasingly available to NGOs for work on HIV-AIDS related issues and will not serve the interests of those directly and indirectly threatened by the disease. Already it seems that "everyone in Kathmandu seems involved, everyone after money, that is" (according to one expatriate commentator). (1995:9)

Likewise, a Nepali policy maker commented on this trend:

> Unfortunately, the disproportionate amount of money that has gone into HIV and AIDS prevention in Nepal compared to other less glamorous diseases like TB and malaria have spread the perception that AIDS is a donor-driven agenda in Nepal and that bigger killers do not get the same attention. This is to a certain extent true, and informal polls of journalists in Nepal show that most reporters and editors believe that AIDS is getting undue attention. Whatever the truth, AIDS organizations are also perceived by some journalists as "dollar harvesters." This has created some problems for organizations dealing with media sensitization, because some reporters seem to think that they are being "used." AIDS organizations and their media advisors need to look at this problem seriously and not underestimate their potential to damage their work. (Dixit 1998)

It seems that Seddon's predictions may have come true.[7] Although the prevalence rate country wide is less than one percent, and various other diseases actually kill many times more people in Nepal than does AIDS, there are currently more NGOs working in the area of HIV and AIDS in Nepal than in these other areas, such as TB and malaria control. The fact is that development in Nepal, including health development, follows a donor driven agenda, and AIDS is currently a hot topic internationally.

8.1.3 The impact of traditional schemata

Traditional ideas also are being reinforced by the NGOs working with HIV and AIDS. Unfortunately, many of these practices are further reinforcing the stigma associated with AIDS. For instance, a worker at one NGO that repatriates and pursues other economic options for FSWs, told me that the NGO he worked for was building a special home for the girls who tested HIV positive and for the girls with "other diseases." When I asked about who else, besides the HIV positive girls, would be kept at the new home, I was told, "Those with tuberculosis and hepatitis B." The NGO Director explained that since these diseases are "contagious" they want to keep those infected away from the other girls. He added, "We don't want the other girls to be victimized." What is most unfortunate is that the HIV positive girls (not a risk to other girls unless sexually active with them) are very susceptible to other infections such as TB. Putting these girls together with TB carriers is like a death sentence for the persons with AIDS (PWAs).

Ideas about the possibility of non-sexual transference of the disease (such as those mentioned in the previous chapters) are also being applied to AIDS intervention work. One NGO director contended that even though there are many organizations working with HIV and AIDS in Nepal, their staff "won't live in the same houses, use the same kitchen or eat off the same plates" as the PWAs. She also gave an example of an international conference she attended in which she was the only female NGO director who was willing to share a room with female PWAs. The ideas of *saruwa* 'transmittable' and *chhichhi durdur* 'separation', although not mentioned by name, are clearly evident in these examples. Again, although various NGOs are working hard to bring HIV and AIDS to the forefront in Nepal, many are participating in practices that are unnecessarily perpetuating stigma and even hastening death.

I found that many of the same ideas reflected in my earlier studies were also in the minds of the NGO workers. For instance, in regard to treatments for AIDS, love, good diet and hygiene were the most common recommendations. One NGO director told me, "If you are healthy (eat well and don't worry) you can stop the growth of that virus. If you are not healthy, then

[7]Comments made by another NGO director (recorded in Sita's text) echo this same sentiment.

naturally, from both the sides—health-wise and disease-wise also—the virus will eat you up."[8] Directors of three other AIDS related NGOs similarly told of the importance of (1) love, (2) good diet, and (3) keeping a positive attitude.

8.2 The role of doctors and policy makers

Nepali doctors and policy makers have also been influential in creating and confirming elements of the wider cultural model. First, through deference to Western education and prevention models (as noted above), the doctors and policy makers have promoted the aforementioned elements (AIDS as fatal, infectious, and sexually transmitted) of the major cultural model. Next, doctors and policy makers have been influential in perpetuating these ideas via the media as we will see in the next section. Finally, doctors have also sent powerful non-verbal messages through their actions that have confirmed many of the traditional schemata associated with AIDS in the minds of the general public. For instance, the common practice of doctors refusing to treat patients once they know they are HIV-positive is well documented throughout the narratives. This practice has also been well documented elsewhere (Dixit 1996; Karki 1998) and we will see further examples of it in the media in the next section. I personally encountered many experiences that further confirmed this practice. Besides the various stories told to me by PWAs, I was told directly by several doctors that they are aware of colleagues who will not treat PWAs. An incident of mistreatment of a PWA also occurred at Patan Hospital during my research that prompted a scolding letter from the hospital director (fig. 8.1).[9] Some members of the Emergency Room staff had refused to treat (or even touch) a patient once their HIV status was revealed. One NGO director told me of different incidences of mistreatment, in which she had taken her HIV positive girls in for treatment, but they had been told to go to another location. After arriving at the recommended location, they were also refused treatment by medical professionals. Another NGO director told me of her friend (a female medical doctor) who refused to touch her when the doctor discovered that a PWA had vomited on her. It seems that fear is prevalent among many in the medical community.

The findings of two different KAP studies done among doctors in Nepal (Bhattarai 1999; Beine 1999) suggest that the knowledge of the majority of the doctors surveyed was adequate in many areas of HIV

---

[8]Note the application of the eating schema.

[9]In my estimation Patan Hospital offers the best care to PWAs available in the whole country. This was also the place of choice among PWAs to be seen. They felt more compassion is given to them at Patan Hospital. This was a rare incident at Patan, but I use it to illustrate that if this kind of practice is taking place at the best hospital, one can only imagine what is happening in other places.

transmission. Nevertheless, there were certain areas where a surprisingly large number of doctors seem to be following the Nepali cultural models of AIDS rather than biomedical knowledge as it relates to HIV and AIDS. For instance, in the first study, 44.5 percent of the doctors agreed that it was necessary to fumigate the bed and the room occupied after the discharge or death of any AIDS patient (Bhattarai 1999:6).[10] Likewise two-thirds of the doctors agreed that gloves need to be worn while feeding an AIDS patient or wiping saliva from his or her mouth and only half responded that HIV positive patients can be kept in wards with other patients (Bhattarai 199:7). Wearing gloves while feeding AIDS patients, and keeping patients in separate wards, are both medically unwarranted practices (Bhattarai 1999:22).

---

[10]HIV cannot be transmitted through exposure to anything (including feces, urine, sweat, etc.) that would be left behind by an AIDS patient, therefore, fumigation of a patient's bed or room would be medically unwarranted (Bhattarai 1999:22).

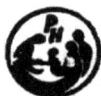

Patan Hospital

5-22278
Phone: 5-22266
5-22295

Lagankhel, Lalitpur
NEPAL

G. P. O. Box 252
Kathmandu, Nepal.

To: Patient Hospital Doctors, Health Assistants, and Nurses
From: Dr. Mark Zimmerman, MD
Date: 8 October 1998

Concerning: **The care of HIV positive patients**

Dear Colleagues,

HIV positive patients pose a number of clinical, social and emotional problems. From time to time, we all need to be reminded about their appropriate care. Recent incidents with two such patients lead me to write to you at this time.

- <u>Examination and referral of HIV positive patients</u>

At Patan Hospital, we expect that all doctors, health assistants, and nurses will provide the same excellent care to HIV patients as they do to all patients. Because of the extremely low likelihood of a medical care giver ever getting HIV from a patient, and because protective equipment is available to all who work in this hospital, there is no excuse for anyone to refuse to see a patient who is HIV positive or to limit the care given.

- <u>Writing and speaking about the "HIV" status of the patient</u>

Universal precautions mean that all blood and body fluids should be treated as if it were positive for HIV. Because more than 90% of the HIV in a community is likely to be unrecognized, it is essential that you take appropriate protective measures for all patients whose body fluid may come into contact with you.

The policy of Patan Hospital and its Infection Control Committee is that we DO NOT label specimens, patient charts or lab slips as being "HIV", "HBV", or even "high risk". If we take special precautions with these few patients, it leads to carelessness with other patients (some of whom will be positive, but unrecognized.)

You should take measures to assure confidentiality about the patient's disease. DO NOT write boldly "HIV" on places where this might be seen by non-staff. It may be best on rounds to speak of a patient's "immunodeficiency virus" rather than saying "HIV" in front of visitors. As with all diseases, a particular patient's HIV status should not discussed outside the treating team.
Thanks for your help in this challenging area.

Sincerely,

Mark D. Zimmerman, MD

FAX: 977-1-225559   eMail: patan_hospital@npl. healthnet. org

Figure 8.1. Hospital Director's letter to address mistreatment of PWAs at Patan Hospital. (Used by permission)

Likewise, 56.7 percent of the doctors responded affirmatively or undecidedly when asked if AIDS is a problem of moral behavior (45.4% yes, 11.3% undecided) and 31.9 percent answered affirmative or undecided when asked whether they would feel uncomfortable inviting someone with HIV and AIDS into their home (Beine 1999). Although the questionnaire was a "tick the box" type, one respondent even wrote in reply to this question, "I know I shouldn't, but still I hesitate."

I also asked questions regarding two popular rumors that were circulating around Nepal during the time of my research. The first had to do with a rumor that people were using HIV-infected needles to "pump up" raw chickens with water before their sale in order to increase their profits. According to the rumor, people were eating the chickens and becoming infected with HIV. The second had to do with PWAs (the newspapers labeled these people "AIDS junkies") leaving "infected needles" hidden in the cushions of movie hall seats where an unsuspecting victim would later enter (in the dark) and sit on the needles, stabbing themselves, thus becoming infected with the HIV virus.[11] It must be noted that the HIV virus is generally very weak and would not likely survive cooking nor even being out of the body long enough to be put in a syringe and stabbed through cushions into another person. In fact, the odds of an infection developing from blood transferred directly from body to body via needles (such as inadvertent medical needle sticks) is only one in two hundred and fifty (Bhattarai 1999:24). Suffice it to say, that the chicken rumor is virtually impossible and the movie hall rumor, although theoretically possible, is also extremely unlikely according to medical professionals. Yet it was surprising to me that 17 percent of the medical doctors expressed belief in the possibility of transfer of AIDS via eating chicken (4.1%) or were uncertain about the possibility (13%) of this mode of transmission. One Western-trained medical school professor commenting on the question volunteered, "We have been teaching this in our environmental health course, but the evidence is not conclusive." Likewise, 59.3 percent expressed belief in, or were undecided about, the possibility of contracting HIV through a needle stick at a movie hall (36.4% yes, 22.9% undecided). It seems that a surprising number of medical doctors are acting, in part, on the cultural model of AIDS as it relates to *saruwa rogs* 'transmittable disease' (including the concept of *chhichhi durdur* 'separation') rather than trusting the biomedical knowledge on the subject.

I should make the point that the figures above suggest that the majority of Nepali doctors do not share these opinions and seem to be treating AIDS patients appropriately. I should also point out that these types of irrational

---

[11]This story made the headlines in several magazines and newspapers as well as in the leading English daily newspaper. In a follow-up investigation, however, no basis was found for the rumors. Interestingly, the local movie hall owners accused the local video storeowners of instigating the rumor in order to increase their profits at the expense of the local movie hall owners.

beliefs (medically speaking) are not restricted to Nepali doctors or even to doctors working in the developing world. A KAP study conducted among primary care physicians in New York State in 1988 demonstrated that 11 percent of the medical doctors surveyed believed that it was either very likely or somewhat likely that a person could contract the HIV virus by being coughed on or sneezed on by a PWA (Gemson et al. 1991).

Although it is clear from the figures above that the number of medical doctors who hold these opinions comprises a minority, the impact of this minority's beliefs and actions upon the wider cultural models of AIDS is great. Many stories about doctors refusing service to AIDS patients have been published in the media. A doctor treating an AIDS patient is not "news" while one who refuses to treat a PWA is "news." The result is that only stories about doctors not treating or mistreating PWAs are published, thus generating a perception among the general public that normalizes the practices of the minority. And since they are doctors, the general public, not being privy to the majority view, defers to the understanding of their "developed" countrymen. Thus, some doctors further perpetuate a cultural model (based on the application of traditional schemata). I will talk more about the role of the media in the creation of a cultural model in the next section.

Doctors' refusals to touch and treat PWAs also have had an impact in the creation of a cultural model in the village area. In a discussion regarding the modes of transmission, I asked one villager why he believed that AIDS could be spread through touch. He responded, "Even city doctors are not touching people with AIDS. We read about it in the paper. They are educated people! What do we know? We are simple villagers. They are the developed *(bikaasi)* ones." Here we see that the doctors' actions have been used to confirm the application of traditional ideas regarding *saruwa rogs* to AIDS. And as can be seen by the figures above, the doctors' beliefs about the separation of AIDS patients from others confirms the traditional concept of *chhichhi durdur*. We also see again the impact of the deference displayed toward those considered more *bikaasi*.

Medical doctors also have contributed to the element of blame in the wider cultural model. First of all, in response to the question about which groups of people in Nepal have the highest prevalence rates, prostitutes and drug addicts were the two most frequent responses. Although these two groups are, in fact, the two most affected groups, they are also traditionally considered "bad people" as has been previously noted. The association of AIDS with these groups, therefore, has inadvertently created the image of AIDS as a "bad people's" disease, thus warranting blame. And a little less inadvertently, a surprising number of doctors (as noted above) considered AIDS a problem of immoral behavior. This certainly perpetuates the idea that AIDS is a "bad people's" disease, which creates societal blame and hate and further stigmatizes those with the disease.

It is clear that some of the doctors are employing a cultural model of AIDS that is a product of both imported Western ideas (fatal, infectious and sexually transmitted) and the activation of traditional schemata *(saruwa* and *chhichhi durdur)*. The view of these doctors is then spread via the media and deference is shown to their opinion by lay people who use the actions of these doctors to construct and confirm a cultural model that includes the above-mentioned traditional schemata. Thus, we see how doctors are contributing to a wider cultural model of AIDS that displays fear, hate, and blame as major components.

When investigating why this "irrational fear" exists among some Nepali doctors it was suggested that the fatal nature of the disease is the key. For example, one NGO director who had many doctors turn her PWAs away told me the doctors were not absolutely certain their textbooks could be trusted:

> The doctors say one thing, but do another because they don't want to die. I think that even though they read about how AIDS can and cannot transfer in their medical books, they are just not sure. They passed their exams by reading the books, but they are just not certain. AIDS is fatal. They don't know if they can trust the books. They don't want to die.

Another doctor, when asked why doctors would be acting against their medical knowledge, replied, "Because death is the final trump card." It seems that fear of death is, indeed, a powerful force that is influencing the cultural model of AIDS in Nepal creating much fear. The biological basis for this will be discussed later in this chapter.

In updating this chapter it must be noted that I have not done any recent follow-up work on this earlier survey. Jha and Madison (2009) however, seem to confirm that some of the earlier findings are still a reality for many in Nepal:

> Health professionals were perceived to lack knowledge and sensitivity in providing health care to often marginalized and stigmatized injecting drug users, sex workers and HIV-positive people. Stigma and marginalization seem to interfere with doctors' and other health professionals' decisions to voluntarily treat persons who they perceive to be at high risk for HIV infections. Doctors and other health professionals appear suspicious, even unaware, of contemporary biomedical knowledge as it relates to HIV. The fear that certain marginalized groups, such as injecting drug users and sex workers, would be infected with HIV has further intensified stigma against these groups.

These same ideas are reaffirmed by Jha, Plummer and Bowers (2011) as well. And a recent article, written by a Nepali medical doctor for the

Kathmandu Post, provides further confirmation that these things are still happening:

> A while ago, when on a visit to Achham, I had the opportunity to talk extensively with locals, and the conversation revolved mostly around HIV infection. I discovered that a whole host of misconceptions abounded in the area regarding the disease, even to an extent amid community health workers. Many, for instance, feared that they would contract HIV/AIDS by sheer contact with patients, and wanted my advice on how to deal with sufferers in their communities, if there was some way to keep them isolated, away from everyone else... I was struck by how—despite all the 'awareness programmes' targeted toward these communities that are conducted regularly—a lasting impact is yet to be seen, and sufferers continue to face ostracisation in society...
>
> It was also while in Achham that I received a call regarding an HIV positive woman of thirty-eight, who was suffering from a prolapsed uterus. I was informed that she had been taken to a private hospital in Kathmandu, but when practitioners discovered that she was infected, they had immediately refused her any further services. It came as a real shock to me that medical officials in the capital would be so ignorant and so callous as to have done this, particularly given the fact that Kathmandu is where most of the organizations working to elevate HIV awareness are themselves based. (Uprety 2012)

This sort of ignorance does not just exist in treating one person or a single case however—ignorance echoes around the country. After all, if health workers at a private hospital in the capital could demonstrate such erroneous, and downright ludicrous, attitudes toward HIV and AIDS sufferers, is it any surprise then that misconceptions and ostracisation of such patients is prevalent in more remote areas? What such attitudes do, ultimately, is create an environment of fear, detrimental for both sufferers as well as the remainder of their communities. The fear of being discriminated against will naturally discourage people from getting themselves tested, and the more untested people there are, the more the chances are of the HIV virus spreading unawares from person to person.

Who will be responsible in this scenario? I am, of course, not excluding myself here. I too am among the smug percentage of the population that is so sure we're making a difference by providing training and programmes in remote areas. I am a member of national and international organizations working on women's health and HIV and AIDS issues, and have written many an article on these concerns as well, but how effective can any of it have been when a woman is still refused treatment by a health worker for being HIV positive? Perhaps this World AIDS Day, instead of counting our meager achievements, we should make it a point to stop being so complacent about what we have done and look at where we have failed instead.

Besides providing confirmation that there are still problems among health workers when it comes to treating HIV, various of the other issues I have spoken to thus far (e.g., traditional beliefs regarding the spread of the disease, the belief in the need to isolate, the incompleteness of awareness campaigns alone, the short-sightedness of NGOs, etc.) are all wonderfully illuminated by the experience of Dr. Uprety (2012), a provider for PWAs, in the article quoted previously.

While it is clear from these examples that problems remain, my own personal experience, based on discussions with HIV sufferers, is that PLWHAs generally face a lesser degree of discrimination or stigma than those I interviewed ten years ago. And, regarding the doctors, if the fatal nature of HIV (i.e., the "trump card") is the basis for this earlier discrimination (as I suggested previously), then as new knowledge (namely, ARVs as treatment) is disseminated to doctors (at least the ones who continue to educate themselves medically), then there would be less reason to continue acting on the traditional cultural model of AIDS as fatal, rather than the biomedical model in which HIV is a chronic treatable illness, and I would expect such behavior to subside. I will speak more to the influence of the media in the next section.

8.3 The role of the media

Various authors have examined the role that the media has played in the construction of a social understanding (cultural model) of HIV and AIDS in various countries (Albert 1986; Baker 1986; Herzlich and Pierret 1989; Lyttleton 1996). As in other countries, the media has been instrumental in the creation and confirmation of the widely held cultural model of HIV and AIDS in Nepal. In this section I will examine several phases the media have passed through in their representation of HIV and AIDS to the general public and I will discuss the role the media have played in the creation of a cultural model of AIDS.

8.3.1 Early media representations

It is notable that early on, doctors and policy makers identified and targeted the media as a valuable vehicle for the creation of public awareness about HIV and AIDS (Karuna 1998). The initial information going out to the general public about AIDS via the media contained ideas (e.g., fatal, infectious, sexually transmitted) passed along to the media by the policy planners, who had developed these messages under the influence of Western models. The use of the media as a vehicle for creating awareness regarding AIDS has been very successful to date. Various studies (including my rural study in chapter five) have confirmed that the media (mainly Radio Nepal) have been the major source of AIDS information (Karmic Society et al. 1998; New Era 1997; Maharjan et al. 1994).

The first phase of the media presentation of HIV and AIDS focused on the issues mentioned above. Because of the association with sexual transmission, the dialogue on HIV and AIDS quickly became subsumed under the girl trafficking discourse. Early articles focused on the association between AIDS and commercial sex work, and FSWs began to be blamed for the advent of AIDS in Nepal. For instance, in 1991 a leading Nepali magazine published an article that featured the story (including picture, name and village) of a woman named Geeta (fig. 8.2). In the article she was identified as a prostitute returning home from Bombay and carrying AIDS (Janmanch 1991:12). Later that same year the director of the NGO where Geeta had been living in Kathmandu returned with her to Geeta's home village. The director describes this visit:

> When we stepped down from our jeep in Melamchi, people surrounded us and stared at Geeta. We soon felt that they were silently blaming her for her condition as they held out their copies of Janmanch magazine. Geeta was thirsty and weak from the trip, but when she attempted to get drinking water from a shop, she was refused. This was her first experience of contempt and segregation in her own community, but not her last. As we walked to her father's house, a large crowd followed us over the bridge and up the narrow path.
>
> We soon met Geeta's father along the track, but he stood expressionless before his daughter. We tried to talk to him about his daughter's health and needs, but he turned from us. Further up the hill, we met Geeta's mother. She asked us to take Geeta back to Kathmandu: she told us she did not want her home. Only then did Geeta cry out in anger and humiliation. (Dixit 1996:58)

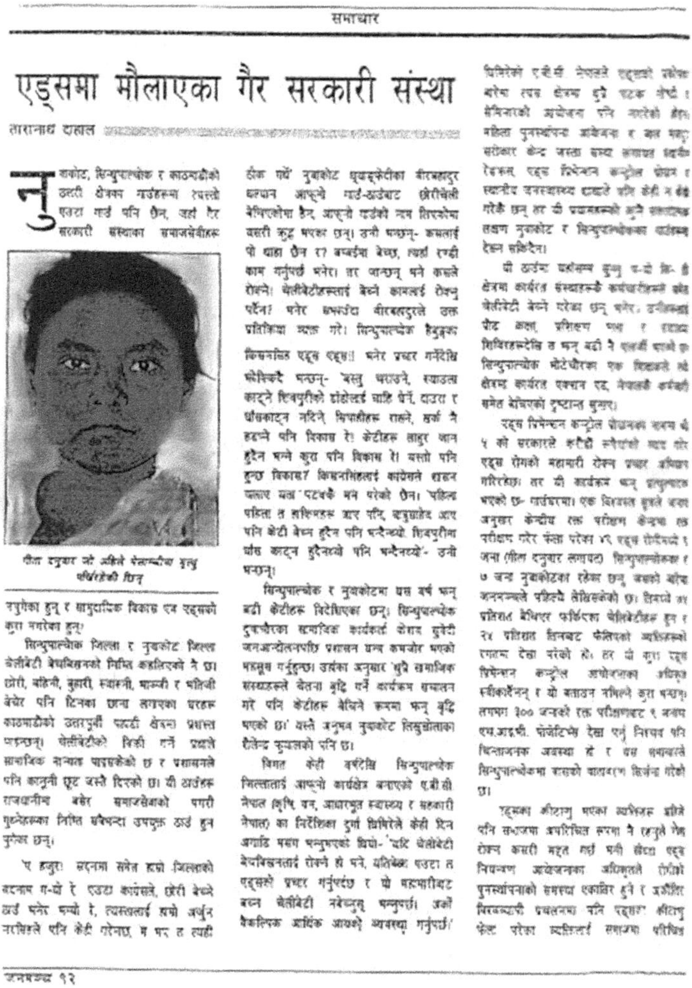

समाचार

एड्समा मौलाएका गैर सरकारी संस्था

तारानाथ दहल

Figure 8.2. Geeta's story, featured in *Janmanch* magazine (1991:12), showed her picture, gave her real name and the name of her village, and prompted much ostricization by her family and other villagers.

Later in the article, the NGO director describes a second visit to Geeta's village after Geeta had reluctantly been allowed to live there again:

> They [Geeta's family] believed that the disease could be contracted
> through casual contact... Geeta's relatives were reluctant to accept

responsibility for her...They still feared that casual contact of almost any kind would transmit the virus.

The community was still very wary and hostile toward Geeta. She
had been restricted from using the road or going to the bazaar. In
other words, she was effectively quarantined. At home, her family
still believed that casual contact with Geeta could make them sick.
She was forced to use a separate comb for her hair, a separate plate
and glass, and she was not allowed to touch or hold her younger
brothers or sisters. In her small world, she was kept apart by fear,
and there were no avenues for simple expressions of love and affec-
tion. Geeta was frustrated and hurt by how she was being treated
and she wanted to leave the village.

I organized another meeting with Geeta's family members to discuss these problems. The family explained their actions. They said
that the community would outcast them if they allowed Geeta to
remain with them. But their own beliefs, I knew, would have pro-
pelled them to treat Geeta like this even without community sanc-
tions. (Dixit 1996:58)

From this example we can see the impact of (1) an association of AIDS
as fatal, infectious, and sexually transmitted as promoted by the media,
and (2) the application of the traditional *saruwa* 'transmittable disease' and
the embedded *chhichhi durdur* 'separation' schemata and *randi* 'promiscuity—including blame' and *ghrinaa* 'disdain' schemata. Unfortunately, this
sad scenario was played out in village after village as FSWs returned from
India with *AIDS rog*.

In 1996 one major media event further supported the association of
HIV and AIDS with the girl trafficking discourse. One hundred twenty-
eight Nepali girls were repatriated to Nepal from the brothels of Bombay
(Ghimire 1997). The underage girls had been rescued from the brothels during police raids and held in various rehabilitation centers while the Indian
Government discussed repatriation of the girls to Nepal. At first, the Nepal
government was not responsive, but after much pressure they agreed to
repatriation (Ghimire 1997). Ghimire writes of the harmful impact a radio
interview had on one of the girls:

We did not receive favorable coverage from the media. The media
has started to publicize the issue, but in many cases some media
only want to publish the victims' names and photographs, which
creates a negative impact in the society. One of the rescued girls
from Bombay was working in a destitute home for widows and displaced women. One day she was interviewed on a radio program.
Immediately after the broadcast other destitute women living in

> the center recognized her voice and came to know about her sto-
> ry. Immediately she was forced by the other members to leave the
> center. They told her that she would continue the same business
> (prostitution) and defame those working in the center... sometimes
> the publicity of the victim creates a lot of problems for the rehabili-
> tation of the rescued girls as well as HIV positive cases. (Ghimire
> 1997:18)

This repatriation made major headlines in various Nepali mediums and
the association of AIDS with commercial sex work was further solidified in
the minds of the general public. And again, the elements of fear, hate, and
blame are clearly evident in this example. It is also evident that the application of the *randi* 'promiscuity' schema results in the labeling of those with
AIDS (due to the strong association with commercial sex) as "bad people."

During the second phase of the media's development of AIDS, the cultural model grew to include other "bad people" (drug users) as carriers of
AIDS. Again, when the findings of the early AIDS studies in Nepal began
to confirm that many injecting drug users (IDUs) were contracting AIDS,
the policy makers began to channel messages to the media that made a
strong association between drugs and AIDS. The media in turn passed the
information along and more stories about AIDS and drugs joined the stories
about prostitution. The association of AIDS with another group traditionally
branded as "bad people" further stigmatized the disease.

The findings of a six-month media study (Beine 2000) confirm that stories that promote fear, hate, and blame (the major elements of the widely
held cultural model) are still being widely circulated via the media. Tables
8.1 and 8.2 display the findings of the media study. Over a six-month period, the leading English daily newspaper published, on average, two and
a half stories weekly about HIV and AIDS. Sixty-six percent of the articles
were related principally to AIDS in Nepal and were published in the "local" section of the newspaper (table 8.1).[12] The other 34 percent of articles
related to AIDS internationally and appeared in the "international" section
(table 8.2). The articles in both sections can be grouped by focus. Forty-four
percent of the "local" articles centered primarily on sensationalizing the
AIDS epidemic in Nepal. Twenty-six percent of the articles would be considered more or less "educational" stories. Nine percent focused primarily
on condom use. Nine percent focused primarily on drug use. Seven percent
focused primarily on girl trafficking or commercial sex work issues. And 5
percent focused on political economic issues associated with AIDS. Of the

---

[12]The Valley/Nation section (local news) which usually fills one page, covers
the numbers of fatalities from the latest cholera epidemic, various bus accident
fatalities, and numbers of Maoist guerillas killed by the police in recent attacks. I
affectionately refer to this page of the newspaper as the "death" page. Again, it is
no wonder that AIDS is perceived by the general public as fatal.

international stories 73 percent were sensationalizing articles, 2 percent were primarily educational stories, and 4 percent focused on a trafficking discourse about AIDS.

Table 8.1. Local AIDS-related articles from a six-month analysis of the *Kathmandu Post,* listed by their focus, title, and association with the wider cultural model

Focus: Sensationalize AIDS	Fatal	Infectious	Sex	Drugs	Other
Over 25,000 Nepalis HIV +	X	X	X		condoms, western anti HIV drugs
Big Dilemma as AIDS Cases Increase		X	X	X	condoms
Tainted Blood Supply	X				
HIV Scourge in Morang	X				
TB Snowballing into Serious Threat	X	X			
Man Tricked Into Marrying AIDS Victim					"dreaded disease"
Rude Shock for Bridegroom with HIV	X	X			"killer disease"
Health Workers Unknowledgeable about AIDS	X				
Nepal Will Have 50,000 AIDS Cases By 2000	X	X	X		
AIDS Claims Seven	X				those who go to foreign countries
Health For All By 2000: A Distant Dream	X	X			
Children Suffer from AIDS Due to Parents Mistake	X	X	X	X	tied to "flesh traders"
HIV and AIDS Alarming in Developing World	X	X			

AIDS And Tuberculosis: A Bloody Tie	X				food: "but if the food and atmosphere are good, they may live longer"preference to attribute death to TB rather than AIDS
Blood Screening on the Agenda Due to HIV	X	X	X		transfusion
HIV to Orphan 40M By 2020	X	X	X		
As Ill Luck Would Have It, She Came Back with AIDS Virus	X	X		X	transfusion
HIV Tainted Needle Attacks—Rumor or Reality?	X	X	X	X	
Hospitals Facing Blood Shortage		X			blood related
Focus: AIDS education and awareness	**Fatal**	**Infectious**	**Sex**	**Drugs**	**Other**
Only Way to Arrest March of AIDS	X	X	X	X	condoms
Talk on HIV and AIDS	X	X			
Workshop on HIV and AIDS Ends	X				
Collective Efforts to Combat AIDS Stressed		X			
Awareness about Aids Vital		X			
Children's Move against AIDS	X				
AIDS Training Ends			X		

AIDS Awareness Workshop in Heteauda		X	X		
Awareness on AIDS Vital				X	"dreaded disease"
In Aid of AIDS (Quiz)	X	X	X	X	foreign origin
Workshop on HIV and AIDS Concludes		X	X		
Focus: Girl Trafficking/ FSW					
The Development Journey		X	X		
Sex for Sale		X	X	X	
They Went to the Land of Dreams to Seek Fortune but Found Only...	X	X	X		foreign tie
Focus: Condoms					
Condom Users on the Rise		X	X		
NGOs Promote Condom Use	X	X	X		
Condom Day for Community Mobilization		X	X		
Thanks to Condom		X	X		
Focus: Drugs					
50 Percent Pushers Are HIV Positive				X	"AIDS junkies"
Needle Exchange Helps Worsen HIV and AIDS Menace	X	X	X	X	expresses compassion toward drug users tied to foreigners
Drug Addicts Contract AIDS Due to Syringe Sharing	X	X		X	compassion expressed "ruined"
Focus: Political Economy					

All's Well at AIDS Meet but Grass Roots Voices Ignored		X	X		girl trafficking/ FSW discourse development discourse
1 out of 5 HIV Patients in Asia	X				new drug therapies economic issues of AIDS

Table 8.2. International AIDS related-articles from a six-month analysis of the *Kathmandu Post,* listed by their focus, title, and association with the wider cultural model

Focus: Sensationalize AIDS	Fatal	Infec-tious	Sex	Drugs	Other
Man Charged for Not Informing of AIDS	X	X	X		
Children Innocent Victims of Africa's AIDS Epidemic	X	X			
Doctor Accused of Trying to Kill Mistress with AIDS Injection	X	X	X		
HIV Cases Rose 10% in 1998: WHO		X			
South Africa Has Fastest Growing HIV Epidemic	X	X			
HIV-infected Mother Hangs Disabled Son					
AIDS, Poverty Destroy African Respect for Dead	X	X			
US Govt. Urged to Collect HIV Positive People's Names		X	X		tied to gays
Homosexuals Have Highest Percent of AIDS Infections			X	X	tied to gays
Death Takes a Holiday in the Gay Community	X	X	X	X	tied to gays new drug therapies
New Rulers	X	X	X		
AIDS Day Observed Amid Alarm in Developing World	X	X	X		isolation new drug therapies
820,000 Asians Contracted HIV in 1998: UN		X	X	X	
Urban Poor Women Face High Risk of Acquiring AIDS		X	X	X	

AIDS Virus Affects 7000 a Day	X	X			breast feeding
Indian State Heading for AIDS Disaster		X	X	X	
Focus: AIDS Education and Awareness					
Global Call to Action against AIDS	X	X	X		economic issues condoms
Clinton Marks World AIDS Day	X	X			
Mandela Hits Out at Silence on AIDS		X			
Anti-AIDS Substance in Urine Identified		X			
US Takes a Hard Look at Blacks, AIDS	X	X	X	X	tied to gays condoms
Focus: Trafficking Discourse					
AIDS, Poverty Spur Child Trafficking		X	X		economic tie

The majority of articles in both the local and international groupings sensationalize AIDS (54% of the total). These stories create fear that consequently spawns blame and hate toward PWAs. One exemplary article, titled "Big Dilemma for Nepal as AIDS Cases Increase," suggests that people with other medical problems will suffer more, as a consequence of the increase in AIDS cases:

> Nepal's health infrastructure may not be able to cope with the increasing number of HIV and AIDS patients who are certain to seek scarce hospital beds when they reach the stage of full-blown AIDS. In that case, people who need immediate medical attention, for example: appendicitis patients or patients with broken limbs will be the sufferers...If the number of people with full blown AIDS suddenly increases, a lot more people with HIV negative will also be sufferers. (Silwal 1998:2)

Such articles certainly play a role in the creation of fear, blame and hate toward PWAs in Nepal.

Although the articles are grouped by primary focus, it should be noted that associations between AIDS and various other topics were also made throughout the articles as is demonstrated in tables 8.1 and 8.2. The strongest associations throughout the articles were: (1) AIDS is infectious (mentioned in 78% of the articles), (2) AIDS is fatal (mentioned in 57% of the articles), (3) AIDS is sexually transmitted (mentioned in 54% of the articles), and (4) AIDS is drug use related (mentioned in 25% of the articles). It is clear from these findings that the media is strongly promoting the major elements of the wider cultural model (e.g., AIDS as a fatal, infectious, sexually transmitted disease). It is also easy to understand how the media's association of AIDS with CSWs and IDUs has stigmatized AIDS as a "bad people's" disease. The association made between AIDS and gays (another "bad people" group in Nepal) in four articles further adds to the image of AIDS as a "bad people's" disease. And, of course, societal blame and hate is traditionally warranted against "bad people" as a form of social control.

Besides these major thematic associations, several articles also made associations between AIDS and various issues we saw reflected in a few of the earlier narratives. For instance, in chapter six I noted the belief expressed by one PWA that an HIV positive diagnosis could turn to negative. One article (*Kathmandu Post* 1998a) commenting on the plight of children in South Africa, states that "two-thirds of babies who test positive for the AIDS virus at birth later test negative." Likewise, several narrators (chapter six) commented on the possibility of new drug therapies to cure AIDS. As noted in table 8.3, three articles included comments regarding the availability of these new drug therapies in the West. Other themes familiar in the narratives, such as a foreign origin of AIDS (four articles) and the association between good diet, positive attitude and health (one article), are demonstrated in table 8.1.

The theme of societal compassion for drug users that was evident among the male urban PWAs in chapter six is also expressed in two different articles. For instance one article tells of an "unfortunate young lad who fell into the clutches of drug abuse" and claims that "the very society which could have rescued him from the horrors of drug abuse was one way or the other responsible for pushing him into the present misery" (*Kathmandu Post* 1998b).

The director of the National Center made the following comments in his evaluation of the media's recent portrayal of HIV and AIDS, which included advice for future use of the media in the fight against HIV and AIDS in Nepal:

> In the Nepali media today, we see a qualitative improvement in the coverage of HIV and AIDS. It is fairly rare to see newspapers and magazines publishing pictures of people living with HIV, or their names. The articles are factually more accurate, fairer, they address the root issues and not just the sensational elements of an HIV and AIDS story. Radio and television have also seen improvements, with the introduction of an adolescent sexuality hotline on FM radio as well as longer issue-based coverage of the disease on community radio and Radio Nepal.

But still, the lack of accurate and up-to-date information on the scientific, sociological, developmental or human rights aspects of the
disease still hobbles the media's handling of HIV and AIDS coverage
within Nepal. If the press and public relations firms are going to be
used as vehicles for awareness creation, it is still necessary to sensi-
tize mainstream media professionals regularly about HIV and AIDS.
Media seminars on HIV and AIDS cannot be one shot affairs, they
have to be regular and sustained. Otherwise, instead of awareness
we're going to have more confusion in the Nepali public.

Aside from the mainstream media, the tabloid press still by and large
treats HIV and AIDS either as a titillating sensationalist news item to
boost circulation, or as an excuse to stereotype, stigmatize or victim-
ize people living with HIV. This has only served to scare the public,
alienate infected people, and perpetuate prevailing ignorance.

Sensitizing media will check the negative side effects of inaccurate
information and help move on to spreading mass awareness and ultimately bring about the behavior change that is needed to halt the
epidemic. It is clear that if Nepal and other South Asian countries
are to tackle a rapid spread of HIV there has to be a radically new
approach to using communications for awareness building. Present
efforts within Nepal for instance may be inadequate to meet the
challenges of this looming crisis. (Karki 1998)

In this section we have seen the interplay that has existed between three
unique groups (NGOs, doctors and policy makers, and the media) in the
creation of a cultural model (I) of HIV and AIDS in Nepal. AIDS has entered
the public conscience of Nepal, in part, via the messages of these various
groups. Because AIDS is a new disease, the formulation of a cultural model
of HIV and AIDS has been strongly influenced by the preliminary messages
about the disease. Once enough information existed, the disease was categorized (through the schematization process) and relevant associated cultural
schemata were applied. The messages of "fatal," "infectious" and "sexually
transmitted" communicated by the NGOs and doctors and policy makers via
the media were enough to evoke associations of AIDS as a *saruwa rog* (requiring the practice of *chhichhi durdur*), and as a disease affecting primarily
those who are *randi*. These various associations have produced a cultural
model of AIDS in Nepal that has, in turn, created an atmosphere of fear,
hate and blame, which is directed at PWAs in Nepal.

8.3.2 Recent media representations

For comparative purposes I conducted another six-month analysis of HIV
and AIDS-related articles published in the *Kathmandu Post* for the period

from November 2012 through April 2013. There were eleven such articles published during this time period and the titles of the articles and the various embedded elements are noted in table 8.3. As can be seen from the data, the elements most referenced were the issues of migrant labor and organizational assistance (seven references for each). The elements referenced in the remaining articles, in order of decreasing occurrence, were the fatal nature of AIDS (six references), hope and available treatment (five references), the remaining problems for PLWHAs, such as issues hindering availability to ART treatments (four references), association with sex and stigma (three each), and drug-use and the infectious nature of HIV (two each). Even though the "fatal nature of AIDS" was frequently referred to, this element often appeared in the same articles that also spoke of available ART.

This is quite a change from the focus of media articles from the same publication some ten years earlier. At that time the majority of articles focused primarily on the infectious nature of AIDS, followed by the fatal nature of the disease, and then on the issues of sex and drug use respectively. In these recent articles, while the infectious nature of AIDS is still noted in two articles, it has dropped to the bottom of the list. This could certainly have the impact of lessening the associated schema of *chhichhi durdur* in the long run. And while the concept of death (i.e., fatal) is still strongly associated with HIV as it was ten years earlier, it is now more in the context of the past tense; most of the articles that mention death do so in the context of people who are now successfully "living with HIV," while their husbands had "died of AIDS years ago." Thus, though the cultural model still includes the concept of death, it is only as a fading memory, now giving way to the current era of "living with HIV" and hope.

In the previous study, sex and drug use were the third and fourth most common elements respectively. Now these two round-out the bottom three (along with infectious association). This should certainly have the long-term impact of lessening the association between HIV and *randi* and "bad persons" as well, which could also subsequently result in less application of the *ghrinaa* and *hela* schemas toward PLWHAs. And while migration was certainly part of the earlier discourse, it was usually in reference to male migrants (with secondary reference to sex). Now migration co-tops the list, but it is in the form of the wives of migrant laborers with no reference at all made to sex. And the idea of hope, associated principally with ARV, but also perhaps associated with help coming from organizations, is developing quickly as a major element of the discourse. Hope was conspicuously absent in the previous study, but it has made its debut to the list of elements in the new cultural model.

Table 8.3. HIV and AIDS-related articles published in the *Kathmandu Post* for the period from November 2012 through April 2013, listed by their date and association with the wider cultural model

Date	Title	ARV/Hope	Fatal	Infectious	Drug-user	Sex-related	Migrant-related	Stigma	Organizational help	Problems
04/19/13	All in a Song	X			X	X	X	X	X	
04/04/13	From HIV Victims to Independent Women	X	X				X		X	
03/16/13	Workers from India Prone to HIV/AIDS		X				X			
02/26/13	HIV-infected Women's Drive against AIDS	X	X				X	X	X	X
01/19/13	Children with HIV Get Helping Hands								X	
01/07/13	HIV-infected Struggling to Earn a Living	X	X				X			X
12/13/12	Fund-raising Campaign for Children with HIV Begins								X	

Date	Title								
12/06/12	Intervention Major Reason for Decelerated HIV Spread Rate	X			X	X	X		
12/03/12	AIDS Awareness Out and About		X	X		X			
12/30/12	VOICES: WORLD AIDS DAY: The Price of Ignorance		X	X				X	
11/17/12	HIV Takes Its Toll On Dalit Settlement		X			X	X	X	X

It is as if the prior media model has been turned on its head. Many of the elements that were at the top before are still in the model, but now at the bottom; and a few new elements have been added. It would seem that, if the media is successful at continuing the promotion of this new model (and as people begin to take in these media representations of HIV and AIDS and integrate them into their own personal model) we may see a shift in cultural models. Fear, hate and blame (the key elements of the earlier model—and the driver of remaining stigma) could be lessened. It must be cautioned, however, that the media plays only a part in the creation of a cultural model, but they are an influential player; and while this certainly impacts the urban areas of Nepal, the rural areas (where media is less influential) will likely be slower to change.

8.4 A comparison of cultural models— implications of underlying biological schemata

The research presented in this book affords good opportunity to compare the emerging cultural model of (I) AIDS with other models around the world. For instance, Paul Farmer (1994:805) identifies the key elements of a Haitian village cultural model with certain shared understandings: (1) AIDS is a new disease; (2) associated with skin infections, drying up, diarrhea; and, most strongly, with tuberculosis; (3) resulting from sexual contact with the carrier, from voodoo, or both; (4) caused by a microbe; (5) transmitted through contact with contaminated blood; and (6) associated closely with larger political-economic issues. Besides this list, Farmer identifies, but leaves unspecified, other key elements of rural Haitians' understandings about AIDS as fatal, which produce much "personal fear" (1994:805). Likewise, Herzlich and Pierret (1989) have demonstrated how the media were influential in the construction of a cultural model (I) of AIDS in France that socially constructed an understanding of AIDS as (1) fatal and infectious, producing great fear; and (2) sexually transmitted, and tied to a group considered deviant (i.e., homosexuals), thus creating an atmosphere of moral judgment and blame. Albert (1986), studying the media's involvement in the creation of a cultural model (I) of AIDS in America has demonstrated that fatal and infectious were two major elements (due mainly to the initial "unknown" nature of the disease) that produced much fear. And because of the "fear of contagion" and the association with the gay community, a major theme of the media was blame, usually in the form of considering AIDS as a punishment of God. And Lyttleton (1996) has demonstrated how AIDS in Thailand (via the media again) was associated with the much feared "other." Like in Nepal, the major association was with prostitutes and drug users (societal deviants).

Although many specifics differ between the Nepali, Haitian, French, American, and Thai models, there are some striking similarities between the models (in form) as well. For instance, all of these models first associated AIDS with marginalized groups. In Haiti, America, and France, this group was homosexuals, while in Thailand and Nepal, it was prostitutes (i.e., those considered *randi*) and drug users, both classified as "bad people" groups who were marginalized by the wider society. Next, both models display the extension of traditional ideas to the new disease. In the case of Haiti, traditional ideas suggest that AIDS can be contracted through voodoo. In Nepal, AIDS, which is considered a *saruwa* illness, can be contracted through the same means as other *saruwa* illnesses (like TB[13] and leprosy). In France, it was pre-existing understandings of STDs (particularly genital herpes) that were influential in shaping a social understanding of HIV and AIDS. In America, ideas about the great plague of the Dark Ages (since "plague" had been popularly presented as an image schema for AIDS) were extended to AIDS. And in Thailand, AIDS was likened to other diseases and so it was associated with the feared "other."

Blame is a common feature of all the models although the object of blame differs from culture to culture. For instance, in the case of the American, French, Thai, and Nepali models, marginalized groups are targeted, while in the case of Haiti, Farmer (1994) demonstrates that blame is directed toward perceived agents of hegemony.

The positing of dualistic explanations for the disease (although they can differ from culture to culture) is also common to various models. For instance, as noted earlier, *karma* (past actions) and drug use were both cited in Nepali texts as possible causes of AIDS. Likewise, Farmer notes the dualistic explanations of AIDS as the possible result of "germs" and "voodoo." Closely related to the idea of dualistic explanations for illness is the notion of multiple causes for disease. The understanding of AIDS being the result of a viral infection or a punishment for sin is common to the American (Giblin 1995:136) and French (Herzlich 1989:1237) models.[14] The notion of multiple causation of illness has also been noted in general models of illness in Brazil (Price 1984:328). In all of these cases we see multiple notions of disease causation that combine traditional beliefs regarding illness with modern understandings of Western biomedicine.

---

[13]Interestingly, in Nepal and France, AIDS is most closely linked with tuberculosis. Farmer quotes one informant as saying, "tuberculosis and *SIDA* (the local and French term for AIDS) resemble each other greatly. They say that TB is *SIDA*'s little brother, because you see them together." I also heard this same analogy used in Nepal. The common association is probably due to the fact that TB is the most common opportunistic infection that affects PWAs in these two countries.

[14]It is also possible that the attribution of multiple causation to disease is universal. Sontag (1991:44) has demonstrated how disease in the Iliad and Odyssey is attributed both to supernatural punishment and natural causes.

In all the models we see the common themes of fear, blame, and hate, because of the association of AIDS with "bad people." In many cases, the common themes have produced common responses. For instance, the early American model, chronicled by several other authors, shares many striking similarities with the Nepali model. For example, Giblin (1995) demonstrated various reactions of fear by the general public against PWAs: people didn't want to sit with PWAs or use utensils of PWAs, morticians refused to embalm the bodies of PWAs, and doctors began wearing masks to treat PWAs or refused to treat them altogether. All of these reactions have also been noted in Nepal.[15] Likewise, Flynn (1996) demonstrates how the early model in America (AIDS as a "gay" disease) was created by the media, and how those infected were branded as "bad people" (1996:14). Flynn also discusses the various rumors that PWAs were deliberately infecting others (1996:14), a product of the extreme fear associated with the disease. I have previously described similar events in Nepal.

Anyone familiar with AIDS research in any given country might recognize themes commonly expressed elsewhere, in the findings of this research. It seems that there are some universals associated with AIDS around the world, for instance, the association of AIDS with "bad people" and blame. Sontag (1991:59) writes, "Any important disease whose causality is murky, and for which treatment is ineffective, tends to be awash in significance... First the subjects of deepest dread (corruption, decay, pollution, weakness) are identified with the disease." Addressing blame specifically, Sontag (1988:101) suggests, "It seems that societies need to have one illness which becomes identified with evil, and attaches blame to its victims." The association between AIDS and STDs with blame prompts an association with strange beliefs of contagion. Sontag (1988:112) explains, "Infectious disease to which sexual fault is attached always inspires fears of easy contagion and bizarre fantasies of transmission by non-venereal means in public places." Sabatier (1989) suggests that blame as well as prejudice are common associations made with STDs worldwide. He concludes that "the process of attributing blame does not always require evidence, and tends to focus on people who are not considered 'normal' by the majority, especially on minorities or foreigners" (1989:66).

Janet McGrath (1991) proposes that all cultures exhibit universal responses to epidemic disease. She suggests that that if an epidemic is evaluated as acute, then direct actions, such as flight or extraordinary preventative measures like quarantine and isolation, are implemented as common adaptive strategies. If an epidemic is perceived as non-acute, then indirect action,

---

[15]One NGO director told me that when they have taken bodies to be cremated at the local temple, they are often refused or charged double once the priests learn that the person was a PWA. And one of the leading doctors treating PWAs in Nepal told me that once he discovers a person is HIV positive he will wear a mask or only speak through a glass window.

such as ostracizing and scapegoating those who are considered at risk, or resignation toward the disease (fatalism) are displayed as common responses. McGrath suggests that these responses are common themes throughout the epidemic disease. Further, she suggests that these responses are mostly biologically adaptive.[16] Interestingly, in Nepal, both direct action (quarantine and isolation *'chhichhi durdur'*) and indirect action (scapegoating—e.g., strong blame of prostitutes [those who are *randi*]) are common responses toward those with AIDS.

As an interesting side note, although McGrath doesn't mention "schema" by name, she acknowledges that a process (similar to the schematization process described in this book) underlies the production of these common responses to epidemic disease. For example, she suggests that the first response to epidemic disease "is based on a familiar response derived from previous experience" (1991:408). This is akin to the idea that schemata created from past experience serve as a kind of template that functions to make meaning of new events that are perceived to be similar. She suggests that "behavioral responses begin with 'normal practice.' That is, the earliest responses to epidemics are those that have been used successfully in response to other crises" (1991:409). McGrath's proposal of the application of "familiar responses" (1991:412) in order to control epidemic disease implies the application of underlying biologically based schemata. This would certainly help to explain, at least in part, the *chhichhi durdur* 'separation', *saruwa* 'transmittable disease', and *randi* 'promiscuity' schemata that have been so easily associated with AIDS in Nepal.

The striking similarity between various cultural models of HIV and AIDS might partially be a result of the application of various universal schemata that produce the universal similarities noted. These universal schemata, in turn, play a part in the social construction of meaning associated with HIV and AIDS, as they are embedded as fundamental elements of particular cultural models of HIV and AIDS. For instance, I propose that in Nepal, biologically based schemata (like Shore's PIMS) are embedded in higher level schemata, such as the *saruwa* schema, and these schemata are in turn embedded in higher level schemata (cultural models).

Other such universal schemata might be (1) a "sexually transmitted disease" schema that posits the possibility for strange methods of transference as noted above, and (2) a "survival" schema. It seems that some sort of basic survival schema exists that causes us, when a disease is understood as fatal and infectious, to act in a way that would assure maximal safety. This would explain in part, the "fatal trump card" idea spoken of earlier as well as the doctors' preferences to act on the conclusions of their cultural model rather than their biomedical knowledge. According to Flynn and Lound (1995:55),

---

[16]McGrath demonstrates that although these responses are believed to be biologically adaptive, under certain conditions they have led to social disintegration.

many irrational fears and actions of people toward AIDS are a result of the fear of AIDS, which in turn, is a result of the fatal nature of the disease.

Herzlich and Pierret, although unfamiliar with the schema concept, have written that it is customary to compare AIDS to other diseases, and to associate AIDS with the oldest and least familiar disease, the plague:

> As an instance of this, let us examine the likening of AIDS to cancer, the plague, syphilis, and leprosy. Such comparisons give rise to what can be called a system of second degree metaphors. AIDS was associated successfully or simultaneously, with all of these diseases, each of which had served as a metaphor at a certain epoch. Although AIDS condensed all of these into a single metaphor, it would during its construction, tend to be most likened to the oldest of them, the disease most distant from and strangest to us. Although the first articles in 1981-1982 mainly compared it to cancer, the prototype of 'modern' illnesses, it would then be likened to diseases—usually the plague—that have vanished in the West. In fact, the comparison was more frequently made with the plague than syphilis, a disease more like it and closer to us... AIDS, as stated, has been the subject of a discourse about the 'other', who is as far as possible from ourselves, as foreign and strange as possible. This discourse works by repeatedly making a cleavage between one's self and others. This is not new: foreigners have always been accused of bringing epidemics. (Herzlich and Pierret 1989:1241)

This comparison of AIDS with other diseases, based in the specifics of the French cultural model, also provides the explanation for the application of various schemata associated with AIDS. We see other illnesses used schematically as a prototype to understand AIDS, and we see, in part, the explanation behind the application of AIDS as a foreign disease and its association with marginalized groups (i.e., those we consider strangest). Although not all of the questions are answered by my proposal that underlying biological schemata inform higher level schemata, and therefore ultimately cultural models, I hope my proposal does shed some light on the connection between cultural and biological phenomena in the creation of a cultural model of HIVf and AIDS in Nepal.

9

Conclusions

In this book I have illuminated a cultural model of AIDS in Nepal and have examined underlying illness schemata. We have seen that the way people make sense of AIDS is through the application of cultural models that, in turn, are made up of various cultural and biological schemata. I have used a methodology that combines cognitive anthropological methods with discourse analysis in order to study meaning construction of HIV and AIDS in Nepal.

Based on the findings of the various studies, I have proposed several group specific cultural models of HIV and AIDS as well as a larger over-arching cultural model of AIDS that encompasses fear, hate, and blame as major elements. And in this second edition I have suggested that some modifications have taken place to this cultural model in the years since the first edition. I have also examined various cultural illness schemata that are embedded in the different cultural models as well as proposing various biologically based schemata that are embedded as constituent elements in these cultural illness schemata. I have also examined the many factors, both cultural and biological, that have contributed to a dominant cultural model of AIDS, and to various sub-group cultural models, in Nepal. In this final chapter, I conclude by reviewing the findings, discussing the implications of the findings, and discussing a few remaining issues.

9.1 Review of the findings

My objective in writing this book has been to examine and describe cultural models of HIV and AIDS in Nepal in depth, both the past and emerging models, as well as to describe the current AIDS prevalence in Nepal. In the preface to the first edition, I introduced the topic, including the structure of the book. In chapter one, I introduced Nepal, explaining how many aspects of her geography, economy, history, educational system, and religion have played a large part in fostering the AIDS epidemic in Nepal. Throughout the later chapters we have seen the impact of these various factors: the impact of geography upon poverty and migration, the influence of Western development paradigms, the influence of hegemonic educational systems, of Brahmin domination, and of the religious caste system (based on the pollution-purity foundational schema).

In chapter two, I examined AIDS as a social and biological phenomenon. I discussed various cultural models of HIV and AIDS worldwide and elaborated on the dynamic nature of cultural models. I also discussed HIV and AIDS as an economic issue in which the first and third worlds are experiencing an ever-widening gap.

In chapter three, I discussed the current AIDS situation in Nepal in depth. I presented the epidemiological facts associated with the epidemic in Nepal and examined further much of the literature on HIV and AIDS in Nepal. We have seen that various structural factors, such as poverty (in many ways related to geography), have created a "push factor" that forces many men to seek work in areas where HIV is prevalent, and forces many women into commercial sex work. We have seen how many cultural beliefs and issues of agency have also further predisposed individuals to HIV infection. Furthermore, I examined the impact that the Nepali emphasis upon Western development has had in the development of various prevention paradigms in Nepal. And I examined the emerging AIDS discourses, concluding that AIDS in Nepal is, indeed, a socially constructed disease with a biological basis.

In chapter four, I described the theoretical framework for the projects conducted to illuminate cultural models and embedded schemata. I examined cultural models as both producers and products and introduced the ideas of schema theory, including what schemata are (and the various kinds), how they are proposed to work, the various characteristics of schemata, and I introduced recent modifications to the schema concept that have guided this research. I also discussed the various cognitive methodologies of systematic data collection and narrative analysis employed in this research and promoted the value of a combined methodology.

In chapter five, I presented the findings of a rural cognitive study that illuminated an emerging general cultural model of HIV and AIDS and provided insight into the many changes that have taken place in regard to illness beliefs and practices over the past twenty-five years, in a rural village in central Nepal. The findings illustrated two major cultural models of HIV and AIDS (one incorporating the other but then adding to it), both of which were produced by combining information obtained from prevention messages (based on Western prevention paradigms) and by applying traditional schemata.

In chapter six, I presented the findings of a narrative analysis study that confirmed the findings of the rural study (i.e., illuminated an emerging wider cultural model) and refined the specifics of certain sub-group models. I noted differences between the cultural models of rural and urban dwellers and between male and female city dwellers. I have identified various traditional schemata regarding worry and health, separation of people with transmissible diseases, and sexual promiscuity that are being applied to AIDS by all of the various sub-groups because of the messages about AIDS that people are receiving. Beyond this, schemata regarding *karma*, drug use, and the importance of good diet and positive attitude are evident in the narratives of city dwellers. Schemata about eating and the shifting nature of illness were exclusive to the rural narratives. And gender-specific schemata regarding drug use and the expected unfaithfulness of men (including a fate schema) are being applied by city males and females respectively. Using an explanatory model (Kleinman 1980), I also examined the various signs and symptoms, causes, treatments, pathophysiologies, and prognoses people attribute to HIV and AIDS in Nepal. Besides further illuminating a wider cultural model and refining the various elements of particular sub-group models, the narrative analysis study allowed me to confirm the validity of the use of the narrative analysis method cross-linguistically.

In chapter seven, I presented a composite dominant cultural model of HIV and AIDS based on the findings of the rural cognitive study and the narrative analysis study. I also further examined some of the underlying illness schemata, proposing a foundational schema of "purity and pollution" that informs various aspects of Nepali culture including people's understanding of HIV and AIDS.

In chapter eight, I examined the role of various cultural and biological factors in the creation of a dominant cultural model of hate, fear and blame. I discussed the role that NGOs, medical doctors and policy planners, the media, and underlying biologically based schemata have all played in the creation of this dominant cultural model of HIV and AIDS in Nepal.

9.2 Implications of the research

What are the implications of this research? Throughout this book we have seen the result of current prevention strategies that are in place in Nepal and I have suggested that in many ways, these strategies have contributed to growth of the problem rather than to the reduction of HIV and AIDS. A thorough understanding of all of the complex factors involved in the spread of disease should guide prevention and education strategies for any disease. AIDS in Nepal is no exception. In this book I have described the process (schematization) and the resultant schemata and cognitive models that people employ in making meaning of the thing called "*AIDS rog*" 'AIDS disease'. It is these cognitive models that ultimately determine people's responses to AIDS. An understanding of the various cognitive schemata applied to create the dominant cultural model of AIDS (and sub-group models) leads me to suggest a few changes to the current AIDS prevention strategies. For instance, although I agree that "awareness building" is vital to the prevention and control of HIV and AIDS in Nepal, the content of the messages should be different. First of all, I suggest that prevention planners stop associating AIDS so directly with sex in the public prevention campaign materials. The policy planners have thus far implemented a Western approach (advocating the open discussion of sex) dispersing condom ads and talk about AIDS and prostitution all over Nepal. Condom distribution has become the number one priority for the HIV and AIDS education/prevention program in Nepal. In Nepal, many things are not necessarily considered "wrong" until they are exposed.[1] Because sex is traditionally a taboo subject for public discussion in Nepal, the open display of condoms and discussion of sex in public has had the result of making sex appear sinful. The current campaign's emphasis on sex (condoms) has further stigmatized AIDS, making it a "bad people's" disease. As a result, people are even afraid to get checked (and certainly will not tell anyone if they suspect they are positive) and I imagine the problem will grow. Statistics show that men still aren't using condoms! I believe that materials that further stigmatize AIDS will only hurt the cause, not help it.

Likewise, the strong association of AIDS with sex has activated the traditional *randi* 'promiscuity' schema, causing women to avoid protecting themselves:

> The prevailing notion of a woman of "good character" in Nepal prevents women from taking measures to protect themselves from STDs and HIV. By discussing sex generally or condom use in particular, women define themselves as sexual beings and thereby call into question their own character and fidelity. (Shresta et al. 1998:1)

Also because AIDS has been strongly associated with prostitution in the media and education campaigns, the application of traditional *randi* schema to those with AIDS further stigmatizes PWAs (persons with AIDS) as "bad people." This stigmatization only reinforces non-reporting. The Western agencies like UNAIDS that are leading the fight against AIDS in Nepal thus far are promoting a media campaign that openly emphasizes these sexual issues. I realize that the association between AIDS and sex is direct and so educational materials need to include that element, but the "public face" of AIDS should be presented more euphemistically, as is the custom in Nepal, rather than so blatantly. Nichter (1989) has demonstrated (in a South Asian context) that one can be sensitive to cultural taboos and still find a way in any culture to talk about any topic. I suggest that advertisements targeting

---

[1]Parish (1991) describes the Newar model of the mind, which includes the concept of *lajya* 'moral shame' or 'embarrassment experiences', when one is caught lying or doing something considered socially improper.

men that talk about "taking care" when "walking with the girls," etc. should be used rather than the current slogan, which is "let's wear condoms and chase away AIDS."

Next, because current campaigns focus on the fatal and infectious nature of AIDS, it is being classed in traditional categories known as *thulo* 'big', *saruwa* 'infectious' and *antim* 'fatal'. Associated with these categories is the idea of *chhichhi durdur* 'separation' of an infectious person. Many PWAs with whom I talked told me that they are voluntarily living separate from others in order to "save them." There are cultural features at work here that perhaps could be built on and worked into the media campaign to target PWAs, perhaps focusing on "responsibility" of PWAs to protect others rather than the focus on "safe sex" and "condoms." Inherent in the idea of "responsibility" is sexual responsibility, but again, to make that explicit is unnecessary and actually might be counterproductive.

Various cultural ideas could be easily built upon in the AIDS prevention campaign. For instance, the idea of low places as places to avoid could be built on in AIDS prevention campaigns. Migration to the Terai or India is a major risk factor for Nepali men. Keeping people out of areas of high HIV and AIDS prevalence will help minimize the spread of AIDS in Nepal.

Likewise, the cultural idea of the importance of not worrying and keeping optimistic (for PWAs) is a positive value. A positive outlook does, indeed, increase one's lifespan: negativity predisposes one to illness.[2] Building on this belief could encourage a longer life for PWAs. And the healthier they can stay, the less of a drain they will be upon the already stretched Nepali medical system.

Another cultural feature that could be built upon is related to the concept of *karma*. Once people discover that they are HIV positive they begin talking about stopping the bad actions and doing good works in order to build their *karma* for the next life. Again, this can be worked into the "responsibility" theme and PWAs can be encouraged to protect others through responsible actions (e.g., abstinence or safe sex). This concept can also be built upon by encouraging PWAs to build good *karma* by being involved in AIDS prevention education with their peers.

Sabatier (1989:65) has suggested that while "education programs and messages designed for the industrialized countries are often inappropriate in the Third World; traditional customs and beliefs may be effective vehicles for indigenous campaigns." Likewise, Nichter (1989) has argued for a more creative use of traditionally appropriate analogy in modern health messages. He advocates the use of cultural metaphors and analogies to exact a closer fit between health concepts and

---

[2]Various studies have demonstrated that positive responses to stressful life events (such as an HIV positive diagnosis) are linked to positive immunologic and health outcomes. For example see Bower et al. (1998) and Kemeny et al. (1995).

prevention messages. Gaenszle also suggests that if metaphors and analogies are already in place to express illness, then logically, healing should be expressed in the same way:

> In recent works in medical anthropology frequent use has been made of the concept of metaphor as an analytical tool. It has been pointed out that bodily processes, and particularly illnesses, are very often described by metaphorical expressions—not only by lay persons (e.g., in patient-doctor conversations) but also in the discourse of medical experts (e.g., textbooks, scientific literature). Whether these are "dead" metaphors, like when we speak of the body as having a kind of military immune-system (red blood cells, anti-bodies "attacking" or "fighting" intruding bacteria), or whether these are "living" metaphors, for example when one attempts to describe stress symptoms by comparing the nerves with weak current cables (Sebus and Oderwald 1991:120), in both cases a psychological process is expressed in terms of a more tangible imagery from another (non-psychological) domain.
>
> So, if illness is expressed metaphorically, it logically follows that the removal of illness, healing, also is expressed in such terms (i.e., "medicine X strengthens the body's defenses," etc.), and, as one expects, the metaphors of healing usually correspond to the metaphors of illness. This is also what the ethnologist observes in traditional societies: the healers diagnose illness in the local idiom—and expel it according to the same logic. (Gaenszle 1994:256)

Throughout this research I have illustrated various metaphoric schemata that are used to make meaning of illness in Nepal. I have also illustrated that the main slogan of the current prevention campaign employs a borrowed Western military schema ('chase away') that seems inappropriate. I would advocate the use of more appropriate health related analogies in the AIDS prevention campaign in Nepal. I have previously mentioned several schemata that could be built upon, but there are probably many other cultural metaphors associated with illness (such as 'eating') that could and should be exploited.

The most important recommendation I have is to provide education by appropriate analogy. Use the familiar to explain the new. For those interested in what this might look like, I have proposed a model that incorporates these ideas into a comprehensive HIV prevention program for Nepal (Beine 2011), that along with being a better fit for various audiences, might at the same time help to reduce stigma. The interested reader is strongly encouraged to consult this resource.

9.3 Final issues

During my research a few questions arose that I have not yet addressed. For instance, there is the issue I raised in the introduction as to why I encountered less display of emotion (depression) by the PWAs during the interviews than I had anticipated. We have seen the strong influence of the *karma* schema throughout the research. The data demonstrate the belief that AIDS can be the result of bad *karma* 'deeds done either in this life or the last life' and the need to earn merit in preparation for the next life (chapter six). And at first I wondered if the less emotional responses were perhaps a product of the Vedic worldview of reincarnation. Heinrich Harrer (1992:205) suggests that "Tibetans do not mourn for the dead in our sense of the word. Sorrow for the parting is relieved by the prospect of rebirth, and death has no terrors for the Buddhist." Although many of my informants were Hindus rather than Buddhists, both of these world religions—based on the same Vedic worldview—teach the concepts of *karma, dharma* 'one's duty in life', and reincarnation. Although this is a plausible explanation, it seems, after further research, that the observation might be due to a combination of factors, including the belief in reincarnation. First of all, it is clear from various narratives that deep depression was the initial reaction for many (several contemplated suicide), followed by anger and a desire to "hurt others," especially those who had infected them. So, perhaps the stoic reaction (by this I mean a matter of fact way of telling the story) is as much a feature of Nepali discourse as it is a true statement of psychological condition. Having said this, however, it is also clear that PWAs soon focus on the positive and begin to think about "doing good things" to make up for the "bad." For instance, the director of one Nepali NGO who witnessed the death of four girls from her own NGO during the last year of their lives, told me, "At first they were depressed. But after two or three days they were normal, they forgot about it. From then on they behaved like a normal person." So, depression would seem to be the initial reaction, but it is soon superseded by the application of the good *karma* schema. Perhaps the application of the worry-leads-to-disease schema also discourages an individual from focusing on the negative and becoming depressed. There was a strong sense throughout the narratives that negative thoughts would only bring one down (to use an American schema), and cause sickness. Perhaps these factors combine to explain the less emotive reaction noted.

Many things I saw during my stay in Nepal also left me wondering if people might actually infect themselves with the HIV virus in order to get financial gain. I was told that people had lied about their HIV status in order to try to get a job with Prerarna (the NGO that employs many PWAs). The phenomenon of purposeful infection has been documented elsewhere. Merrill Singer (1999) writes of people in Africa seeking to become HIV infected. In that case it is "the dance with the cruel bureaucracy that leads people to want to be sick, to literally want to die later to survive a little better right now."

In the Nepali case, life for the average villager is a daily struggle for survival and foreign aid is a major industry. These villagers are smart—they have figured out that in order to get the money associated with a development project a community need only to identify its number one "felt need" (the new development "buzz word"), the thing which the organization asking is able to provide. If a health development organization asks, "What is your greatest felt need?," then clean water and medical help are the main answers. If technological or agricultural development is the thrust of the NGOs work, then electricity or help with crops becomes the major "felt need."

As has been previously noted, AIDS has become the hot topic in Nepal and there are many organizations with lots of money that are now focusing primarily on HIV and AIDS. Many of these organizations work exclusively with former FSWs, helping them start small businesses or teaching them skills such as sewing. The average villager is unable to access any of the money associated with these projects unless s/he is a member of the target group the NGO has identified. This begs the question: will the average poor villager, suffering under the weight of poverty (and unable to access the huge amounts of foreign aid money because s/he is not in the target group), begin to pursue prostitution or an HIV positive status in order to be eligible for resources found exclusively among the girl trafficking and HIV and AIDS focused organizations sponsored by international donors? [3] Only time will tell, but it has already been confirmed that some have arrived at the doors of Prerana carrying with them a fictitious HIV positive status, seeking jobs that are reserved for the HIV positive members of the organization.

This fact should serve as a gentle reminder that there are many major problems facing Nepalis at the end of the twentieth century, and NGOs need to avoid "bandwagon" or "current trend" thrusts, and seek to help all those in need. If this message is ignored, it is very possible that organizations seeking to combat problems such as HIV and AIDS will inadvertently promote the growth of the problem by encouraging people to become members of the target population in order to avail themselves of resources they could not otherwise access.

There are also issues remaining regarding the language of AIDS. As I discussed in the preface to the first edition, the verb *phasnu* 'ensnared' was often used to describe a person's experience with AIDS. The verb *lagnu* 'captured' or 'possessed' was another common verb used to describe their condition.[4]

---

[3]In 2010 there was a proposal before the government to allocate (from the national budget) 3,000 Nepalese rupees (about 40 U.S. dollars) per month to about 3,000 HIV positive widows and 1,000 infected and affected children (Sharma 2010).

[4]*Phasnu/lagnu*, therefore, might be identified as a cultural illness schema in Nepal. Although there might be some semantic domain overlap between the Nepali *phasnu/lagnu* concepts and the western war schemata used for illness, the Nepali

Both of these verbs associated most frequently with AIDS in Nepal (*phas-nu/lagnu*) were spoken only in the passive form. Watters and Rajbhandary (2000:120) suggest that *lagnu* is a verb commonly associated with various physical ailments in Nepali and that sentences using this verb are most often spoken in the passive. The use of the passive sentence construction,[5] a prevalent feature in the Nepali language, has been identified as a linguistic feature common throughout many of the other languages of South Asia as well (Masica 1971). Although various linguists have addressed the issue of the function of passives linguistically (Comrie 1989; Foley and Van Valin Jr. 1984), few have dealt with the question of what the cognitive implications for such a linguistic feature might be.

It seems to me that the use of the passive has cognitive implications for reducing the level of personal responsibility associated with the contraction of disease. Instead of "I am sick," the preferred Nepali phrase is "I have been captured by sickness." Responsibility for one's own situation is lessened and blame can more easily be deferred to fate. Perhaps this preference for the passive is a result of an overarching attitude of fatalism prevalent throughout Nepal (Bista 1991).

In conclusion to the second edition of this book, I want to focus on a few remaining issues that should continue to draw our attention in relation to HIV and AIDS in Nepal. First of all, housewives of migrant laborers now make up the largest single group of HIV-infected persons in Nepal (Sarkar 2010). Despite that fact there remain few programs specifically tailored for these women (or for wives of migrant laborers in general). Regarding the disparity often afforded women in HIV programs, Stephen Lewis (2006), UN Special Envoy for HIV and AIDS in Africa has commented:

> The single most intractable dilemma has been the excruciating vulnerability of women, the huge and disproportionate numbers of deaths they face, their overwhelming responsibilities for the sick and orphaned, and the apparent inability of African Governments or the international community to do anything decisive about it...

> Let's be frank about it: the United Nations' record on women is abysmal. It's been abysmal for sixty years. Both internally and externally, the United Nations has continuously failed the women of the world.

Nepal would not seem to be an exception to this. As reported earlier, most resources to combat HIV and AIDS have been allocated to "high-risk

---

schema implies a spiritual dimension as well (one is also captured by spirits), not included in the western war schema.

[5]In active sentence construction the subject is typically the actor (e.g., John hit the ball). In the passive sentence construction the subject is the recipient of the action (e.g., The ball was hit by John).

groups," and wives of migrant laborers have not yet been identified formally as such.

Next I turn my attention to the remaining problem of ARV availability versus accessibility (as described earlier). The fact is that despite the achievements over the past ten years, progress has not been socially, economically, or geographically distributed equally across Nepal. Much work remains to be done in this arena in the coming years.

And given the worrisome connection between HIV and tuberculosis,[6] continuing diligence is essential. In 1998 tuberculosis was noted as the most significant opportunistic infection affecting HIV positive persons (Suvedi 1998:55) and a follow-up study done ten years later (Dhungel et al. 2008) confirms that tuberculosis is still the most common opportunistic infection affecting HIV positive persons. Lack of such attention could prove disastrous for a country like Nepal that has finally just begun to get a handle on its TB epidemic.

And finally, what are the wider implications of this research? First of all, in regard to the wider application of the cultural model concept to other illnesses, Blum, Pelto and Pelto (2004), drawing on the illness cultural model concept I introduced, have applied the model to better understand vitamin D deficiency in Northern Niger. So, now the model has been tested and proven cross-linguistically (as noted earlier), across disease categories, and across continents. Secondly, "fighting" (the Western warfare schema) seems to be the predominant schema being used to understand and communicate about HIV and AIDS in the Americas, Europe, Africa, Asia, and the Pacific (e.g.,"fighting AIDS" appears to be the universal slogan for the prevention "campaign"—another warfare term). I have seen evidence of this from each of these places. And in regard to the use of the war schema elsewhere around the world, currently animated condom imagery (like that of Dhaaley Dai in Nepal, carrying a shield) appears in prevention campaigns in forty-one languages (The Body 2005) last time I checked. What are the implications of this? Are there similar cultural schema, such as the *randi* schema, in operation in these cultures? Will the HIV and AIDS prevention efforts be negatively impacted by this approach as a result? It will take anthropologists more familiar with these particular situations to address the appropriateness of this approach in these particular contexts, but I think it is important to raise the question.

In this book I have presented the various faces of the AIDS epidemic in Nepal. I have examined the the epidemic, the various responses to the epidemic through time and by various groups, and illuminated cultural models

---

[6]Tuberculosis is one of the leading causes of death (co-infection is common) in HIV-infected people. HIV compromises the immune system and increases the likelihood of people acquiring new TB infection. Likewise, it also promotes both the progression of latent TB infection to active disease and causes the relapse of the disease in previously treated patients.

and underlying illness schemata that are influencing people's understandings of the disease and their responses to it. We are now entering a new era for AIDS in Nepal. We must consider the facts and work for a better understanding of the multitude of disparate factors that have come together to propel the spread of the epidemic. It is my sincere hope that this examination of the social and cultural issues associated with the disease will serve to further educate those involved in the fight against HIV and AIDS in Nepal and enhance the success of future prevention and intervention measures. And above all we must not forget that there are people behind the various faces of AIDS in Nepal. The last chapter of this book is dedicated to hearing the stories of those most affected in their own words.

Part Four

In Their Own Words

10

In Their Own Words

In this final chapter I let those with HIV and AIDS tell their own stories. These stories represent a selection among those that were used to develop the research findings presented in the earlier chapters of this book.[1] The interviews were conducted in Nepali and then transcribed and translated using the methods described earlier. In many of the interviews I also asked questions. These questions are also included and bolded. It is my hope that as you read these stories the problem of HIV and AIDS in Nepal will become a human problem rather than just a statistical pandemic that plagues another of the world's third-world countries. All personal names and village names have been changed for the protection of the story teller.

10.1 Sita

Long ago, I lived in the town of Lagankagl.[2] As I have heard it, we had six members in our family. But I only ever saw four. Out of the four of us, only two are left. When my sister died, my mother started gambling because of the pain of my sister's death. She started selling things to get money. She even sold the utensils with which we ate. Now, what could we kids do? At that time, we started to visit our aunt very often. We would arrive at our aunt's and she would give us three hundred rupees[3] (about $4 dollars by today's standards) per month. And she would give us that money. We would

---

[1] These are the narratives collected prior to 2003 and as such they reflect only the themes that were prominent at that time. The later narratives (2012) are not included here for the sake of brevity, but will be published in full in at a later date.

[2] This interview was conducted with the first HIV positive person (a young woman) identified in Nepal. The interview was also conducted with the assistance of the NGO director who interspersed comments at various points during the text. The NGO director's personal comments are marked as such.

[3] The rupee is the currency of exchange in Nepal. Today the value of rupee is near 75 rupees to $1 USD.

buy meat and rice, but the next day, it would all be gone. Our father would also send us rice from the army barracks. Our mother would get angry and say, "It's not right for us to only eat rice." We would eat rice, and the following day, it would all be gone. It turns out that our mother had sold it for money. My aunt also once gave my mother money for us to be able to go to school. She took the money from our aunt promising that she would also buy us new clothes. But mother wasted it gambling, so we weren't even able to study. Then my mother died. She died of excessive smoking and drinking. She even used to drink beer. Even though she had a fever, she needed to drink beer. She was addicted to it. She continued her addiction even though she had asthma, and the disease had gotten worse in her. At that time, Patan Hospital[4] was not yet built. There was only the mental hospital. So I carried my mother there myself. At that time, I had my mother admitted and it only cost twenty-five piasa (1/4 of a rupee). They asked me where we were from, and I replied that we were from Lagankagl. "Do you have a father?" they asked. "No, not here in town," I said.

After that, she was admitted to the mental hospital. For twelve or thirteen days, I had to sit by my mother's bed and watch for leeches on my mother's head. If I didn't stay and watch, my mother would scold me, so I was bound to do it. I did so to please my mother. But after she would fall asleep, I would go out to play. And after some time, I would come to my mother again, and I would tell my mother, "I'm hungry." But what could she give me to eat? We had rented our house out, so I went to collect the rent money. But when I arrived, the tenant said, "How can I give you money? It's the off season and our business is not running well." And they didn't give me any money.

Then I told my mother what they had told me. After that, my mother died. And after her death, I went to live with my aunt in the area of town known as Dobighat. Meanwhile, there was no work to do. My uncle would go to work around two o'clock in the afternoon and return around two o'clock in the morning. Then, since I didn't have any work to do and no money to purchase the things that I needed in Kathmandu, I felt that I should tell my aunt that I would go look for a job. I went to the place where people carry stones and bricks for money. During those days, most of the people who did that kind of work were men. They probably looked for a man, but there was none available. I was the only girl there. Of course, there were other girls there, but they were women. The women were given seven rupees while I was only given six rupees, fifty piasa. Then, afterwards I counted my money and realized I was actually only given six rupees, while others were given seven. Then, I asked why this was so. The boss replied that it was because I was small. "Oh, that's why. I'm small," I said. So from that time, I only carried two bricks, one in each hand. And after that, they

---

[4]Patan Hospital is a Christian Hospital run by the United Mission to Nepal.

asked me why I had carried so few bricks. And I answered, "Oh, it's because I'm small." They all laughed.

After that, I didn't go back to work. Then, my father came back from the army. He stayed in Dobighat for one week. And after that, he wanted to leave, taking me with him. He said, "Let's go, daughter." He took me to the town of Dhanagadhi. First he took me to Hetauda and we stayed there for six days. And then he took me to Dhanagadhi. At first, I didn't want to go, and I told this to my father and my aunt. My stepmother also said, "Come on daughter. I won't beat you anymore. I'll take you wherever I go and will not let your father beat you."

What could I do then? Since I didn't have my own mother, I thought, "Well at least my stepmother will care for me." When we reached my stepmother's, however, my father began to listen to her. I was very small. My stepmother told me to carry heavy things. And when I couldn't, my stepmother complained to my father. My father told her to beat me severely. I cried and cried. I had never carried such loads. One day, I was compelled to carry ten large baskets of corn. I couldn't even walk straight. My legs began to shiver constantly. So at last, I dropped it in the street. My mother complained to my father about it; that his daughter had disgraced her, weeping in the street. My father scolded me, telling me that I needed to be beaten. In this way, my father continued to scold me. What could I do? There was no way out.

Sometime after that, my aunt arrived from the East. She called me saying, "Niece." I said, "Yes." "Would you like to become a Buddhist nun?" she asked. "I said, "Yes." But my father didn't want to let me go. I was his only daughter. There was no one else to look after the cattle, and he wouldn't agree to let me go. But he told me he would let me go in the days to come. We set a date and that date finally arrived, but my father left to Kathmandu. He told my stepmother not to send me until he returned. Now, what could I do? They wouldn't let me go be a Buddhist nun.

Then, when a brother from the monastery came, he asked me if I would like to study Buddhism. I acknowledged that I would, and he took me to teach me Buddhism. (The brothers) asked me to take a vow to become a nun. They required us to take a vow stating that we would remain unmarried, and also that we would not listen to our parents. They asked us whether we would leave the practice if our parents forced us to become married. I said, "No." They would say, "When your parents ask, 'Are you ready to leave (the monastery) or not?'" They would ask how we would answer. And we were to say, "No." Such vows we were to make. We would take vows like this. I had taken the vow one month and shaved my head the next. This is also required to become a Buddhist nun. Then, after shaving my head, I was not allowed to see the face of boys for twenty-two days. During that time, I was also not allowed to sit, even on a wooden chair, and I slept on the ground. Finally, after twenty-two days, I was allowed to sleep in a bed.

Before he had become a monk, one of the brothers in the monastery had been married. His wife was in the town of Jharlang. Her mother-in-law would frequently chase her out of the house, because she didn't have any babies. My brother would frequently ask me to go and to retrieve her. After his mother would throw his wife out of the house, he would send me to retrieve her. Sometimes when I was there, her mother would ask me where I had come from and where I was going. I would tell her I had come to sell meat. Indeed, I was only pretending. In reality, I was there to collect my sister-in-law. She would again ask me to tell the truth. "Have you come here to get your sister-in-law?" And she would ask, "Where is your brother?" I told her that I didn't have any idea about where he had gone. She would ask me, "Are you the husband of my daughter?" To this question I didn't know what to say. I couldn't say anything. So, I returned to the monastery without her, and I told the brother she wouldn't send her with me. Rather, she would ask me why I went there. When I said that I have come to receive the sister-in-law, she scolded me, saying, "Are you the husband of my daughter?" Then my brother also scolded me saying, "Well, why didn't you bring her secretly?"

Much later, when the sister-in-law was not there, he called me during the night. When he called me by name, I responded and he said, "If you come and sleep with me, only then I'll teach you. Otherwise, I won't teach you." I kept quiet and didn't say anything to him. Finally, I said, "If you don't want to teach me, then don't teach me." After that, I sent a letter to my aunt, asking her to come and get me. They sent my uncle, and my uncle had come to receive me. But my uncle took me to my father's house. Again I escaped from there. After escaping from my father, I came back to my aunt's. Even though I was in my aunt's home, my father continued to pursue me. I wanted to stay with my aunt. Then, my father rebuked me saying, "Who's more important? Your own father or your aunt?" I was torn. I needed the support of my father, but every time I was around him, he would always pursue me.

At that time, I set up a little shop. I would cook beaten rice, curry, breads, and I would work. My aunt would go to her job. My cousins would also go to their jobs, and I would be left all alone. Still my father didn't stop pursuing me. He would pursue me in Dhanagadhi as well as here too. My father threatened me that he would take me with him. There was one man who would come to take tea and wine at my shop. And he asked where my home was. I replied, "Lagankagl." He asked again whether I have any parents or not. I said, "I've got a father. No mother. Just a stepmother." And he asked me, "Does she treat you well?" "No," I said. Then he continued, "I've got a sister in India who has two children. I could get you a job. Your only job would be to bring them from school." So I agreed. I did not want to appear before my father. I thought that if I went far away from him, he wouldn't be able to find me.

So that man took me to India, and he sold me there. I don't know how many rupees he sold me for. I didn't understand much over there. Sometimes they say Mumbai and sometimes Bombay. I stayed there for twenty-two months. After twenty-two months, I became sick. They (brothel owners) brought the shaman into the home to treat me, but it didn't heal me. Rather, he told me that I was possessed by an evil spirit. Then they also brought a doctor in, but his treatment didn't work either. And then, I don't know what they were thinking, but they took me to the temple too. They thought that that would cure me. They made me wear copper bracelets too. The bracelets made me afraid at night, but if I took them off, they would scold me. So, I took them off at night and put them on again in the morning. So I would put them on in the morning and take them off at night, but still I didn't recover.

In the brothel, there were six or seven other Nepali girls. We never really talked about where each one was from. The brothel owners didn't like us talking very much. They would scold us severely. They wouldn't even let us see a magazine. What could we do? They would scold us. One of the brothel owners had gone to Kathmandu, where she was caught and imprisoned. Because she was imprisoned, her husband had to make frequent visits there. Since I knew how to cook, they asked me if I wanted to go to Kathmandu, and I agreed. They took me up to Gorakhpur Station where I was to go to Kathmandu by train. The brothel owners had cooperated with the police to send me away. The police in India cooperate with the women (owners) in the brothels. Sometimes when they get enough money, through cooperation, then they buy the one woman they like, paying them money, and they'll even make them their wives. Then, the husband will go to work for the whole day, and he'll return when evening falls. We never see how much the police pay for these women. They don't let us know anything. They do it all in secret. They cover the money with a cloth, and we don't know how much they take.

After that, I came here. When we got to Gorakhpur, the fellows that had brought me there ran away. I don't know where they went. I had a lot of leg pain, but at that time, I was still able to walk some. Then a cycle rickshaw came by and carried me to the bus, and I took the bus to Kathmandu. And then I went to my aunt's house. Following that, I had been brought to the hospital for a checkup. Later on, I was admitted to that same hospital. Sometimes, my aunt would ask me where I had gone and why I had gone so far. When they (my aunt and uncle) asked where I had gone, I simply told them that I had gone to India, but I didn't tell them the things in detail. After I was admitted to the hospital, I didn't know anything about my condition. And then one lady asked me. She said, "Sister." I replied, "Yes." She said, "Do you want to go to this sister's home?" (the home of the NGO operator). "I don't know; let me think about it," I said. And then, when this sister came, I told her that I would like to go to her home. Once at her home,

I became a believer (Christian). Now once I became a believer, I wondered whether I would still be allowed to observe *Dashain* or not, and I wondered whether I would be allowed to observe *Maghe Sangranti*[5]. These are the kinds of things I worried about. At last someone told me that it was okay for me to observe such things even as a believer. So knowing this, I consented to go with my sister (the Christian NGO operator).

Interview questions

Where did you go to?
To Kupondal.

How did you feel when you discovered that you have this disease HIV/AIDS)?
I felt extremely sorry.

Did you know anything else regarding this disease before?
No.

Did your family take care of you?
No.

How did you feel at that time?
Very upset. Now what could I do? That rascal took me there to India.

Did you tell your family that you are HIV positive?
No.

Why not?
I don't know.

Do you have other brothers and sisters?
I don't have any younger brothers, but I've got my aunt's sons. They're like brothers. But they've only come one day to see me here. That's all. Only my younger sister came here to help look after me.

Does that family know that you are HIV positive?
Yes, they do. Whenever I go to the village, sometimes I hear people say things like, "Don't drive her around," or "Don't let her come in the house." These are the type of things I've heard.

---

[5]Both *Dashain* and *Maghe Sangranti* are traditional Hindu festivals.

How do you feel when people don't accept you or won't let you come inside of their houses?
It's painful, but we remain quiet. A few days ago, my sister asked me why I hadn't gone to the village lately. I said, "What to do? It's seems that I have forgotten the way." What else could I say? I just told her that I had forgotten the way, then finished the conversation.

In your opinion, do you have HIV or AIDS?
I'm not really sure what to think. All I know is that it gives me pain. But whatever it is, no medicine can cure it. I think the only thing that's needed is love.

So right now, you don't feel as if you've got any certain disease, but you're getting love continuously.
Yes.

What do you think about HIV and AIDS? What is the difference between the two? If a person gets HIV or AIDS, will they die? What are their symptoms? What information do you know about these things?
Somebody says I have HIV, but I actually don't know. It was said that Nanumaya had AIDS, and at the last moment of her life she discharged stool while she was trying to urinate. That was one case. That might be what happens to people. Another was Phulmaya who only had one hole to discharge urine and stool. Also worms came to her badly. That may be another symptom. We had to take care of her daily.

Did she ever recover from her tuberculosis?
No, she didn't. I felt much sorrow a few days back when I was in the hospital, because I was the one who was sick, but you had to suffer too (talking to the NGO operator). When you had to stay on the floor, it made me very sorrowful. Do you remember?

Where did the nurses come from in Patan Hospital?
From Nepal. Some nurses wear gloves while working with me and some don't. At the time of urinating, some will wear gloves and some don't.

At this point, the NGO operator began to talk:

> It doesn't do any harm for me not to wear gloves, because after the death of Nanumaya, we went to the hospital for an HIV checkup, because Nanumaya had vomited all over my head. I had to clean up after her. One nurse said that she could stand the stool and the feces and would be ready to clean it up but couldn't bear the sight of cleaning up the vomit. So she told me to do it myself, and she

left and I had vomit all over my body. There was blood and vomit, all the contemptuous things. So after that, the two of us here went to Patan Hospital again for a checkup.

Sometimes she (Sita) doesn't think that she has HIV. We make her feel this way because we live together and eat together and so on. But we shouldn't have fear of such things. I might have gotten it because of the earlier situation. Therefore, we went to a checkup. But, no HIV was seen in my body. I would like to get checked up once more. I am willing to go for a checkup again. I know that HIV doesn't shift to each other by living together, because I've already gone for a checkup three times. For this girl, she doesn't feel so much pain because of the impending pain caused by HIV/AIDS. She feels more pain because people neglect her or despise her. It makes her sick.

What do people do when they find out that you are HIV positive, or in your case (to NGO operator) that you work with people who are HIV positive?
(NGO operator) In some places they'll totally reject us. They'll neglect us like anything. For example, when we went to Beijing, others did not even want to ride with us on the same bus. Because of these types of things, I feel very sad. In Beijing, there was a world women's conference. I was invited to attend. At that time, we (Sita and I), like mother and daughter, went with another Nepali sister working with another AIDS NGO. But she didn't want to even travel on the same bus on which we traveled and didn't want to walk where we had walked, and she didn't want to come into the room where we were sleeping. There were three of us sleeping in this room: myself, this girl (Sita), and another HIV positive girl. We pushed the beds together and we slept together on the bed. These girls didn't understand the English language, so I needed to stay with them. Although she (Sita) is like my sister, she also resembles my daughter. And this was the first time she was going abroad besides India. And it was not right for me to leave her alone. Greater is my love for her than is my fear of contracting HIV/AIDS. According to her experience, she found that other HIV positive girls remaining in NGOs were just there for money; they were not receiving love and care. She felt very sorry for that.

Do you know how the other sister might have got HIV?
(From this point on Sita answers all of the questions.) I've heard that she was also taken for the same task (prostitution). She was also taken for the same work.

Do you know how else HIV spreads?
(Through) sexual relationships, while using needles with blood, and then from other instruments that contain one's own blood. These types of

instruments should be boiled in hot water. Pregnant women can also shift AIDS to their children. It's good for HIV positive pregnant women to abort their babies.

What do you think the different types of treatments are for HIV? For example, many people have come here saying that certain incantations, or wearing amulets, or other charms will be good treatments for HIV/AIDS. What's your opinion?
Yes, I've heard that. They say that amulets are available. But, I don't believe in such things. It is God's will as to whether he heals this disease or not. I don't need anyone else. There is no greater power than the Lord to heal.

How do you think the HIV disease works inside the body? How do you feel right now? Normal or abnormal?
Right now I don't feel anything serious with me.

But in other people, do you understand the way that HIV/AIDS works?
Some people say that after getting such disease, one suffers from fever and the cold from time to time. And when I get a cold, I pray to the Lord and know that I am in his hands. My only hope is in prayer.

When you first discovered that you were HIV positive, did you feel that your life was finished?
No.

Why not?
Because I realized that now I have a chance to get love from my mother (the NGO worker). That she would show love to an orphan like me.

(Then the NGO operator asked,) What I wanted to ask you is that when you first came to us (to the NGO) you weren't a believer; however, as soon as you discovered that you had HIV, you didn't feel like you were going to die very soon. And also you didn't feel like there was no one to take care of you because you had found us, and we were looking after you with care and service. Is this right or wrong?
(Sita replies) At that time, I didn't know you were believers, or I didn't know anything else about it.

The NGO operator commented, "She didn't know that we were believers (Christians). The only thing she found here was care. She felt that she had been cared for with great food. She understood that much—only we would feed her five times in a day."

Did you know very many things about the disease when you went to the hospital for the HIV checkup, and at that time, did they tell you that you were HIV positive?
(Sita) No, they didn't tell me. But they would put on gowns and gloves if they needed to give me an injection, and they would take them off if they didn't need to give me an injection. That much only I could discern. I didn't know anything else about the disease. They didn't tell me anything about the disease, but I only could see them changing their clothes and treating me carefully.

Didn't the doctors and nurses in Patan Hospital teach you about the disease or did you only come to know something about it here?
I learned about it from here only. There are some small booklets put out by them.

The NGO operator added, "We taught her these things slowly, with counseling, from the small booklets that we use here."

Do you still have fear or not?
No I don't. One should not make mistakes, but there is no point in fear.

The NGO operator asks, You've been living with us for five or six years. What do you think will happen to you? Have you ever thought that 'My family hates me and my friends despise me so what will happen in my life?'
(Sita replies) People say that when a person gets HIV, they will die within five or ten years, but I think I may live a long life. Recently, I gained six kilograms.

To this the NGO operator added, "We admitted her to the hospital for eight days, and at that time she had lost seven kilograms of her weight, but six kilograms have been recovered. I've given her permission to eat whatever she likes."

10.2 Prabita

I am an HIV positive woman. When I was small, I was very talented. When I was small, I was very interested in studying, and I enjoyed sport as my hobby. I was born in the village, and when I was small, I couldn't study at an early age. I was admitted to class one when I was nine years old. I studied very well from class one to class five. I would finish in the first or second position among all my classmates. But by the time I reached class five, I was getting older, and I didn't study quite as well. In the village, the grass needed to be cut for the cows and other animals, and I needed to help with the farming so my studying began to suffer. But I went on studying, through sixth class, seventh class, and up to eighth class. But in the later years, I did not study as well. I also began to put more emphasis on sports at that time, around class eight or nine. I even played at the national level when I was in ninth class. I enjoyed *kapadi*[6] and running races very much. Those are the kind of sports that I used to do. But since I was interested in studying too, I concentrated only on studying and playing games during my childhood. I didn't have too much interest in other things. As soon as I reached class nine, marriage proposals began to reach my home—because I was born in the village, and this was the village custom to marry at a young age. My parents wanted to force me to marry.

I told my parents, "I don't want to marry right now. I want to study, and I'm interested in sports, and I want to make a name for myself in this country." But my parents and my grandparents said, "It's our tradition to give our daughters away in marriage at a young age. When people marry late, other people will talk behind our backs saying we weren't able to give our daughter away in marriage and so on. So you should marry," they said. However, I went on rejecting all the proposals. But in the end, my attempt to escape marriage failed, and I had to be tied in the tie of marriage. I was under compulsion. So many proposals came to me. I thought to myself, "After I get married in the village, the rest of my life will be spent cutting grass and leaves, and doing farming." But I wanted to continue my studies and do something in this country.

Knowing this, my aunt talked to me, and she said she would search for a boy for me to marry from Kathmandu. She figured if she could find a boy from Kathmandu for me to marry, there I would be allowed to study and be involved in sports too. She said, "There you can become great and you can do anything you want." When I heard this I thought, "Wow, people in Kathmandu are really educated and quite understanding; because they are literate, they will allow me to study too." Liking this idea, I agreed to marry.

So, I agreed to marry, and I got married in the year 2052[7] (1995/96), right after passing class nine. After marriage, I started class ten and began staying in my father's house. While I was staying with my parents in class ten, I used to go to my husband's on the weekend. I would go on Friday, stay there all of Saturday, and return to my parents' home to begin my classes on Sunday morning. In that way, I studied. So, I continued studying that way, sometimes staying with my parents, sometimes with my husband. But, by contact with my husband, I conceived a baby in my belly. And at that time, it was time for the test exam. Then, I was eight months pregnant. Because I was so concentrated on my studies, I didn't care about my prestige. In spite

---

[6]a popular South Asian sport

[7]Nepal follows the *Bikram Sambat,* a traditional Hindu solar calendar that is approximately fifty-seven years ahead of ours (the new year begins in mid April).

of my big belly, I continued in school, wearing school dresses, and even covering with shawls. It was my thought that I should work hard for a year, and after a year I would bear a child. And then, I would study well, and my child would also be in a better condition. I thought I would be able to complete my studies and keep my child at my parents' house. I went on studying, so that I could make my child's future brighter. The behavior at my husband's house was not quite as modern. They were not very understanding. So, I studied, but when the exam came nearer, I couldn't go to see a tutor. And as the test grew near, I was in my ninth month. And when I came home to my husband's house, after finishing the test, the baby was about to be born. So, in this condition, I passed the exam.

So, I passed the test, but near the time of delivery, things got worse. We had very little money. When the time for delivery came, my husband's family made us live on our own. We were separated from them because of a conflict between my husband and his parents. Living on our own, we didn't have much money. I was studying, not working; I was only a student. I was studying, and my husband was a drug addict. He had started using drugs when he was sixteen years old. Now, he's thirty-one. This was a secret to me, and I didn't know it at the time (of our wedding). Only after five months of marriage, when he got arrested in Kathmandu did I come to know this. Had I known this secret earlier, I probably wouldn't have married him. But now, the baby had already been conceived and was in my belly. I guess this was simply my fate. Then, the time came, and the baby was born. But we still had to live apart. We were not even getting food to eat. My husband went on using drugs and didn't have too much concern for me.

At delivery time, I went to the hospital. None of my husband's family cared for me while I was in the hospital. They didn't even bring me food. Since I wasn't being taken care of by my husband's household, the doctors and the nurses at the hospital took care of me. They saved me from embarrassment by providing me food and clothes for three days. During this time, neither my mother-in-law nor father-in-law came to take me home. Because my husband was busy taking drugs as well, there was no one to take care of me. Because of that situation the doctors helped me very much. And finally, my own parents had to come and take me to my house. They returned me to my husband's home after taking me to the hospital. But my in-laws didn't even give me food. They only have one son, and now they have a new star, their grandson. They should have thought of making their grandson good, taking care of him, even though their son had been involved in bad company. But they didn't have that sort of mentality. They got mad at me, and I had to go on living with that family in that way.

Anyway, I brought the new baby boy home. According to our Nepali tradition, a woman who has delivered a baby should not go to her parents' house before eleven days have passed, and her brothers, and grandfather, and maternal uncles should not be able to see her face until after that. These are our traditions. But, because I had been in such a difficult situation, my grandfather himself had come to the hospital to discharge me and to arrange for food for eleven days. The eleventh day after a baby is born, we Nepali people call in the priest to perform ritual ceremonies and to purify both the child and the mother. Only then are we able to return to our parents' house. In the parents' house, our maternal relatives present clothes and gifts to us. This is our custom in our culture. If anyone from the maternal home sees my face before eleven days however, they are not supposed to hold this festival, this custom. Even though this is the cultural rule, and my family had seen me before the time, they brought the priest from their side and performed all the ritual ceremonies. And they performed the name-giving ceremony on the eleventh day. Everyone in the family had come, and they had brought me back to my parents' house.

I stayed there with my parents and my family for three months. When I returned to my husband's home after staying at my own home for three months, I had many confrontations with my mother-in-law. Nepalese mothers-in-law are naturally very terrible. They are very strict. They torture and treat their daughters-in-law very poorly, differentiating between daughters and daughters-in-law. They treat their daughters as dear, while they are very harsh with their daughters-in-law, overloading a great deal of work on them, as if they were a plowing ox.

I was getting stronger and my health was being restored from the pregnancy. We were still living separately from my in-laws, but when I needed better food, I went to my in-laws' and I was able to recover. I had to work for them. Anyway, I came to their home and stayed there. I stayed together with my in-laws. We had been made to live separately until the time of delivery. But after (the baby was born), I came to live with my in-laws. At that time, my husband had been sent to our ancestral village. I couldn't eat alone; therefore, I lived together with my husband's family.

After that, there were three months left before my SLC[8] examination. I took the SLC examination and it was okay. If I had had a chance to get a tutor, I would have passed it with really good marks. Because of the baby, I didn't get much opportunity to study in the house. Also, my in-laws didn't allow me to study because they said if anyone reads or studies at the time of delivery, they will suffer from headache or eye pain or these kinds of things. Therefore, I didn't have much opportunity to study. But on the basis of my studying class nine and ten, I went ahead and took the SLC exam. That year, I failed the science portion of the exam, but I tried it the following year and passed it. And now, I still have the will to go on in my studies, but I don't think I'll get the chance to study. Even if I get the chance to study, my

---

[8]School Leaving Certificate

condition is so poor now. So, I took the SLC exam and passed. But I don't know that I will have opportunity to study higher.

After passing the SLC, I came to an organization called LALS[9] in the year 1998. There they collect old syringes and give new syringes to drug users so that they will not get HIV. My husband used to come and exchange syringes frequently. Before that, I didn't know that he would do this. Later, he took me there, and I knew, by the contact with the nurses, that his blood had been checked. HIV positive had been seen in his blood. Until that time, I had no idea what HIV was, or how it transferred, or what the disease was. When I heard about AIDS for the first time, I guessed that it must be the name of a bird. That means I didn't have any knowledge about it. There was an organization called *Prerana*[10] that was established from the place called WECOM BP Memorial.[11] The people at LALS told me I should go there to gain information about AIDS. When I first learned that my husband was HIV positive, I thought that my life was totally ruined. I would be better off dead, but the sisters at Prerana counseled me a lot.

They counseled me saying, "This is how the disease shifts. So, you might not have got it. You need to go get your blood checked. Don't be hopeless, because there may be nothing to fear." I began to go to Prerana for counseling. When I began coming to Prerana, since January 1998, I had missed three to four months of my science classes, so I gave up studying science to come, and I began to work at Prerana as a volunteer. After I began to come here, I got a lot of information about HIV. I felt there must be a lot of people who have the same pain that I have. For example, my husband is an addict. I didn't know that. For instance, I am an innocent girl from the village. I thought that an educated man of the town would have a gentle behavior toward me, and I married him, thinking that I could also become great and contribute something toward the country. When I lived in the village I was naïve. I didn't know what drugs were all about. I had never heard about AIDS as well. Only after five months of marriage did I learn that my husband was a drug addict, and that he was involved in such habits. I came to know that when my husband was arrested, and, at that time, I was already pregnant, with a baby in my belly. And I didn't have an abortion either.

Now, I was married. After he had put *sindoor*[12] on my head before the society, I had to stay with him since I was his wife. Therefore, I continued to stay with him, living in that house, keeping my feelings to myself. Later,

---

[9]Life Giving and Life Saving Society of Nepal, an HIV/AIDS prevention NGO.

[10]*Prerana*, founded in 1996, is an organization of people living with AIDS. *Prerana* offers counseling and educational services and operates a AIDS hotline. *Prerana* means 'inspiration' in Nepali.

[11]Another AIDS prevention NGO.

[12]*Sindoor* is a red powder traditionally worn along the part of a married woman's hair.

at the end, we again lived separately from my in-laws. And my in-laws don't know. The fact that we are positive is limited to us. I know he's positive, and that it could be shifted to me. But he's still my husband and I have all the knowledge about HIV now. If I follow safe methods, I won't get it. I have to stay with my husband. I have to help him. He doesn't have anyone except for me. He's been taking drugs since he was sixteen and now he's thirty-one. Recently, he's not been taking drugs. He tells me that he's taken it (drugs) since he was a little kid. His mother used to sell the drug called brown sugar near their home, and he got knowledge of it from there. Sometimes his mother would send him there to sell it. One day, he asked a man who was buying it what it was. The man lied to him and said, "If you take this, you will reach heaven at once. And in a day, you will meet God." So that day, he began to take it. Then he was sixteen. Now, he's thirty-one. Until this time, he's been addicted and unable to give it up. If my in-laws had told me about their son's habit before marriage, I wouldn't have married him. They thought if he got married, he would become better. They tried their best to make their son better. They even put him into prison to try to make him better, but it didn't break the addiction. Now I, once a free and innocent girl, am ensnared. I've been badly ensnared by the actions of my in-laws. They knew their son had been involved in bad habits, so why should they put another's life in danger? If they had thought like that, my life would not be in danger. Or if I had known about drugs and AIDS, I could have got married with good information about it. Now, we've been kicked out of their home, and are despised intensely. We've been given only a small room, and we are living there, hiding our bodies. It's been difficult for us even to have enough food. I have a small baby, but I've left him at my parents' house so that he won't be infected with HIV as we have been. However, we haven't checked his blood yet. That's our current condition. It's all because of my husband. I don't have any fault in it. At first, I didn't know. Because of my husband, I've got it. I've got it. I hope that the other women of this country might not get it.

Now, all the government and NGOs should get together and should start teaching about HIV in different places. Go into the schools and talk to the students about HIV and sexual diseases, STDs, and those kind of things. Put the information in textbooks, such as the science books, the math or English books. And children should be taking classes. We ought to inform them about it. For example, if I had known about it while I was in school, I wouldn't have become ensnared, and my life wouldn't be in danger. The main thing is that education about HIV and STDs should begin first at home. I've seen many who have HIV. They have double problems. If they remain quiet and don't inform their family about the disease, there's the danger of them shifting the disease to other members of the family. But if they inform their family, they'll be kicked out of the home with a vigorous hatred at a time when they need a good diet, counseling, love, care, acceptance, and sympathy. In that kind of situation, where do they go? If they are cut off from family and society? It is their own country. Had they known about AIDS, they could have been careful. They would have been careful and not done such practices had they had information about how the disease infects, and the effects it will have on this life. They've destroyed their life without knowing anything.

So now, we have to think carefully about these things and give this much attention in our coming days. Many people in the urban area probably don't even know the words "AIDS" and "HIV." These days however, the Nepali television broadcasts information about condoms and protection from AIDS. This doesn't mean that everybody has a television, because many don't have. And since they don't, they might not know about HIV. And the man who only watches television once in a while doesn't understand immediately. Even for us, it was difficult to understand. We came to understand only after coming here many many months and hearing the explanation of counselors. Not everyone knows about it. Therefore, we have to explain about AIDS to urban inhabitants. That's the main thing. The members of parliament need to take an interest in clearly explaining the subject throughout Nepal.

First of all, it needs to publicized more in the schools. If we are able to go to classes and tell the students about it, they'll return to their families and tell them that such a disease is emerging. They can explain how the disease shifts. This is the only way we can prevent it. Many people feel shame when they talk about condoms, the process of using one, and even when they just see one. If children ask their parents what a condom is, they hesitate to tell them. But one day in the future, they will certainly know. When they get to the point of having sexual relationships, they'll ultimately know about them, and recall their childhood curiosity. If they understand about sexual disease, HIV, and so on before the stage of having sexual relationships, it may prevent them from getting HIV and STDs, and they can be safe from every kind of disease. Because our country of Nepal is very small and poor, all of us must be united for the development of our country. Many of our brothers and sisters in Nepal, because of the poor conditions in the house, because there are many children, and there's an economic crisis, etc., are bound to go to foreign lands, especially India, to earn money. And there, they usually have unsafe sexual relations.

Moreover, many Nepalese girls from the villages are being trafficked and sold to foreign countries. Then, when they get HIV or STDs, they're sent back to Nepal. Prestige is very important to Nepali girls. When they lived in the villages, they didn't have enough to eat in their homes, so they eloped with boys without knowing anything about their conditions. These girls are led by a strong desire to come to Kathmandu, desiring the good foods, and good clothes. But then, they find themselves in Bombay. And when they return from Bombay, in that condition, they can't go to their home. The society itself despises them, and they are afraid of the society. They are afraid of their parents and their brothers and sisters. Therefore, they can't return back to their homes. And they are forced to spend the rest of their lives selling their bodies, as if they are cattle. They continue to look for customers from street to street. They don't care a thing about who AIDS shifts to and who it does not. Why should they care about such things? Anyway, they have to eat; they have to go on earning money. They have to live. In that way, they go on living day by day. Men have been involved in sexual relationships with these women just for pleasure. The men probably don't know that they're from Bombay, and many of these girls probably don't know about their own condition.

For these reasons, HIV has been spreading rampantly throughout Nepal as well as other countries. Let's not only talk about Nepal; HIV has been spreading through the whole world and it's a death sentence. Currently, there's no cure for this disease so the main thing we have to do is forget what's happened up to now and focus on the children, the children of the future. We need to take control of this disease, informing (school) classes about HIV and STDs from the very beginning. We should do door-to-door counseling through cooperation of the NGOs and the government. This is how the situation is. The problem can't be solved by just telling one or two people or going to one or two houses and villages. The message needs to be spread throughout the country, other countries too, and all over the world. Not only in Nepal but also in other countries of the world. Many people probably don't know what HIV is. Which bird's name is it? What is this? They don't even know what a virus is. The main thing is it needs to be explained. The main thing is that people who are well known, such as the people in the government and others, should be attentive to the problem.

For example, HIV came to me, undeliberately. I got it, and I've got a baby. Both of us, my husband and I, are HIV positive, and we're uncertain about whether our baby has HIV or not, and what will happen to his future. The child is dependent on us. If both of us die, who will look after him? Today the situation is hard in the world. It's hard enough to provide for oneself. It's not always possible to provide for others. Tomorrow, that baby may become tossed by the weather, or ramble aimlessly weeping and begging, and become a street boy. Now the question must be asked, "In the future who will care for this child?" Because, when we die, we leave this world. But those who remain are left to handle the problem. The problem will be theirs to handle.

For example, we've been noticing that many in Nepal have HIV. They've been coming to us and calling in on hotlines too—they were kicked out of their home, or were not telling the fact that they have HIV; there's the possibility of their wives getting HIV as well, or husbands will get angry with their wives if their wives demand they use a condom. They say, "If we tell, we won't get food from our parents. We won't have a balanced diet;" or, "thinking that we would receive family care, we told them. But it went opposite. We were expelled from the home. Now we're wondering where to go." Many parents, both father and mother, are HIV positive. Many of them still have dependent children. We need to begin to think about these children. Right now, we're getting help from the organization known as Prerana. We get counseling. Many people call on the hotlines. We are meeting together once a week. People who are positive bring their families, and we teach them about the disease. We train them with the kind help of doctors, who are helping us very much. This is how the training has been going. It's a matter for us to all think about. Take my life as an example. When I was told that my husband was HIV positive, had I known about these things, I would have practiced safe sex and not lived with him carelessly. But, I got HIV. And if I didn't know about AIDS, I might have fed my baby from my breast. When my husband got his blood checked, I checked right after him and found out I was HIV positive. If I had not discovered this, I would have continued feeding my baby from my breast. And there's a thirty-five percent possibility of shifting the disease through breastfeeding. Therefore, I have stopped feeding the baby breast milk. So, I think the best thing to do is let others know about HIV. I don't want others to suffer as I have.

10.3 Raju

I have gotten the terrible disease known as HIV, and now, at this stage, have come to be at Prerana. If you want to know about me, it would be good to talk about my past history.[13] So I will tell you how, little by little, the incident of my becoming HIV positive. When I was one year old, my own mother died. After that for some time, for three or four years, I lived with my aunt. And then later, after my father's second marriage, I again came to live at my father's house. At that time, my father used to go out of the home frequently for work. And in the house, the family environment was not so good. I also kept company with some bad friends. That might have made things worse at home. Also, because I didn't have my real mother, I began to behave badly.

Having passed tenth grade, it was time for the school leaving certificate exam. After the SLC exam, I began to be involved in bad habits with my friends and became a drug addict. Up until that time, my family didn't know about it. I used drugs for about seven or eight years. Meanwhile, I left my own home because my stepmother was not very supportive. My father was also working away. In one sense, I was despised in my own home, and I had to leave my home and go out on the street.

---

13 Raju is a young man.

Then, I managed to pass the ICOM and passed at the certificate level. And I also took a job thinking that I would stand on my own two feet. And again, three or four years passed in this way. After that, my painful memories, so to say, went away, because I was taking drugs. I needed to earn money for drugs. I had to buy my own food. I could not even get love from my own family. At that time, I lived alone. I also didn't take very good care of my own health. I was taking intravenous drug injections. Because of this, I got HIV from another person. Perhaps while I was taking drugs, I got HIV. But I don't know for sure. At that time, I did not have my blood checked.

I got fed up with the drug life and went for medical treatment to a drug rehab center. I went for treatment but still did not get my blood checked for HIV at that time. I went to a rehabilitation center and was there for about one year. Then, I got a little sick. After six or seven months, I got a little fever. I also had bad diarrhea and had to go for a medical checkup. I also had other problems. A few glands were also swelling in a few places. Since men do not normally have problems with swollen glands, and also I had the fever and diarrhea, I went for a checkup at Patan hospital. I told the doctor my being a drug user. Then, I told him that I had just come from the rehabilitation center. He did lots of tests and checked other things too. He checked my urine and skin, thinking the swollen glands to be a symptom of tuberculosis. However, that wasn't the result of the tests. At last, he suggested that I should get tested for HIV because I was an IV drug user. At that time, I was not mentally ready for the test. I was in a dilemma. What would happen if I had HIV? I wasn't ready so I decided not to do the test at that time. But the glands continued to grow. If I had to work or got wet in the rain, I would have fever. And also I would lose my appetite. I thought about it again and decided to go and get a checkup. Now I felt that I was mentally ready for the results. I felt that this was important for my life. Why should I worry about whether I have it or not? It only increases the mental anxiety, the worry.

After preparing myself mentally, I went to the same doctor in Patan hospital. I gave my blood for an HIV test. After that, the results came back and they diagnosed me in two ways. One was the ELISA test and the other was the spot test. Both of them revealed that I was positive. Now how can I tell you how I felt at that time? HIV is incurable. There's not been any medicine discovered which will cure it even though the world is trying to discover the medicine. I became extremely depressed. At that time, I was living at the rehabilitation center, where my every move was watched carefully by people who cared for me. "Now what to do?," I thought. Evidently, I'd gotten it. Now, I became mentally depressed, and evil thoughts of evil deeds came into my mind. At first I wanted to die in that very moment, because I thought, "Now my life is finished; there's nothing left. Therefore, I should die."

But the counselors at that center who had done my medical treatment inspired me, saying, "Now brother, why don't you spend the rest of your life doing something good? Whatever may have been the past life is done. You only have your whole life ahead. If you'll keep healthy, eat well, live well, do good things, and don't take drugs again, you may live another eight to ten years. You still have a long life ahead of you. At least for the sake of your future, live in a good way and you will find goodness in life. Human life is a gift. According to our Hindu religion, human life can only be gotten by eighty-four thousand rebirths. So then, why do you want to destroy the rest of your life?" they asked.

They said, "Whatever is past is past. The wrong you've done has been done. Now, think of the coming days in a nice way and live a good life." I thought about what they said and felt that it was better to spend the remainder of my life well than to stay involved in taking drugs and remain a bad person, spoiling my own health. I thought, I'll at least do some creative work, do some good things.

Slowly, that feeling took over my mind. After that, I came to know that there was an organization called Prerana, which helps those who are HIV positive and has a counseling service. After that, I came to Prerana. After coming to Prerana, I met people here. They saw my qualifications and talents. They said, "Please, come and work here. Come at first as a volunteer. We need people like you who can promote Prerana—leading us in the right way." So whatever remains of my life, at least of the rest of my life, I can spend with those guys who are using drugs. At least I can advise them. I can tell them, "You ought not to use drugs. Even if you think you can't live without them. And if you are unable to stop using drugs, then at least clean the syringes properly, so you won't get AIDS." So I decided to spend the rest of my life on behalf of Prerana doing counseling and teaching those who don't know about AIDS, and talking to those who are at high risk, telling people how they can be saved from AIDS and spreading awareness about AIDS. I managed to get AIDS. At least the coming generation may not get it. If we teach them, they will become a bit literate and alert about AIDS, and they may teach others too. For this reason, I joined Prerana. Now, my sole aim of life is to help those who have HIV, to help as much as I can and spread awareness about it. That's all.

I've already told you about my family background. I don't live with my family, even today, because I am unwanted at home and now I have to live by myself. I am doing well. I've not relaxed into drug taking again and have been living a good life. Still, my family won't accept me. Even the society will treat me in a different way after they know I have HIV because of the structure of our society in this country. It's like that; if anyone has AIDS, then they will behave toward that person in a very bad way. Many people have the idea that AIDS only comes by way of prostitution. Even though the society thinks this way and despises people who have AIDS, I mustered up all my courage and have come before everyone to say, "Yes, I've got AIDS. This is my reality. Why should I run away from reality? Because of my work, because of my willingness to admit it, you may not get it. Or others may not get it. I want to do something great. I want to spread awareness to others."

As far as my family's non-acceptance of me, well, that's just the way it is. I can live by myself. I don't want to get married. It's not right to destroy another person's life. Such type of sinful things should not be done. Instead, I'll spend the rest of my life in some productive work in the field of HIV/AIDS. I'm keeping that kind of thinking, and I'm going forward. Perhaps God will certainly help me. Needless to say, God will help me to do good work. Having this idea, I'll go forward.

10.4 Indra

My story is that I used to use drugs.[14] Years back, drugs were cheaper. They were much cheaper, available for ten to fifteen rupees. At that time, I took drugs. We didn't know then that the drugs would become so expensive later on and that the laws would become so strict in the future. Anyway, I used drugs. I used them for almost twelve or thirteen years. After that, for one year I took TDGC (a type of drug). Whenever we would go out into public, we were caught by the police. It became difficult to go outside.

After that, we got sent to a treatment center, or the Freedom Center.[15] One day, while living at the Freedom Center, I went to the hospital for a checkup. It was there the doctor suggested that I should get tested for HIV. When I did my blood checkup, it was reported back to me that I was HIV positive. HIV appeared in me. However, I didn't believe so much in it. Therefore, I went to Teku Hospital (a government run hospital) and got checked there too. The test at Teku appeared positive too. The HIV appeared and I felt a little sorrow in my heart. I was so upset I didn't want to live. I felt it would be better for me to die taking drugs. Then, I went back to Freedom Center and sought advice from the brothers of the center.

They counseled me a lot, saying, "You shouldn't take such steps. One day even the people who do not have HIV will also die. It's not only those with HIV who die. Even people who do not have HIV will also die. So, even if you do have HIV, you do not need to worry so much. You might live five years or ten years, or even twenty years. You can do something great with your

---

[14]Indra is a young man.

[15]Freedom Center is a Catholic-sponsored drug rehabilitation center on the outskirts of Kathmandu. The center was started by an American Jesuit, Father Gafney, who was murdered in 1998. The Center continues to be run by Father Gafney's Jesuit associates.

life with the time you have left. Let's show society some great works and do good." That's the kind of suggestion they gave me.

I went to the doctor at Patan Hospital too. There, the nurse also gave me good counseling. And because of the counseling I got there, I haven't felt too much sorrow even though I do have HIV. Of course, I do feel pain, but I'm not so sorrowful that I want to die anymore. Now, I do hope to manage the rest of my life well and handle life in the proper way. The only problem is that I don't have any family to help me. Since I don't have anybody in my family, I will have a problem. Right now, I have to stay in others' homes. I even have to depend on others for bus fare. This has me a bit depressed. I don't have a mother or a father. My father died when I was very young. As to my mother's death, it's been fourteen or fifteen years. And after my mother's death, I was ensnared in drugs like this. A while back, I lived here at Freedom Center. But now, I am living in Baktapur. I've got sisters as well as a brother, and a sister-in-law. They don't take much care of me, however. My brother has to work and take care of his own wife and children. He struggles to support them and so is torn between looking after me and looking after his family. It's really difficult. Because of these facts, I wonder how I should spend my life. I haven't told my brother or my sisters that I am HIV positive. I am in this state because of my own irresponsibility and carelessness. I didn't even care that I may infect my friends. When I became extremely addicted to drugs, I would go through withdrawals, and I would grab any available syringe. It didn't matter who it belonged to. There wasn't money to buy syringes. At that time, I would stick myself with any syringe that I could get. It's because of my own carelessness. How can I say it appeared to me? It's an impossible matter. It's really hard to say. To say it is impossible. As for how it feels, it's hard to bear, or intolerable.

From now on, I won't take drugs as long as I live. I'll live in a nice way. I'm planning to live a good life. Perhaps I'll live for five or ten years. And if by chance any medicine appears by that time, it would be great. If not, what to do? The thing that I shouldn't have done, I've already done. And since that's the case, there's no advantage to be gained by worrying about it. There's no value in worrying from now on. It would only harm the health. Therefore, I don't worry so much. Of course, worry still comes. Saying this doesn't mean that it doesn't come. I think there's no more things to tell you.

10.5 Akash

HIV and hepatitis B have come to me because fifteen years ago, I was a drug addict.[16] I took drugs for pleasure. I would go with my friends, roaming here and there in the evening, enjoying the pleasure of drugs. In the early days, we didn't worry much. At that time, there were only whites (a slang

---

[16]Akash is a young man.

drug name). Because at the time we used whites, we didn't know about such things as AIDS and there was no fear of getting the disease. We continued taking drugs. After some time, we stopped using whites and began using brown sugar (another slang drug name). Once brown appeared, we used it for four to five years. We shared needles with our friends when we did brown. And up until then, we didn't have the slightest knowledge about HIV. When stronger drugs such as browns appeared, we gave up using whites and started using browns. The same way, we chose to use brown rather than inject TTGC (another type of drug).

We went on injecting. And at that time only, we came to know that there's a disease called HIV that transfers through using syringes, and sexual intercourse. However, at that time, we were addicts, and we didn't care. We figured nothing more than death could happen. We just figured that eventually we would die, whether by using drugs or HIV. We didn't care at all. And we used to share our syringes with friends. Sometimes when there was no water, we would use our spit to clean the needles, and we would use the same needles.

And now, let's talk about sex. We became more degenerate, moving from one pleasure, abusing drugs, to another pleasure, sex. We began going to prostitutes and having intercourse with them without using condoms. And we had no idea where these girls were from or what types of girls they were. At any rate, we went to the prostitutes and spent the night with them just for pleasure. And when we were fully satisfied, we would return back from there. After returning from there, a particular type of fear would enter the heart. But the fear would not last long, and again, we would need sex again just like we would need drugs again. After using drugs, we would seek sex pleasure immediately. We would go back the next day.

After some time, I stopped that and I came to Freedom Center. When I finally got fed up with using drugs, I came to stay at the Freedom Center for treatment. I came here to change my attitude toward drugs and my habit of using them. While I continued staying at Freedom Center, I learned that drugs are not our problem, but it is our habit that is our problem. At that time, I began to have physical problems. I found that I needed to go to the doctor to get a checkup. I went to the doctor and openly told him about my background, during the checkup. When I told him plainly that I had once used drugs, he suggested to me that I should have my blood tested—and I asked why.

He said, "Because you used drugs, there may be some reasons." So I agreed, and then I came back to the center. After coming back to Freedom Center, something like fear arose in me. After returning to the Freedom Center, I talked with the brothers, and they gave me a suggestion. They gave me the good suggestion that if I wanted to get better, or more healthy, I would need to have a checkup. They suggested that I should get a blood test. They told me that I needed to be mentally prepared in case I did have

HIV or some other disease. They said I needed to be mentally prepared to accept it. After staying at the center for three or four days, I was mentally prepared. When I was mentally prepared, I was ready to accept any bad consequences of the bad things I had committed, and I went to the hospital and gave my blood. After giving blood, I had bad feelings in my mind for one or two days. I stayed here trying to understand my own feelings. After four days, I was called to come and pick up the report of my blood test. I went to Patan Hospital where I had tested my blood. There I had a friend. He's a close friend who works there. He met me when I arrived there.

He said, "You know such and such thing may happen. How prepared are you regarding this matter?" I told him my feelings. "Yes, these things may happen, but I'm prepared." Then, after talking with him, I collected my report. Then I went to the doctor and he asked me whether I could listen or understand the things that he was about to tell me. Since I was prepared, I was able to listen. He said, "You know that a man who has HIV can live a long time. If one takes care of their health, they can live a long life. A person doesn't die immediately after getting HIV." He consoled me saying such things. Then he told me the reality. He told me that I was HIV positive and had hepatitis B--I didn't even feel the ground I was standing on. What he said had suddenly shaken me severely. For a moment I thought, "How can I go on living? Why should I live? If this is indeed the case, it would be better for me to die. I'd rather die using drugs."

That day, my friend helped me a lot. He brought me back here to Freedom Center. If I hadn't had my friend's help, I probably wouldn't have come back. He brought me back to Freedom Center and I talked with the other brothers here. While talking with the brothers, it was very difficult for me to accept the fact that I was HIV positive even though I thought I was fully prepared to hear the news. At first, I could not decide why I should live, or what I had to live for.

After returning here, I talked to the brothers and told them the same thing. The brothers gave me good suggestions. After listening to their counsel, I have been controlling myself, so far. The things of the past are now gone. I had done many stupid things. As a result, I am suffering today. So why not spend the rest of my life in a good way? Perhaps because I have the disease, my inner heart is being hardened, and my resolve for not using drugs has been strengthened. In one sense, I've gotten inspiration from this experience. On the other hand, I've had some hard things too. I didn't know how to tell my household that I've got it. I didn't know whether my parents would support me or not. Such fears came to me. We talk about these kinds of things in group meetings. We share the feelings too, and we try to remain positive. Then one day, the situation arose that I needed to go home. And the brothers said to me, "You can now go to your home and tell your parents about it, for it's necessary for you to do so."

After that, I went home. In the beginning, it seemed like I was afraid to tell anyone. The first day home, I tried to tell my parents, but I couldn't. The whole day passed in vain; I just couldn't tell them. In the night, a different thinking came to my mind. I realized it would be worse if I didn't tell. The next day, as soon as I got up, I talked with my parents. I sat in front of them. I told them that I had gotten such kind of disease and perhaps I wouldn't recover from it. This is the kind of conversation we had. We talked for a long time. My mother wept suddenly when she heard such things. My father also cried. My father had hoped to accomplish many things through me. The hope that my father put in me all broke into pieces. I myself also felt sorry. Even I cried. Then, I tried to comfort my household. "Anyway, now I've got it, and you ought to accept it too." Such things I told them. Then I got strong support from my home too. "Alright my son. The things you shouldn't have done, you've already done. That's finished. Now do good things. Don't be away from us as long as you live."

We talked in such ways, and I felt strong support. And I came again to Freedom Center from home. And I've been staying at the center until now. From time to time, physical problems appear. It's not that problems don't appear, but the main thing is that we should not be afraid. In the beginning I thought that I was the only one who had it. But now, I've seen outside that many others have also been living with HIV. If they can live with it, why can't I? Now I want to spend the remaining days having faith in God and being good.

Interview Questions

This disease that you've been suffering from, what do you call it, HIV or AIDS?
I don't give it any particular name. This is an unknown disease that can be shifted to anyone else.

Do you prefer to think of it as AIDS or HIV?
Now, I think I've got HIV. Because, as far as I've heard, if anyone gets AIDS, many problems begin to appear. But, because I don't have those kinds of problems yet, I'd call it HIV.

What sort of symptoms did you get when you first had HIV?
In the beginning, my glands began to swell. It first appeared in the neck, and then in the armpit. After it appeared in the armpit, I went for a checkup, and only after that did I know that it was one of the symptoms of HIV. Otherwise, I would have just thought that it was normal, that the glands just were a bit swollen. But afterwards, I knew.

What are the different ways of becoming infected with HIV?
First of all, needles, and then sex, and next wounds. If anyone has HIV in his blood, and is dripping, and another person has a wound in the hand or

another part of the body, and if the fresh blood of the person having HIV falls on the wound of the person who does not have it, it can be spread. And next, it can be shifted while donating blood.

What are available treatments for HIV?
I feel the main treatment for HIV is to care for one's own health and to do nothing else that harms one's health. For instance, if a person has HIV, they may get a disease like tuberculosis. And the patients of tuberculosis should not smoke. If anyone smokes, it may harm him worse.

What sorts of treatments did you try after the disease appeared?
Since it appeared, I haven't tried any sort of treatment yet. But the support from home and friends is needed. And if we can get good support, it will be good for us.

Who gave you advice on treatment?
Freedom Center. First of all, I got information from one of my friends. And now also, from the one friend who helped to bring me here. And also, I'm grateful for the help of Freedom Center. I'm getting nice treatment. I'm very happy to have been able to come to Freedom Center.

How does HIV work inside the body? What does it actually do?
As I have heard it, it slowly, slowly makes a person feel hollow. Then, slowly, slowly one loses their energy. Their bones begin to hurt. This and many other things.

How did you contract HIV?
I'm not quite sure about it because it also might have been because of drugs, or because of prostitutes because I have experienced both of them.

Which way do you think was more probable, through the needle or through sex?
As far as I think, it's more possible that it came from sex than from syringe because I have not shared syringes with too many people. There were only four or five people sharing in our group, and they're all okay up until now. So, I guess it's more probable that I got it from prostitutes.

How did you feel when you learned that you have HIV?
For a while I felt that I was good for nothing. Then, I reached a decision to commit suicide. Then, all of a sudden, I got help from one of my friends who brought me to Freedom Center. I thank him very much. I probably wouldn't have come here on my own, and after coming here, I've had a lot of opportunities to change my feelings. This is how things

have been going up until now. In the same way, I will try to live well in the coming days.

Did you think that only you got AIDS and not other people?
Well, in the beginning, for two to four days, I thought so. Why did it come to me and not to others? But it was purely my fault because I was the one who did the risky things. If others did the same risky things, no doubt they would catch AIDS too. Therefore, it's far better not to do such things deliberately.

But there are other people who go to the prostitutes and are IV drug users, yet they have not gotten AIDS or HIV. Why do you think that this is?
In this case, they probably used or followed safe methods. When I was taking drugs, I didn't think like that. I just wanted a quick fix. Perhaps I am now suffering from the disease because such things should be done with whole consciousness and thinking. Isn't it so? Having sexual intercourse with a prostitute is taking a high risk. Because a prostitute has sexual relationships with so many people, we cannot say that they don't have HIV or AIDS for sure. They may have it, but it may not transfer if one has adopted safe methods.

How did your friends and family respond after you told them that you were HIV positive?
Well, as far as friends are concerned, they're behaving nicely toward me while I'm staying at Freedom Center. I did tell one or two friends, and I got comfort from them. They've said things like, "Well now at last you've got it. Anyway, don't make yourself more depressed from it. Many other people may also be suffering from it. Therefore, keep these things in your mind. Don't take it so seriously." And now, I've been getting good support from my home too. In the beginning, I suspected that my household wouldn't accept me because I have the disease. I have found however, that everyone in the home supported me.

10.6 Gopal

When I was ten years old, my father died.[17] After that, no one in the house was able to control me. I began to have bad habits and behaviors. Slowly, I began to hang around the wrong kinds of friends who also were practicing the same behaviors. By the time I reached high school level, I started smoking. No one at home laid strict rules for me. There was no one in the home to stop me. My mother was busy with her work and my sisters with their work. I was home alone. I would go to school and come back home. I didn't care

---

[17]Gopal is a young man.

about rules too much. Therefore, I started smoking cigarettes. In my school days, I began hanging around the same types of friends, and I gradually started smoking hashish. After I began to smoke hashish, I was still studying in classes seven to nine, but my studies completely deteriorated. And since I was getting involved in such practices, I started getting entangled in drugs. After that, I gradually started taking Nikson. Then at last, after four years of using TBGC, I found myself ensnared in brown sugar for about two years.[18] At that time, I created a lot of problems for my family and a lot of suffering. Sometimes, I would steal money from my own home. Sometimes, I would sell my own clothing and did many other things because I had to get money from wherever I could—because of my intense addiction to drugs. In the course of my addiction to drugs, I completely screwed up my life.

When I realized that I had ruined my life, I began thinking, "Well, what should I do?" And, I learned from some friends that there was a place called Freedom Center, run by Father Gafney. [19] They said, "Go there and it will be good for you." After about a month of that, I became extremely upset and thought, "What can I do?" I realized that I must give up drugs. Unless I give them up, I can't do anything. So, I decided to give up drugs and went to the Freedom Center and stayed there. It was fun to stay at the Freedom Center. I learned new things. After about three months of living there, the glands of my neck began to appear swollen. I felt lethargic, and I couldn't be very active. After a while, I went to visit the main counselor and talked to him. I told him I had been suffering from these things and asked him what I should do—whether I should go in for a checkup, or try something else. After I talked to him, he suggested that I go for a checkup the following day.

I went to Patan Hospital the next day, in the morning, for a checkup. When I went to the hospital, my glands were still swollen, so I told them my history, that I was a drug addict. When I told them I was an injecting drug addict, they made me take many blood tests, such as a VDRL, HBC, HIV, etc. After three days, the report was returned. When the report was returned, I was not given it at once. They delayed me there; they wouldn't tell me for about a week in the Freedom Center. And finally, they told me that I was positive. At first, I was utterly hopeless, thinking that I wanted to kill myself. I thought, "What can I do now? And how am I going to live?" I felt the vanity of life and wanted to die. Then, I got some counseling. There in the Freedom Center, I was treated really well. The time passed from one week to two, and, after the second week, I wasn't in as much despair. While I was staying there, I came to know about the organization called Prerana, that it had been made for HIV positive people, so I came here.

---

[18]Nickson, TBGC, and brown sugar are the names of several popular illegal drugs.

[19]Freedom Center is a Catholic sponsored drug rehabilitation center for men that was founded by Father Gafney in 1976.

Interview Questions

What did your friends do when they discovered that you were HIV positive. Your mother, friends, and neighbors?
The neighbors don't know. I don't think it's necessary to tell them. In certain circumstances, it's necessary to tell people, but it's not necessary, nor fair to tell everyone because the environment of Nepal isn't like that. I tell where it's needed. I'll go on telling like that. Of the members of my family, only my mother knows, but my brothers and sisters do not.

To what do you attribute your illness?
I call it *"karma,"* in our Buddhist tradition. It is caused by the things which I have done before in my life, the very bad things which I have done, but I'm not sure what those things are. Not just things from this life, but the things from last life which I've done bad. Any bad things that I have done, this is the major cause. So, according to our Buddhist religion, I got this disease because of my previous life. It's all because I might have done something wrong, some sin that I don't know about. This is most likely the cause.

Why did HIV come?
Because of the injection. I used to take drugs from the syringe.

But what about your other explanation, about bad *karma*?
In my previous birth, I might have committed some acts of sins and so on. I think it is the consequence of previous life's sins that I am suffering now.

What are the symptoms of HIV?
For more than a month, I've had fever and diarrhea as well. These are the minor symptoms. Then next, the glands beside my mouth appear. If you're asking how it transmits, it transmits by injecting drugs or having sexual relationships. These two ways, taking drugs in injection and having sexual relationships with many are the main causes for the transfer of the disease. HIV is not like other diseases. It appeared suddenly. Right now, no cure, no medicine is available. It may be a kind of punishment for sin. It may be the cause of previous bad deeds. That may be why it's affecting me so badly at this time. Therefore, it's my guess that it's the consequence of the previous life's deeds that cause such an incurable disease like HIV in this life. It is my belief that I might have done something wrong, some bad works in the last life, of which the consequences I am bearing now. In my previous life, I might have done something like that, and now I'm bearing the result. Thinking this way is the only way I can bear the feelings. Actually, HIV has not infected me because of that reason, but because I injected drugs. But this is a self-satisfying answer for me. And now, when I think about how it

infected me, there is no way out. Previously, I might have done that sort of thing. Therefore, it infected me. Just for self-satisfaction I desire to believe this way.

How are people who know that you are HIV positive treating you?
Up until now, my friends have been treating me well. At least those who know me well. Perhaps they don't know that I'm positive. And my neighbors, I think they will probably hate me when they come to know that I have HIV. Thinking that I am positive and got such a disease and it's incurable and there's no medicine available, I am sure they'll hate me.

What kind of treatments have you tried?
Up until now, I haven't tried any medicine. Until now, I've simply been living with self-control. For me, it's a good thing, because a medicine has not yet been discovered. The main treatment for HIV is to make one's heart happy, strong, and have positive thinking. I've been living in this same way. The old things are in the past. The things that I did in the past are gone now. There's no point in worrying about that. Well, the main thing is to think of what's happening to me right now, and to focus on that. I have to think of what's happening right now in my life. One shouldn't worry about the future too much either, thinking, "The disease has caught me," and "What will happen to my life?," or, "I will die soon," or so on. We should not worry about the future in this way. Rather we should live happily while we are on this earth, disregarding the future. The future is not so important, but to live happily in the present life with a positive attitude is important and necessary too. If anyone does so, I think it is the only way of treatment for HIV/AIDS, because the more a person feels happy, the more he gets good things in his entire life. Even if a normal man lives being unhappy, he will get sick.

What will the virus do to you?
What will the virus do to my body? It will make my immune system weak. And when the immune system of the body becomes weak, it decreases the fighting capacity against any disease, and gradually one can be infected by another disease. And finally, I may die having another disease.

What will happen to you?
The main difficulty now is when we are feeling sick. At times like that, we feel only negative feelings. Feelings like "Now I will die," "Now I'm dying," or these kind of feelings. Nowadays, we can fear whether we will die soon, or tomorrow, or the day after tomorrow. That kind of thinking appears now and then. At times like that, we need a friend. We need to help each other, to treat each other kindly. It helps to share our feelings and problems with each other.

Do you have someone like that?
Yes. Yesterday he left for Denmark for six months. After six months, he'll come back.

So what will you do in the meantime when you are feeling depressed?
I'll come here and I'll share it.

10.7 Shoba

Previously, we lived in India.[20] By India, I mean Babai Village. Altogether there were six in our family: my two brothers, two sisters, myself, and my father. My father had lived in this village for a very long time. He went with my mother to the foreign land of India when they were very young. After they went to this foreign land, my father began to work there, and they settled down there, my father and mother and all. We were also born in India, in the village of Babai. It is said that after my birth, when I was three years old, my father died. At that time, my brothers and sisters had been studying.

After the death of my father, my mother (stepmother) alone could not support the family for there were five dependent children. After that, my brother and sister who had been studying decided they should go to work to earn money, and in this way, they gave up school. One of my sisters and my eldest brother had to support our family. When our brothers were older, they began to ask where our family originally was from. They desired to return to our family's home place. At that time, we packed up and came here to Kathmandu. In those days, we were still small. Much time has passed since then. I've become bigger and my younger sister is also grown. In fact, she is now taller than me. I enjoyed staying in the home and preparing food rather than doing other kinds of work. My sisters found some work in the garment factory, and so they went to work. And after that, I also went to work in the garment factory. And I also continued the work at home.

There was a friend of my brother-in-law, my sister's husband in Darjeeling. My brother-in-law loved him very much. They were very close friends. Unfortunately this boy was a drug user. Since my brother-in-law's friend was a drug user and since he loved him very much, he had fear that he would become worse if he continued to stay there in Darjeeling. He thought it might be better if he came here and stayed with us. He thought if he brought him here, he might become better. After he came here, he didn't take drugs anymore. In his past, he was not only a drug user but also a rough boy. By rough I mean he used to chase girls daily while he was in Darjeeling. It is rumored that one day he chased four to five different girls, and sometimes he used to sleep with them too. Actually, we didn't know

---

[20]Shoba is a young woman.

why he did these things. After he had become good, what happened is that we ended up getting married even though I was not willing.

This is how it happened: My parents didn't give their consent to a marriage. He used to always tease me. He used to always say that he was going to marry me, and he would ask for my consent. I thought that he was making fun of me. One day he grabbed me by the arm and asked, "Well, will you marry me or not?" I told him not to keep joking all the time. I said, "It's not good to always joke all the time." But when I said that, he assured me that he was very serious. And he told me that I should accept his proposal, and that if I didn't that he would kidnap me one day. And I also challenged him back, saying we would wait and see just how much courage he had. Actually, I said this joking. Certainly he thought that I was not ready to accept his offer. He had not only told me these things. He had also told my brother-in-law. He had said, "I will marry her. Certainly I will marry her whether she agrees or not." He had said that if he had failed to marry me, he would not stay here any longer.

We didn't answer yes or no. And because we didn't, he kidnapped me forcibly. I screamed very loudly and all my brothers came running at once. And they told him that he shouldn't treat me like this, but he had to consider me as his own sister, since he had been staying with me in the same neighborhood. Then he said, "I love her. If she agrees to marry me it's alright. Otherwise, I'll kill myself using this khukuri."[21] He was so obstinate. After that, his sister, my sister-in-law, came and took me off. Only after that, did we consider these things deeply. Anyway, he had kidnapped me. Now, after being kidnapped, it's difficult for a woman who's been kidnapped to live in the society, and everyone suggested to me that I must now marry him. He's a fine man. It doesn't matter, but he is a Chhetri.[22] After that, we were married. And we got married in the house of my brother-in-law.

After that, he said, "Let's go to Darjeeling. We'll live there instead. If you don't like it there, we'll come back here and continue to live here." Since he had been a drug user, I didn't know if I could believe him or not, whether he had actually given up drugs or not, whether he had just said he had or whether he really had. I thought perhaps he'll take me there and sell me for drug money. There will be no one for me to turn to there. I didn't have any relatives there. No one I recognized. I thought, "It's better that we go some other time, not now." I didn't know what would happen to me there. I thought like that.

After that, we moved in with his relatives. We didn't go to Darjeeling. We stayed here. After that, we would fight a lot. This was because I hadn't married him because I liked him. I really didn't like him at all. Even though we were husband and wife, we didn't treat each other like husband and

---

[21]traditional Nepali knife.

[22]the next caste below Brahmins.

wife. I wouldn't listen to him at all. If he tried to do anything to me, I would directly threaten him. "If you torture me or scold me, I will kill myself either by hanging or drowning myself, and you will be charged for my murder." And so he wouldn't touch me, thinking that I would really do it.

And after that time, again we went to my brother-in-law's house and lived there. They provided food for us, and we lived together with them. I told them I didn't want to go to Darjeeling because I was fearful. So we stayed in the house of my sister and brother-in-law, but my husband couldn't find any work. There was no work available, so he went to work as a laborer. He said to me, "I'll go do labor work. You don't need to do anything. Just stay home." And he went to work as a laborer. We would eat in the house of my brother-in-law. And in time, the laboring work was finished. After that, he was able to find work in a restaurant. He started working there and enjoyed it.

After a long period, I started loving him, the poor, pitiful fellow. Later on, I grew fond of him and actually liked him, after a long time of staying together. I grew to love him and found him to be a good man. Then, I considered it alright and both of us were reconciled, and our marriage was excellent. Thus, we stayed together. And then he said, "We shouldn't live like this. I'll go to my home and bring money, and we'll buy land." Saying this, he left to his home and went to request money from his family. Arriving to his home, his mother wouldn't give him anything, because she knew he was a drug user, and he had always used to lie, and they didn't believe him. He told them that he had gotten married. "Are you lying again, saying that you're married?" they asked. What type of marriage did you do? We'll accept whatever caste you married as long as it was according to your will. Show your wife to us, only then we'll give you money," they told him. So finally, they sent us money but it was only twelve to thirteen thousand rupees. There was no point in starting a business or buying a piece of land with so little money. All the money was used up in just renting a room and buying all the necessary items. We didn't even have enough to buy food. The amount of money was not sufficient. He was now unemployed.

Sometimes, my husband would have fever, and in the beginning, he suffered having continuous boils. He used to go to the hospital regularly to try to find out why these things were happening, and he kept cutting his boils. Since that time, he began to suffer from the disease. Since the boils would come, he would need to stay home, and when he had diarrhea there was no point in going to work—he needed to stay at home. Even when he had fever, he had to stay at home. There was no use talking about work, about earning money, and eating. That time was really difficult for us to bear. We really had a hard time. We didn't have enough food to eat. To find out what had happened to him, we went everywhere for checkups. But nowhere were we able to get an accurate diagnosis of the problem. Actually, you need to request the HIV test if you want it, but we didn't do that. We did other blood tests, skin tests, and did everything else. But in Nepal, you have to tell them what you want to be tested for. And we didn't know about HIV, so we hadn't gotten tested for that. And so when we left the hospital, they had made no conclusions about his sickness.

After that, we went to many other places, thinking it might be tuberculosis, but they told us it was not TB either. Then my husband decided to go to Darjeeling. He said, "I'll go to Darjeeling. There are quite good hospitals there." He went there and was checked, and it was confirmed that he had TB. So he took TB medicine for one year. He had to take it straight for nine months in a year. Within the nine months of taking the medicine, the diarrhea had also stopped. Before he went to Darjeeling, he was so haggard, and now he returned from Darjeeling feeling as healthy as he was before. And everybody commented that he had become well. And it was almost a year after our marriage. He stayed there for an entire year. After he returned from Darjeeling, he had been home only five days when his problems started up again.

At that time, I had been staying with my brother-in-law. There's no point in staying alone. Where would I get food to eat? So he came and stayed there, and it had only been five days after his return. And again, the diarrhea returned. He said, "I am taking my medicine just like I am supposed to. I don't know why this is happening to me again." Thus, ten or twelve days passed and his diarrhea returned like it had been before. He said, "I have to go there again and find out what is happening. It's not usual that the disease re-infects a person who has recently taken the whole course of medicine for TB." So he went there again. They told him since the bug had apparently been resistant, there was no sense in him taking the medicine for TB again, so he took some medicine for diarrhea. But it gave relief to him for only five minutes. It didn't stop it at all. And he came back again, being extremely haggard. After he came here, he came to my brother-in-law's. After he came to my brother-in-law's, we talked, and we agreed that we should take him to Teku hospital.

At that time, I began to have a suspicion about his illness. I had been reading one of the books from class four. While I was reading, I found there written what HIV and AIDS was. It said the diarrhea continues for more than one week, and everything else I found. And the glands also came exactly around the mouth and nose. There these things were written. So I showed the book and told him that these things were written in the book, and that I was suspicious that he was suffering from this same thing. Then, he replied, "Yes. It seems so. The things written in the book and the things that have been happening to me are the same." After reading the book, he knew the fact, and said that we had to go check and see if he was HIV positive. So we went to Teku and checked. My husband was tested at Teku; he was positive.

After returning from there, he said "I have such and such a disease, and I won't live too long. Since I won't live too long, I want to go home. You do whatever you want to do. I'm going to the village. After my death, I don't know whether anyone will take care of you or not." After that, he went, telling everyone he was going home. He didn't want to stay here at all. He was wondering whether there was medicine for this disease. Thinking that it was possible, he borrowed ten to twelve thousand rupees from home again. After he borrowed the money but determined there was no cure, he thought like this: "I'm going to die anyway, so I might as well go spend money." He went to the market and bought a rope, and he also bought beer and drank too much. He was thinking to kill himself with the rope. He also bought sari and clothes for his mother. Then he came to me and said, "I'm planning to die in the village by hanging myself. What do you want to do? If you also want to die by hanging, come with me." I got extremely mad because first of all, he married me by force, and now he got this disease. I had grown to love him and had taken great care of him. Because I worried so much about him, I also became haggard. One will automatically become worried in such a situation, won't she?

After that, he went home. He left for his own village. My brother-in-law also suspected what he would try to do, so he sent a letter ahead to the village explaining that my husband was coming and that he had planned to hang himself. If we sent a message like this, that such and such was going to happen, then they would prevent it at the other end, and he wouldn't get a chance to kill himself. Because others ultimately knew, he was not allowed to kill himself there. So he was not allowed to kill himself, and he lived a normal life. But day by day, he became more and more sick. And at last, he was confined to his own bed.

Meanwhile, I was here. He was in the village confined to his own bed, and I remained here. Then, I met a nurse. She was from Teku herself. This is how we met. When my husband had gone with his brother to Teku for the checkup, she asked him whether he had a wife or not. So when she asked about it, he said that he had. She inquired where I was living. My brother-in-law had given her the address where I lived. Because he had given her that address, she was able to easily find me on a Saturday. I talked to her, and she showed great concern and counseled me.

She told me, "It may not be only him who is infected, but if fever comes to you, you need to take medicine for the fever. If headaches, you need to take medicine for the headache." She told me, "It'll be alright." She said, "Later on they may discover medicines for this disease. It'll be okay. That will be good. However," she said, "Have you checked your blood or not? You need to do that." She said, "I'll introduce you to a doctor." So I met this doctor. The doctor counseled us, and it was quite nice. Actually, I had been very worried about these things. I figured when he had the disease, I might have it too. I was worried that I had it. I was sure that I had it too (and I was right). After meeting the doctor, I was not fully at peace, and they suggested that I get more counseling. I felt all alone. And even though I felt all alone, the doctor told us that there were other people in Prerana who were also positive. They were starting a new organization. He suggested that I should join the others who were also positive to help start up Prerana. We were invited frequently to come to their meetings about starting the organization and met many different people. We also met many people from different NGOs. At that time when we were starting to build up Prerana, I met many other women, such as myself, that were in the same situation.

After that, I began to stay with them and thought that at least I was not alone. Others were going through the same thing, and I began to forget all the difficulties. I became engaged in the work. Since everybody was busy in the process of starting Prerana, I forgot all my worries. I began to realize that it had not just infected me, but others too. Many different organizations helped us. It's a fact that there were only three of us when Prerana was started. It's now been more than three years since we started the office. However, I've come here daily as a volunteer, and the organization has been formed. Anyway, the donors are now providing. However, these days it's a little difficult. We're not really sure what's happening at Prerana. Some say we're not doing anything, but we come day by day and work. We're not sitting here empty-handed. We're also taking classes. I forget when we started taking classes, but it's been for a while now. We've been getting a total of twenty-six hundred rupees from the national center as salary for doing many things.

Interview Questions

Did you get tested?

I did. When we started Prerana it used to be in the lower part of the LALS building. We were only three in number then. And many people helped us. There were only three of us, and we founded it down there, at the LALS building. After that, I told one of the sisters there, and they agreed to test my blood. The sister was not sure if I had AIDS because she told me that some people wouldn't be infected even if their husbands were positive. "However, let's check it out and see what the result will be," she said. I don't remember the name of the clinic we went to, but we paid two hundred rupees for the test. And we were told that the positives were of two kinds, one and two. At that time when we did the checkup, we were told both one and two. We couldn't understand the things we were being told. What was this "one" and "two"? We had no idea what ones and twos were. All we knew is that when we got checked, I had it. Even though I now knew I had it, I didn't worry too much. I had already taken many classes about it. Positive is nothing. One day a man must die after he is born. People die having all sorts of diseases. Some may simply die having diarrhea. Some die getting cancer. The positive is actually nothing else. It's a kind of virus. There are many who are finding their positive blood to be changed into negative after a long time, if one controls himself or herself, mentally it can be so. That's the thing.

So for three years you've known that you have HIV?
Yes, it's been three years since I knew.

How long ago did your husband die?
It's been exactly two years since my husband died.

And you haven't had any symptoms appearing in you?
No, not yet.

10.8 Thuli

This is how I came to have it.[23] I did a checkup in the Bir Hospital when I had gone there for a small operation. And at that time, I was told that I was positive. At that time, they told me that I should go to Teku. After they told me, I didn't want to go there. I thought, better to die at home than in the hospital. Thinking this way, I came home after being discharged. They didn't even stitch my wounds. Being discharged from the hospital, I went home. They had done this small operation there, and they concluded that I was positive. They told me I should go to Teku, but I refused to go. They found that I was positive, but not my husband. Then I went home. I told them, If I die, I'll die in my own home. I don't want to die in the hospital. And I departed from there.

After that, my husband took me again to Teku for a checkup. And there we did a checkup. I was simply thinking I wanted to die because of the infection. My husband bought a big bottle and a syringe, and, pulling me along, he took me to Teku. Having brought me to Teku, they also told me I had it. After learning that, what was I supposed to do? That's all.

Interview Questions

What was the reason that Bir Hospital didn't do treatment when your test results were positive?
Well, I don't know why.

Is your husband also here? When did you get married?
Yes, he's here. We've been married for four years now.

---

[23]Thuli is a young woman.

Where did you live when you were small?
Here in Kathmandu.

What did your parents do?
My father used to drive a trolley bus. My mother left us when I was very small. She eloped with another man. I met her when I was seventeen or eighteen years old. She eloped and married in Kunta where she is living now. She has children that are all adults now. Her children are also all married.

Is your mother's life well?
Yes, it's fine.

Do you go there often to see her?
I've been there a few times. I went there a few days ago during the Naag Panchami, but I didn't go there for Dashain or Tihar.[24]

And how long has it been that you've been taking TT?
I've been taking TT for two years.

And how long have you been using drugs?
For a long time. I used smack for a long time. I started using it in my childhood, when I was about twelve or thirteen.

Did you have enough money then?
At that time, I had my brother. He was not dead. He also used to take drugs. At that time, he earned and provided for me. I learned about taking drugs from him. At that time, he had a job and we didn't care about getting diseases. We just used drugs and made it our habit. At that time drugs were cheap; we could get them for between ten to fifteen rupees. That's how I started to use drugs.

When you had your first sexual experience, who did you have that with? How did you get involved in this profession? Was it under compulsion of someone else or was it of your own volition?
There was a girl. I worked for her. She was a broker, a girl broker. I didn't know that at the time. Her name was Laxmi. I didn't know the work she did. She kept me there for washing dishes. One day, she brought a boy in a taxi who was also a broker, and I was sent in the taxi. So I went. They said, "You shouldn't work here. You should go work in this other place. They'll give you more money. Better clothes." So I was excited. When I went, it was like

---

[24]These are all Nepali festivals.

this. I was forced. At that time I was only fourteen years old. They forced me in that way.

How many people were there at that time?
There was only one.

Didn't you defend yourself?
At that time, I was all alone and I was afraid. I did scream and shout, but there was nobody there to help me. I didn't even have any clothes, so I grabbed the *kurtha*.[25] And wearing only a *kurtha,* I ran away back to the same man who had brought me there in the taxi. The broker had taken five thousand rupees from the boys. The boys were caught and taken to prison. They were taken to prison in Hanuman Dhoka (this is the location of the Nepali police station in Kathmandu). There they were detained, but the man who raped me was not caught. He had already escaped. That broker was arrested and put in jail for one or two days. I was set free; they let me go. I had a very difficult time for one or two months, and with no other choices after one or two months, I went back to the same man (the broker). I was compelled to marry him, but these days, I'm not doing that kind of thing.

So now you only do between husband and wife.
No, I'm not even doing that.

You also had a baby didn't you?
Yes, I did, but he died.

Was that son from your husband or from another man while you were doing the profession?
He's from my husband.

How old was your baby?
Two years and sixteen days.

Have you ever been to jail?
Not yet. Not this time. I was arrested when I used to take drugs. I was put in the prison for two years and sixteen days.

How long have you known that you're positive?
It's been about a year that I have known that I was positive.

Now you live with your husband don't you?
Yes.

---

[25]a type of Nepali shirt.

Is your husband also positive?
I'm not sure.

When he was tested, it was not found in him was it?
No.

So you stay with your husband even though you know that you're HIV positive through the checkup. Then, what do you do now when you have sexual intercourse with each other?
He uses condoms.

Why?
I got it anyway, but I don't want my husband to get it.

How did you get it, through syringes or by other things? Do you know?
I got it by using syringes. I used the same syringe as my husband's, and others. Whether another of these fellows had it, I didn't know. I didn't know that they had just gotten out of jail. So apparently, it was transmitted from one of them to me.

10.9 Hari

Since childhood, I have grown up under the care of my parents.[26] And then I joined the army. I studied very little, only up to second class. From there, I went to India and joined the army. After that, I came home. After coming home, I started cultivating crops and raising animals. There was nothing else except that. Then in the year 2052 (1996/97), I noticed that my stomach was swelling. I came here to Ampipal hospital. When I came here, I didn't have any money to buy medicines, so I couldn't take medicines. Consequently, the illness reoccurred again this year. That's why I'm here now. Thus far, there aren't a lot of symptoms.

Interview Questions

Then why did you have an HIV test?
I don't know. God may know. Regarding this, I haven't done any mischievous deeds. When we haven't done mischievous deeds, we don't need to worry about HIV. The doctor told me (I have it), but I don't believe it yet. I'm sure that I haven't been entangled in wrong places or done wrong things.

Then how did you get the disease?
I might have got it through eating things, or eating with someone. I really can't guess. People won't tell you if they have it. They won't tell if they have

---

[26]Hari is a young man.

it, and then we eat together. So, while sharing the same plate, if they have blood coming from somewhere, it's ultimately transmitted to me.

From your point of view, how did it come to you?
I don't know how it came to me. I really don't understand.

In your opinion, are HIV and AIDS different, or are they the same?
I don't know about it. I'm an illiterate person. I just don't know.

Do you know of any person in your village who has HIV?
It was found in a girl there. She died here at the hospital. It's said that she used to live in Bombay. She died here. After her death, there was a rumor about her. Now, we're not involved in that sort of thing, so how did it come to us?

How did you feel after getting HIV?
After the doctor told me I had HIV, he asked me how I felt. I haven't found any differences yet in being at home and being here. The only difference is that the disease of asthma has grown more severe here at the hospital. At home the disease didn't bother me, but after coming here, it's grown more severe. That's all.

Then why did you come to the hospital?
I've had a lot of diarrhea. I've had diarrhea from yesterday at four in the morning until today, and I have a knot here inside my stomach. It's very big. Because of the knot, I could not bend down. After having diarrhea for several days, I was carried here in a basket to be admitted. After being admitted, I came here to this department.

Did you first go to the shaman?
No, I don't go to shamans.

Did you used to go to shamans?
No, never went to shamans.

Do other people in the village go to shamans when they're sick?
Traditionally they do. There's an old custom of going to shamans, but I don't practice that. I tried herbal medicines, but it didn't work. When it didn't work, I was serious. When I became seriously ill, the villagers brought me here by carrying me. After twenty days or so in the hospital, the doctors checked my blood. After my consent, they tested my blood. Before testing my blood, the doctor told me that he guessed that I had HIV, and said that I would fail the test. I didn't know.

Now do you know about HIV and AIDS or not?
I don't know what it is; you should explain it to me. But I just know that I'm probably ensnared and will probably die, and I need to make other friends aware of it.

In your opinion, what will happen to you after a half year or so? What do you think will happen to you?
After a half year, I don't know what will happen. I'll meet you and show the results after one year.

In your opinion, will a person who is HIV positive live or die? What will happen to them?
I don't know what will happen. He might die. That's in the last stage.

Well, he might die. After how many years?
I don't know that.

Then, do you feel fear?
I feel no fear at all.

Why?
I don't know why it's so. I don't have any fear of illness and my death. But because of this disease, I can't sleep much right now. If you're doubtful in your heart, disease will catch you. If you aren't, it won't catch you. Illness is a thing caused by psychological attitude. The same is the case with HIV.

Are you married?
I am not only married. I've got kids too. Two kids: one son and one daughter. I've got two grandchildren on my daughter's side.

Oh, you're a grandpa?
Yes.

What about your wife?
She isn't with me now. She went with another man.

Where did she go?
She's gone to Kathmandu.

How many people live together in your family in the village?
My father, mother, brother, and his wife.

Did you tell your family that you've got HIV?
No.

Why not?
Because I am thinking to live away on my own. I'll make my food separately.
I won't let my parents and brother be at risk. Of course, I am at risk.

What about your other villagers?
I won't put them at risk either. I'll separate myself. I'll live separately and
save them too.

Therefore, you haven't told your condition to the villagers.
Not yet.

**What do you think will happen when you tell the villagers about your
condition?**
I shouldn't tell them or they will despise me. If I do tell them, they will start
to neglect me. You'll neglect me. The other fellow will neglect me. So why
should I tell? Isn't it enough to not commit mischievous deeds?

What do the villagers do to a person who is HIV positive?
I don't know. I don't know that.

In your opinion, what is HIV?
This is a fatal disease. Am I right or am I wrong?

How does this disease come to other people?
I don't know.

How does this disease transmit?
I've heard that it transmits from sexual intercourse. I don't know whether
it's right or wrong.

Have you heard of other possible ways of transmitting the disease?
No, I've not.

What will you do after you go home to the village?
I'll do the work of raising animals and cultivating crops.

And will you continue to take the medicine for TB?
Yes, I will take it.

10.10 Ramesh

I was born in Nepal.[27] Later on I went to India and worked there three years. I worked in India for three years in a leather factory doing leather work. The fact is, I used to visit brothels while I was in India. Then, I came to Nepal after being sick and the doctors told me that I had AIDS. That's all.

Interview Questions

After you go home, when you recover from tuberculosis, will the villagers continue the practice of *chichidurdur*?
No, they won't.

In your opinion, how does AIDS transfer? How did you become infected?
I don't know how I became infected. I don't know.

You now know that you have HIV virus in your blood, and the doctors have told you that you have AIDS as well. So how did the HIV virus come into your body?
How to say how it came. I don't know. I used to drink and smoke.

Do you think you got AIDS because you drank and smoked?
All I know is I used to do those sorts of things. I don't know how it comes or how it doesn't.

Do the people of your village know anything about AIDS—for instance, where it comes from?
I don't know.

Do you know how this disease spreads from one person to another?
I don't know.

Before we began this interview, you told me that in your village, people think that this disease perhaps transmits from one person to another from sharing one plate, eating together. Do you believe in such things?
I don't know what to believe and what not to. How to believe and how I shouldn't.

Do you know what sort of treatments for AIDS are available?
How could I know that? The doctors might know. But how do we know?

---

27 Ramesh is a young man.

Do you know what the disease AIDS does to your body? What do you think the disease will do to you? Will it make your body weak or do anything else?
No. I doubt that it will make me weak.

What do you think will happen to you after having the disease AIDS?
What do I think will happen to me? I don't think anything will happen.

Don't you think anything will happen in your life? What do you think will happen to you? Do you think it will do anything good or bad to you? Do you think it will kill you or save you? Do you think it will make you healthy or unhealthy? Or what else?
It'll automatically make me unhealthy.

What do you think might happen after you become unhealthy?
What do I feel might happen? I don't know.

Is AIDS the final disease? Does the disease AIDS kill people?
What do I know whether it kills or saves?

Which city did you work in India?
In Bengal, Calcutta.

Did you ever receive a blood transfusion in your life, while you were sick?
No.

Have you ever used drugs?
No. I've never practiced that sort of behavior.

Do you think that AIDS is a result, starts from a smaller disease?
Before I had malaria fever. Then I went to the malaria center and took medicines.

Do you mean that perhaps you think AIDS first started from malaria?
Yes, I do.

If you have fever or diarrhea, do you think they can change into another disease?
I don't think so.

Do you think you got AIDS because of something you did physically, or because of bad deeds of the previous life, or because of possession of witches or evil spirits?
Now how can I say how I feel? This is all because of my own weakness of blood in my body. If anyone has got weak blood, the disease starts infecting. This is a fact. It's not because of sin, or possession of witches.

Is it perhaps because your planets are spoiled that you have to bear your fate and have gotten this disease?
One must bear whatever things are written on his forehead.

Do you believe that?
What to believe and what not to. I have just heard it. But now, I have been suffering the same.

Could it be perhaps your bad luck?
That may be possible.

If you're weak, is there more possibility to get AIDS or not? If you're weak, will AIDS infect you or not?
How would I know whether I got it being weak or anything else?

Or is it perhaps because of foods or changing climates that you got this disease?
I don't know how I got it.

In your opinion, can AIDS transmit from one person to another because of eating in the same place, or sleeping together in the same bed, or while wearing the same clothes?
Well, I don't know that.

Is wasting a symptom of AIDS?
I don't know. I've not seen such a skinny person.

In your opinion, should the person with AIDS be deprived from the activities of society or be given opportunities to be involved in the activities of the society?
Some do so, while some don't.

Well, what's your personal opinion?
In my opinion, I feel better if they're kept together.

In your village, do people hate those who have AIDS?
I'm not sure what they do.

Then, do they neglect them?
I haven't been neglected yet, but I don't know about others.

Are there any other people in your village who have AIDS?
No, not that I know of.

Will other villagers look down on you if they know that you've got AIDS?
Yes, they might do that.

If they do that, how will you feel? Will you feel that they're hating you or that they're neglecting you?
At that time, I'll feel like I'm despised.

Appendix: Focus Group Interview Questionnaire

Health-related Questions

1. Create a flow-chart starting with the question "What do you do when you don't feel well?" Then ask, "How do you decide when to go to *baidhya*, when to go to the Health Post, when to go to hospital, etc.?" When interviewing someone about his or her illness, ask "*Ke bhayo*" 'What happened?' to elicit symptoms, and someone then gives the interviewee advice. Further questions to ask are, "In your village, who diagnoses most illnesses (e.g., *baidhyas, dhaami-jhaankris, jotise,* medical hall, health-post worker, self)? What kinds of symptoms do you self-diagnose? What kinds of symptoms do you go to others to diagnose? Is there an order to which of these steps are taken, and when?"

2. Distribute questionnaire. Do pile-sorting exercise. (Which illnesses are similar and why?) Expand list to include other words for illness; see "Words for Illness" handout. What kind of categories emerge? Are they symptom based, or (1) physical, (2) fate, luck, and *karma,* or (3) spiritual? (Are these categories heuristic devices or emic realities?) Focus on WHY certain piles were made. What do these piles have in common?

   [My notes suggest that illnesses may not be directly caused by hot-cold imbalance, or bad *karma,* but a person can be more susceptible if these factors are involved. When asked if witches cause sickness, one person responded, "No, but if a person's planets are *bigriyo* 'spoiled', then the witch can take advantage."][1]

Categorization of Illnesses

1. Are some illnesses hot and some cold? Pile them accordingly.
2. Are there inside illnesses and outside illnesses? Which are which and what is the difference?
3. Are there long illnesses and short illnesses? Do you know this concept? Which illnesses are long and which are short?
4. Are there physically caused illnesses? *Karma?* How do you categorize illness?
5. Are there *mailo rogs* 'dirt illnesses'? Which illnesses are *mailo?*
6. *Saruwaa rogs* 'transferable illnesses'? Which illnesses are *saruwaa?*

Causes of illness

1. Can illness be a result of *laago* 'spirits'? Which illnesses can be spiritually caused (or is it that someone is more susceptible to an illness if spiritually attacked, or if spiritually attacked more susceptible)?
2. Which kinds of spirits cause which? *Boksi* 'witches', *kul deutaa* 'clan gods or house gods', *Deutaa* 'Hindu gods', *laago* 'spirits of the dead'? Do *boksi* 'witches' or *baidhya, dhaami,* or *jhaankris* cause these?
3. Can illness be a result of bad *karma?* Which illnesses most likely?
4. Can illness be the result of *bigrieko graha* 'spoiled planets'? Which ones?
5. Can illness be the result of *kiraa* 'germs'? Which ones?
6. Can *din dasaa* 'day unluck' cause illness? Which ones?
7. What are the other ways a person can get illnesses?
8. How can you determine which is the cause of an illness?
9. What does the average villager know about these things? Who would know more?

Greater susceptibility to illness

1. Will mixing certain foods make one more susceptible to illness? Which ones? Or will it actually cause illness? Who is the agent?
2. If *kamjor* 'bodily weak', are you more susceptible to illness? What makes one *kamjor?*
3. Can fear make one more susceptible to illness? Why?
4. Can changing *haawaapaani* 'climate' make one more susceptible to illness? What kind of weather is more likely to promote illness? Which

---

[1]In this appendix, my comments, which were not present in original questionnaire, are in square brackets.

season is one more likely to contract certain illnesses? Cold, hot, or monsoon?

5. Can illness be the result of *sutra laagyo* 'sudden shock'? Which illnesses?
6. Are certain illnesses a result of *laaparwaahi* 'negligence'?
7. What should persons with certain illnesses eat or not eat?
8. Who is at highest risk for getting ill? Why?
9. Are there certain places that one would be more susceptible to illness (e.g., lower down or higher up)? Why? Does going from low to high or high to low make one more susceptible? Why?
10. Why do some people fall ill and others do not?
11. What are other factors that would make a person more susceptible to illness?

Transmission of illness

1   How are certain illnesses 'transferred' *sarnu*? Give me a few examples.
2   Can illness be spread through eating *jutho* 'left-over food, considered ritually polluted'? Which illnesses?
3   Can illness be spread through:
    a. cooking utensils? Which illnesses?
    b. sleeping in the same bed with sick person? Which illnesses?
    c. clothing? Explain this.

4   Which illnesses *sarnu* 'transfer' and from what do they *sarnu* to? (i.e., Which illnesses can change into another illness?)

Symptoms of illness

1. *Suke* 'dryness' is a symptom of which illnesses? What about *dublo* 'thinness or wasting'?
2. *Pahelo bhayo* 'becoming yellow' is a symptom of which illnesses?

Treatment

Which illnesses get treated by the *dhaami* 'traditional healer', and which by Western methods? How is this decision made?

Separation of sick people

1. Which illnesses require the practice of *chhichhi-durdur*? Why?
2. Are people with certain illnesses *ghrinaa garchha* 'despised'? Which ones? Why? Is this good or bad?

3. Are people with certain illnesses *helaa garchha* 'hated'? Which ones? Why? Is this good or bad?
4. Should people with these illnesses be kept away from community involvement? Why?

Further Questions

1. Before going to a specialist (*jhaankri* or doctor), what kinds of home remedies do you try for the following?
   cough
   cold
   fever
   diarrhea
   swollen glands
   runny nose
   headache
   shivering or shaking
   back pain
   others?

2. Is there a belief that once western medicines have been eaten, village medicines no longer work?
3. Which type of medicine has more 'power' *shakti*? Western or village?
4. Which illnesses are best treated by doctors?
5. Which by *dhaami-jhaankri*?
6. Which of the following are available around here?
   medical shop
   health post or sub-health post
   ayurvedic clinic
   others?

7. How have things changed in 25 years? How has having a hospital close by changed treatment-seeking behavior?

Words for Illness

1. What are the levels of illness and what are the characteristics of each?
2. What are all the words for illnesses and what distinguishes between them?
   rog: (*aayo, bhayo, laagyo?*)
   biraami: (*aayo, bhayo, laagyo?*)
   bimaari: (*aayo, bhayo, laagyo?*)
   dukkha: (*aayo, bhayo, laagyo?*)

bisancho
asancho
byathaa
others?
suggested: *byathaa* 'ghost and spirit caused', *mailo rog*

3. Which illnesses are long duration and which are short?

aayo	bhayo	laagyo	dukkha	other

HIV/AIDS-related Questions

General Knowledge about HIV/AIDS

1. What is HIV? Have you heard of it? What have you heard about it?
2. What is AIDS? (If answer is "I don't know," ask them what other villagers say about these things.) Is AIDS one illness or two? If they still don't know, ask who would know these answers, that is, who can diagnose AIDS: traditional healers *(dhaami-jhaankri, jaanne, baidhya)* or doctors, or both?
3. Are HIV and AIDS the same illness? How do they differ? Are they affected by the same factors (i.e., *kamjor,* hot-cold system, etc.)

Categorization of HIV/AIDS

1. Is HIV a hot or cold illness? What about AIDS?
2. Is HIV or AIDS an inside illness or outside illness?
3. Is HIV/AIDS a long illness or a short illness? Do you know this concept? What illnesses are long, what are short?
4. Does HIV or AIDS start first as a smaller illness? Which illnesses?
5. Is HIV/AIDS a physically caused illness? *Karma*? Other? How do you categorize illness?
6. Is HIV/AIDS a *mailo rog* 'dirt illness'? What other illnesses are *mailo?*
7. Is HIV/AIDS a *saruwaa rog* 'transferable illness'? What other illnesses are *saruwaa*?

Causes of HIV/AIDS

1. Can HIV be a result of spirits? What about AIDS? Which kinds? *Boksi* 'witches', *kul deutaa* 'clan gods or house gods', *deutaa* 'Hindu gods', *laago* 'spirits of the dead'? Do *boksi* 'witches' or *baidhya, dhaami,* or *jhaankris* cause these?
2. Can HIV/AIDS be a result of bad *karma*?
3. Can HIV/AIDS be the result of *bigrieko graha* 'spoiled planets'?
4. Can HIV/AIDS be the result of *kiraa* 'germs'?
5. Can *din dasaa* 'day unluck' cause AIDS?
6. What are the other ways a person can get HIV/AIDS? List first, then ask following:
   a. Touching?
   b. Sex?
   c. Blood transfusion?
   d. Sharing clothes?

7. How can you determine which of these is the cause?
8. What does the average villager know about these things? Who would know more?

Greater susceptibility to HIV/AIDS

1. Can HIV/AIDS be the result of 'mixing' *misaaunu* certain foods? Which types? Will mixing certain foods make one more susceptible to HIV/AIDS? Which foods?
2. If *kamjor* (bodily weak) are you more susceptible to HIV/AIDS? What makes one *kamjor*?
3. Can fear make one more susceptible to HIV/AIDS?

4. Can changing 'climate' *haawaapaani* make one more susceptible to HIV/AIDS? What kind of weather is more likely to promote AIDS? In which season is one more likely to contract HIV/AIDS? Cold, hot or monsoon?
5. Can HIV/AIDS be the result of *sutra laagyo* 'sudden shock'?
6. Is HIV/AIDS a result of *laaparwaahi* 'negligence'?
7. What should a PWA eat or not eat?
8. Who is at highest risk for getting HIV/AIDS? Why?
9. Are there certain places that one would be more susceptible to HIV/AIDS (i.e., lower down or higher up)? Why? Does going from low to high or high to low make one more susceptible? Why?
10. Why do some get HIV/AIDS and others not?

Transmission of HIV/AIDS

1. How is HIV/AIDS 'transferred' *sarnu?*
2. Can HIV/AIDS be spread through eating a PWA's *jutho?*
3. Can HIV/AIDS be spread through:
   a. cooking utensils?
   b. sleeping in the same bed with PWA's?
   c. clothing?
   Explain this.

4. Can any other illness *sarnu* to HIV/AIDS? Which illnesses? Can HIV/AIDS become any other illness? Which ones?

Symptoms of HIV/AIDS

1. What are the symptoms of AIDS? Is *suke* a symptom of AIDS? What about *dublo*? How do you decide if someone has AIDS?
2. Is *pahelo bhayo* 'becoming yellow' a symptom of AIDS?

Medical Treatments for HIV/AIDS

1. What kinds of treatment are available?
2. If being treated for AIDS at the hospital, would you also seek treatment from a TMP?
3. Is AIDS best treated by:
   a. home remedies or TMP?
   b. Western medicine? (Hospital)
   c. a combination of both?
   Why?

Treatment of PWA's

1. Should people with HIV/AIDS be separated from others? Why or why not? Should *chhichhi-durdur* be practiced toward PWA's?
2. Are people with HIV/AIDS *ghrinaa garchha* 'hated'? Why? Is this good or bad?
3. Are people with HIV/AIDS *helaa garchha* 'despised'? Why? Is this good or bad?
4. Should PWA's involvement in community activities be limited? Why?

Glossary of Nepali Terms

aakaash devi—sky god; one of the many gods that can affect health

antim—fatal

asancho—not well

ausadhi—medicine

baahira—outside

baantaa—vomiting

baidhya—(gen.) local doctor (spec.) Muslim traditional healer

baulaaune—crazy

bhaepachhi—after becoming

bhagaanu—chase away

bhagaaun—(3rd per. plural of *bhaagnu*) to chase away

bhitra—inside

bidhaami/biraami—sick, ill

bigriyo—spoiled

bikaas—development

bikaasi—developed

bimaari—sick, ill (alt. of bidhaami/birami)

bisancho—not well

byathaa—a great sickness (often spiritually caused)

chhichhi durdur—the cultural practice of separation of those with saruwa illnesses from the rest of society for (1) the purpose of controlling disease spread, (2) as a form of social control over bad behavior, (3) both

chintaa—to be worried, anxious, overwhelmed with cares or saddened by circumstances

chyoba—(Tamang lang.) derogatory term meaning low

dai—older brother

dev—god, spirit

devidasi—slaves of God

dhaal—shield

299

dhaami—one category of traditional healer
dharma—one's duty in life, religion
didi—older sister
dublo—skinny, wasted
dukhchha—(verb) pain
gaaun—village
gharko ausadhi—house medicine, home remedy
ghewaa—(Tamang lang.) Tamang ceremony
ghrinaa—societal hate as a form of social control
graha—planets
-haru—(suff.) plural suffix
hela—despise
jaamaa naag—wet place for snake worship
jhaankri—(gen.) traditional healer (spec.) Hindu healer
jiwan—life
jotise—astrologer
jutho—ritually polluted
jworo—fever
kaam—work
kaamne—shaking
kamjor—weakness
karma—(1) the works done in a past life that either earn merit (if good) or
     punishment (if bad) in one's present life, (2) the works done in this life
     that will either earn merit (if good) or punishment (if bad) in the next
     life
khaanaa—food
khaanu—to eat
kharaab—bad
khattam—finished; in relation to illness it also has the sense of 'fatal'
khola—river
khun—blood
kira—bugs or insects, germs
kitaanu—germs
kshayarog—tuberculosis
kustha rog—leprosy
kyekpama—(Tamang lang.) elder men (alt. *memema*)
laago—spirits
laaparwaahi—negligence
lagaaun—(3rd per. plural of *lagnu*) to wear
maanche—man, person
madesh—plains
madeshi—plain dwellers
masaan—another of the Nepali gods that can affect health

murpa—(Tamang lang.) low place
naag—the snake god
naramro—bad
paakhaa naag—dry place for worshiping snake god
paap—sin
paapsaap—various sins
pahelo bhayo—to become yellow
pahile janam—previous life
parbatiyaa—mountains, mountain dwellers
pichas—another of the Nepali gods that can affect health (evil one)
preranaa—inspiration, encouragement
raamro—good or pleasing
randi/o—(-i fem. –o masc.) a sexually promiscuous person
rog—a disease, illness
saadhaaran—simple
saano—small
sarir—body
sarnu—transmit, shift
saruwa—transmissible, infectious
thulo—big, great
turpa—(Tamang lang.) high place

References

Acharya, Bipin Kumar. 1994. Nature cure and indigenous healing practices in Nepal: A medical anthropological perspective. In Michael Allen (ed.), *The anthropology of Nepal: People, problems and processes,* 234–244. Kathmandu: Mandala Book Point.

Adams, Vincanne. 1988. Modes of production and medicine: An examination of the theory in light of Sherpa medical traditionalism. *Social Science and Medicine* 27(5):505–513.

Adams, Vincanne. 1998. *Doctors for Democracy: Health professionals in the Nepal revolution.* Cambridge Studies in Medical Anthropology 6. Cambridge: Cambridge University Press.

Adhikari, Ramesh, and Jyotsna Tamang. 2009. Premarital sexual behavior among male college students of Kathmandu, Nepal. *BMC Public Health* 9:241. Accessed January 2013. http://www.biomedcentral.com/content/pdf/1471-2458-9-241.pdf.

Albert, Edward. 1986. Illness and deviance: The response of the press to AIDS. In Douglas A. Feldman and Thomas A. Johnson (eds.), *The social dimensions of AIDS: Method and theory,* 163–178. New York: Praeger.

Allen, N. J. 1976. Approaches to illness in the Nepalese Hills. In J. B. Louden (ed.), *Social Anthropology and Medicine,* 500–552. London: Academic Press.

AmfAR (American Foundation for AIDS Research). 1999. *The AmfAR AIDS handbook: The complete guide to understanding HIV and AIDS.* New York: W.W. Norton and Co.

AmfAR. 2010. AmfAR: Making AIDS history. Accessed January 2013. http://www.amfar.org/about-hiv-and-aids/facts-and-stats/statistics--worldwide/.

AmfAR 2012. Statistics worldwide. Accessed January 2013. http://www.amfar.org/about-hiv-and-aids/facts-and-stats/statistics--worldwide/.

Anderson, Jon Gottberg, ed. 1987. *Nepal.* Sixth edition. Insight Guides Series. Singapore: ASA Productions, Ltd.

Asamoah-Odei E, Jesus M. G. Calleja, and J. Ties Boerma. 2004. HIV prevalence and trends in sub-Saharan Africa: No decline and large subregional differences. *Lancet* 364:35–40. doi:10.1016/S0140–6736(04)16587–2.

Atran, Scott. 1990. *Cognitive foundations of natural history: Towards an anthropology of science.* New York: Cambridge University Press.

Baker, Andrea J. 1986. The portrayal of AIDS in the media: An analysis of articles in the New York Times. In Douglas A. Feldman and Thomas A. Johnson (eds.), *The Social Dimensions of AIDS: Method and Theory*, 179–194. New York: Praeger.

Banerjee, Priya. 2008. A comparison of trends in HIV and AIDS prevalence rates and preventive strategies in Nepal and India. Paper presented at Public Health Without Borders APHA 136th Annual Meeting, San Diego CA, October 29, 2008.

Baral, Sumi. 1999. Succesful enabling and educational strategies for sex workers. The findings of a study sponsored by the National Center (NCASC)/University of Heidelberg STD/HIV Project and SEDA. These findings were reported at a talk program held at GTZ, Kathmandu, Nepal. January 1999.

Bartlett, Frederic C. 1932. *Remembering.* Cambridge: Cambridge University Press.

BarnabasAID. 2013. Nepali Christians marked as Hindus in census "manipulation." *Barnabus Aid*, January 08. Accessed May 2013. http://barnabasaid.org/US/Nepali-Christians-marked-as-Hindus-in-census-manipulation.html.

Bastola, Aditya. 2011. Population Mobility, and HIV & AIDS: Review of laws, policies, and treaties among Bangladesh, Nepal and India. Kathmandu, Nepal: CARE. Accessed January 2013. http://www.carenepal.org/publication/_EMPHASIS_Review_Laws_Policy.pdf (no longer available).

Beine, David K. 1996. The 1995 Amp Pipal family planning survey. Manuscript.

Beine, David K. 1999. Doctor's knowledge, attitudes and practices regarding HIV/AIDS in Nepal: A KAP study. Manuscript.

Beine, David K. 2000. Media coverage of the epidemic in Nepal. Manuscript.

Beine, David K. 2001. Saano Dumre revisited: Changing models of illness in a village of Central Nepal. *Contributions to Nepalese Studies* 28:155–185. Center for Nepal and Asian Studies.

Beine, David K. 2002. HIV/AIDS in Nepal: The making of a cultural model. *Contributions to Nepalese Studies* 29:275–310. Center for Nepal Asian Studies.

Beine, David K. 2003. *Ensnared by AIDS: Cultural contexts of HIV/AIDS in Nepal.* First edition. Kathmandu: Mandala Book Point.

Beine, David K. 2006. The cost of conflict: The impact of the Maoist insurgency upon the spread of HIV and AIDS in Nepal. Paper presented at the meeting of the Society for Applied Anthropology and the Society for Medical Anthropology, Vancouver, BC, Canada, March 30, 2006.

Beine, David K. 2011. Causes of HIV and AIDS stigmatization in Nepal: A proposed model to reduce stigma. *Global Journal of Health Science* 3(2):3–9.

Bell, Janet. 1994. Hydrodollars in the Himalaya. *Ecologist* 24:113–115.

Berlin, Brent O., and Paul D. Kay. 1969. *Basic Color Terms*. Berkeley: University of California Press.

Bernard, H. Russell. 1995. *Research Methods in Anthropology*. Walnut Creek, Calif.: Alta Mira Press.

Berridge, Virginia. 1992. AIDS History and Contemporary History. In Gilbert Herdt and Shirley Lindenbaum (eds.), *The Time of AIDS*, 41–64. Newbury Park: Sage Publications.

Bhatt, P., V. L. Gurubacharya, and G. Vadies. 1993. A unique community of family-oriented prostitutes in Nepal uninfected by HIV-1. *International Journal of STD and AIDS* 4:280–283.

Bhatta, P., S. Thapa, J. Baker, and M. Friedman. 1994. Commercial sex workers in Kathmandu Valley: Profile and prevalence of sexually transmitted diseases. *Journal of Nepal Medical Association* 32(111):191–203.

Bignall, John. 1993. Will the Badi Survive? *The Lancet* 324:983.

Bista, Dor Bahadur. 1991. *Fatalism and development: Nepal's struggle for modernization*. London: Sangam Books.

Bjerk, Sunny. 2012. Is "AIDS fatigue" real?: Media coverage of HIV and AIDS has sharply declined, December 6. *Advocate*. Housing Works. Accessed January 2013. http://www.housingworks.org/advocate/detail/is-aids-fatigue-real-media-coverage-of-hiv-aids-has-sharply-declined/.

Blaikie, Piers M., John Cameron, and David Seddon. 1979. *The struggle for basic needs in Nepal*. Development Center Studies. Paris: Development Center of the Organization for Economic Cooperatio n and Development.

Bloomberg. 2010 AIDS "fatigue" may cause lack of funds, former UNAIDS head says, December 1. Accessed January 2013. http://www.bloomberg.com/news/2010-12-01/aids-fatigue-may-cause-lack-of-funds-former-unaids-head-says.html.

Blum, Lauren, Gretel Pelto, and Pertt Pelto. 2004. Coping with a nutrient deficiency: Cultural models of vitamin A deficiency in Northern Niger. *Medical Anthropology* 23(3):195–227.

Blustain, Harvey S. 1976. Levels of medicine in a central Nepali village. *Contributions to Nepalese Studies: Journal of the Institute of Nepal and Asian Studies* 3:83–105. Tribhuvan University, Kirtipur.

The Body. 2005. New global campaign launched to promote condom use: "Three Amigos" animated PSAs use humor to stop spread of HIV. Accessed January 2013. http://www.thebody.com/content/art9165.html.

Boseley, Susan. 2011. Crisis looms as global fund forced to cut back on Aids, malaria and TB grants. *The Guardian,* November 11. http://www.guardian.co.uk/society/sarah-boseley-global-health/2011/nov/23/aids-tuberculosis.

Boseley, Sarah. 2012a. Aids conference forces Washington's epidemic into global spotlight. *The Guardian,* July 9. http://www.guardian.co.uk/society/2012/jul/09/aids-conference-washington-dc-epidemic.

Boseley, Susan. 2012b. HIV Survivors: Alive, but facing poverty, loneliness and prejudice. *The Guardian,* July 27.

Bower, Julienne E., Margaret E. Kemeny, Shelley E. Taylor, and John L. Fahey. 1998. Cognitive processing, discovery of meaning, CD4 decline, and AIDS-related mortality among bereaved HIV-seropositive men. *Journal of Consulting and Clinical Psychology* 66(6):979–86.

Boyer, Pascal. 1990. *Tradition as truth and communication: A cognitive description of traditional discourse.* New York: Cambridge University Press.

Brewer, Paula. 1995. *Harvard AIDS review: AIDS in India.* Cambridge, Mass.: Harvard AIDS Institute.

Broder, Samuel. 2010. The development of antiretroviral therapy and its impact on the HIV-1/AIDS pandemic. *Antiviral Research* 85(1):1–18.

Brown, Judith. 1993. Dry and tight: Sexual practices and potential AIDS risk in Zaire. *Social Science & Medicine* 37(8):989–994.

Brown, Tim and Peter Xenos. 1994. AIDS in Asia: The gathering storm. *Asia Pacific Issues* 16:112-127. Honolulu: East West Center Publication 16.

Browner, C.H., Bernard Ortiz de Montellano, and Arthur J. Rubel. 1988. A methodology for cross-cultural ethnomedical research. *Current Anthropology* 29(5):681–702.

Burbank, Jon. 1992. *Culture Shock: Nepal.* Portland, Ore.: Graphic Arts Center Publishing Company.

Campbell, Ben. 1997. The heavy loads of Tamang identity. In David Gellner, Joanna Pfaff-Czarnecka, and John Whelpton (eds.), *Nationalism and ethnicity in a Hindu kingdom: The politics of culture in contemporary Nepal,* 205–235. United KingdomHarwood Academic Publishers.

Caprara, Andrea. 1993. The perception of AIDS in the Bete and Baoule of the Ivory Coast. *Social Science & Medicine* 36(9):1229–1235.

Casson, Ronald W. 1983. Schemata in cognitive anthropology. *Annual Review of Anthropology* 12:429–462.

Center for Disease Control (CDC). 2012. Socioeconomic Factors Affecting HIV Risk. HIV prevention in the United States: Expanding the impact: Today's epidemic. Accessed January 2013. http://www.cdc.gov/nchhstp/newsroom/HIVFactSheets/Epidemic/Factors.htm.

Center for Disease Control (CDC). 2013. Prevention benefits of HIV treatment. Accessed January 2013. http://www.cdc.gov/hiv/topics/treatment/resources/factsheets/tap.htm.

Central Bureau of Statistics. 2012. National population and housing census. Accessed January 2013. http://cbs.gov.np/wp-content/uploads/2012/11/National%20Report.pdf.

Chakraborty, A. K., S. Jana, A. Das, L. Khodakevich, M.S. Chakraborty, and N.K. Pal. 1994. Community based survey of STD/HIV infection among commercial sexworkers in Calcutta (India) 1: Some social features of commercial sexworkers. *Journal of Communicable Disease* 26(3):161–167.

Chhetri, Damien. 1998. Letter to the editor. *Face to Face* 16:3.

Chomsky, Noam. 1957. *Syntactic Structures*. The Hague: Mouton.

Christian Medical and Dental Associations. 2011. News & Views from the Christian Medical & Dental Associations: June 23, 2011 Washington Update. Accessed June 26, 2011. www.cmda.org.

CIA. 1999. *The World Factbook*. January 1999. Accessed January 2003. http://www.cia.gov/cia/publications/factbook/np.html.

CIA. 2012. Country comparison: HIV/AIDS: Adult prevalence rate. *The World Factbook*. Accessed January 2013. https: //www.cia.gov/library/publications/the-world-factbook/rankorder/2155rank.html.

CIA. 2013. Southeast Asia: Nepal. *The World Factbook*. Accessed January 2013. https://www.cia.gov/library/publications/the-world-factbook/geos/np.html.

Cohen, Jon. 2011. Breakthrough of the year. HIV treatment as prevention. *Science* 334(6063):1628.

Cohen Myron S., Ying Q. Chen, Marybeth McCauley, Theresa Gamble, Mina C. Hosseinipour, Nagalingeswaran Kumarasamy, James G. Hakim, Johnstone Kumwenda, Beatriz Grinsztejn, Jose H. S. Pilotto, Sheela V. Godbole, Sanjay Mehendale, Suwat Chariyalertsak, Breno R. Santos, Kenneth H. Mayer, Irving F. Hoffman, Susan H. Eshleman, Estelle Piwowar-Manning, Lei Wang, Joseph Makhema, Lisa A. Mills, Guy de Bruyn, Ian Sanne, Joseph Eron, Joel Gallant, Diane Havlir, Susan Swindells, Heather Ribaudo, Vanessa Elharrar, David Burns, Taha E. Taha, Karin Nielsen-Saines, David Celentano, Max Essex, and Thomas R. Fleming. 2011. Prevention of HIV-1 infection with early antiretroviral therapy. *New England Journal of Medicine* 365:493–505.

Cohen, Myron S, Charles Holmes, Nancy Padian, Megan Wolf, Gottfried Hirnschall, Ying-Ru Lo, and Eric Goosby. 2012. HIV treatment as prevention: How scientific discovery occurred and translated rapidly into policy for the global response. Health Affairs 31(7):1439–1449.

Conklin, Harold. 1954. The relation of Hanunoo culture to the plant world. Ph.D. Dissertation. Yale University.

Cortazzi, Martin. 1993. *Narrative Analysis*. London: Falmer Press.

Cox, T., and Bal Krishna Suvedi. 1994. *Sexual networking in five urban areas in the Nepal Terai*. Kathmandu: Valley Research Group.

D'Andrade, Roy. 1984. Cultural meaning systems. In Richard Shewder and Robert Levine (eds.), *Culture theory: Essays on mind, self and emotion*, 88–118. Cambridge, England: Cambridge University Press.

D'Andrade, Roy. 1992. Cognitive Anthropology. In Theodore Schwartz, Geoffrey M. White, and Catherine A. Lutz (eds.), *New directions in psychological anthropology*, 47–59. Cambridge, England: Cambridge University Press.

D'Andrade, Roy. 1995. *The development of cognitive anthropology*. New York: Cambridge University Press.

D'Andrade, Roy, and Claudia Strauss, eds. 1992. *Human motives and cultural models*. New York: Cambridge University Press.

Dahal, Dilli Ram. 1994. Poverty or plenty: A case study of the Byansi people of Darchula District. In Michael Allen (ed.), *Anthropology of Nepal: Peoples, problems and processes*, 36–48. Kathmandu: Mandala Book Point.

Dahal, Madan Kumar. 2008. Foreign aid in Nepal: The changing context. *TelegraphNepal.com*. Abridged version of paper presented at a symposium held by Central University of Sikkim in cooperation with Nepal-India B P Koirala Foundation on April 17–18, 2008, Gangtok, India. Accessed January 2013. http://www.telegraphnepal.com/views/2007-05-14/foreign-aid-in-nepal:-the-changing-context.

Deeks, Steven G., and Andrew N. Phillips. 2009. HIV infection, antiretroviral treatment, ageing, and non-AIDS related morbidity. *British Medical Journal* 338(a3172). Accessed January 2013. http://cyto.mednet.ucla.edu/biohiv/2013/deeks%20and%20philips%20review.pdf.

Desh, Pardesh. 2010. Program summary, May 22. Accessed January 2013. https://www.comminit.com/en/node/ 308167/347

Dhalburg, John-Thor. 1994. Facing peril of Aids in Nepal. *Los Angeles Times*, July 4.

Dhungel, Basundhara. 1994. The qualitative community judgement: The role of intermediate health practitioners in Nepal's family health services. In Michael Allen (ed.), *Anthropology of Nepal: Peoples, problems and processes*, 245–255. Kathmandu: Mandala Book Point.

Dhungel, B. A., K. U. Dhungel, J. M. Easow, and Yi Singh. 2008. Opportunistic infection among HIV seropositive cases in Manipal Teaching Hospital, Pokhara, Nepal. *Kathmandu Medical Journal*, Vol. 6, 3(23):335–339.

Dieffenbach, Carl W., and Anthony S. Fauci. 2011. Thirty years of HIV and AIDS: Future challenges and opportunities. *Annals of Internal Medicine* 154(11):766–771.

Dixit, Kunda. 1998. Awareness to behavior change through media. Abstract of paper presented at the Second National Conference on AIDS, Kathmandu, Nepal, August 1–4, 1998.

Dixit, Shanta Basnet. 1996. Impact of HIV/AIDS in Nepal. In ABC Nepal (ed.), *Red light traffic: The trade in Nepali girls*, 49-65. Kathmandu: ABC Nepal.

Dougherty, Janet W. D., ed. 1985. *Directions in cognitive anthropology.* Chicago: University of Illinois Press.

Duesberg, Peter H. 1996. *Inventing the AIDS virus.* Washington, D.C.: Regnery Publishing.

Durkin, Maureen. 1984. Multiple therapeutic use in urban Nepal. *Social Science & Medicine* 19(8):867–872.

Ecologist. 1993. Himalayan "baby" scheme condemned. *Ecologist* 23(6):2.

Economist. 1993. Trekking and wrecking in Nepal. *Economist* 329(7831):35.

Economist. 1997. AIDS treatments will not be accessible to third world AIDS victims. In Daniel A. Leone (ed.), *The spread of AIDS.* At Issue Series, 23–25. San Diego, Calif.: Greenhaven Press.

EIU (The Economist Intelligence Unit). 1996. *Country Profile: Nepal.* London: E.I.U. (The Economist Intelligence Unit).

Erpelding, Anne, and KP Bista. 1997. Assessment of knowledge, attitude and behavior concerning STD/HIV in selected populations: Report of a study from Nepalganj. Kathmandu, Nepal: Ministry of Health, Department of Health Services National Center for AIDS and STD Control, and University of Heidelberg STD/HIV Project.

Fauci, Anthony. 2011. AIDS fight hits hurdle over funding. *Wall Street Journal,* May 27.

Family Health International. 2010. Ek Apas Ka Kura, May 22, 2010. Accessed January 2013. http://www.fhi.org/en/ CountryProfiles/Nepal/res_radio.htm.

Farmer, Paul. 1992. *AIDS and accusation: Haiti and the geography of blame.* Berkeley: The University of California Press.

Farmer, Paul. 1994. Aids talk and the constitution of cultural models. *Social Science & Medicine* 38(6):801–809.

Farmer, Paul. 2006. Haiti violence disrupts health care services. National Public Radio (Morning Edition), February 07. Accessed January 2013. http://www.npr.org/templates/story/story.php?storyId=5193542.

Fee, Elizabeth, and Daniel M. Fox, eds. 1992. *AIDS: The making of a chronic illness.* Los Angeles: University of California Press.

Feldman, Douglas A., and Thomas M. Johnson, eds. 1986. *The social dimensions of AIDS: Method and theory.* New York: Praeger.

Feldman, Douglas A., and Thomas M. Johnson, eds. 1990. *Culture and AIDS.* Westport, Conn.: Praeger Publishers.

Fillmore, Charles. 1977. Topics in lexical semantics. In Roger Cole (ed.), *Current Issues in Linguistic Theory,* 76–138. Bloomington: Indiana University Press.

Fiske, Alan. 1991. *Structures of social life.* New York: Free Press.

Fiske, Susan, and Shelley E. Taylor. 1984. *Social cognition.* New York: Random House.

Fleming, Alan F., Manuel Carbalo, David W. Fitzsimmons, Michael R. Bailey, and Jonathan Mann, eds. 1988. *The global impact of AIDS.* New York: Alan R. Liss, Inc.

Flynn, Tom, and Karen Lound. 1995. *AIDS: Examining the crisis.* Minneapolis: Lerner Publications Company.

Foster, George M., and Barbara Gallatin Anderson. 1978. *Medical Anthropology.* New York: John Wiley & Sons.

Fredrick, John. 1998. Deconstructing Gita. *Himal* 11(10):12–19.

Frumkin, Lyn R., and John M. Leonard. 1997. *Questions & answers on AIDS.* Third edition. Los Angeles: Health Information Press.

Fursad. 2013. HIV AIDS. Accessed in January 2013. http://fursad.com/ads/Aids/pg11.html.

Gaenszle, Martin. 1994. The shaman and the doctor: Conflicting systems of interpretation and diagnosis in east Nepal. In Dorothea Sich and Waltraud Gottschalk (eds.), *Acculturation and domination in traditional Asian medical systems,* 53–60. Beiträge zur Südasienforschung 160. Stuttgart: F. Steiner Verlag.

Gaenszle, Martin. 1997. Changing concepts of ethnic identity among the Mewahang Rai. In David N. Gellner, Joanna Pfaff-Czarnecka, and John Whelpton (eds.), *Nationalism and ethnicity in a Hindu kingdom: The politics of culture in contemporary Nepal,* 351–373. Australia: Harwood Academic Publishers.

Gagnon, John. 1992. Epidemics and researchers: AIDS and the practice of social studies. In Gilbert Herdt and Shirley Lindenbaum (eds.), *The time of AIDS,* 27–40. Newbury Park: Sage Publications.

Gao, Feng, Elizabeth Bailes, and David L. Robertson. 1999. Origin of HIV-1 in the chimpanzee Pan troglodytes. *Nature* 397(6718):436–441.

Garro, Linda. 1986. Intracultural variation in folk medical knowledge: A comparison between curers and noncurers. *American Anthropologist* 88(2):351–370.

Gemson, Donald H., John Colombotos, Jack Elinson, James Fordyce, Margaret Hynes, and Rand Stoneburner. 1991. Acquired immunodeficiency syndrome: Prevention: Knowledge, attitudes and practices of primary care physicians. *Arch Internal Medicine* 151:1102–1108.

Ghimire, Durga 1997. Sexual exploitation of Nepalese girls. Paper presented at the Regional Seminar on Girls' Rights—Societies Responsibility Taking Action Against Sexual Exploitation and Trafficking, Bombay, India, December 1997. Organized by the Center for Population and Development Activities (CEDPA), Washington D.C.

Ghimire, S. 2010. War, social separation and increasing vulnerability of HIV in Rolpa: An ethnographic study of conflcit-affected hill district of Nepal. Abstract of a paper presented at the AIDS 2010 XVIII International AIDS Conference (Abstract no. TUPE0648), July 18–23, Vienna, Austria.

Ghimire, S. 2011. Euphoria versus sufferings: Revolutionary Rolpa in post conflict context. *New Angle* 1(1):104–112.

Giblin, James C. 1995. *When plague strikes: The Black Death, smallpox, AIDS.* New York: HarperCollins Publishers.

Gladwin, Thomas. 1970. *East is a big bird.* Cambridge: Harvard University Press.

Global Fund. 2013. About the Global Fund. The Global Fund to Fight AIDS, Tuberculosis, and Malaria. Accessed January 2013. http://www.theglobalfund.org/en/about/.

Good, Byron. 1994. *Medicine, rationality, and experience: An anthropological perspective.* New York: Cambridge University Press.

Good, Byron J. 1977. The heart of what's the matter: The semantics of illness in Iran. *Culture, Medicine and Psychiatry* 1(1):25–58.

Goodenough, Ward. 1956. Componential analysis and the study of meaning. *Language* 32:195–216.

Goodenough, Ward. 1957. Cultural anthropology and linguistics. In Paul L. Garvin (ed.), *Report of the Seventh Annual Round Table Meeting on Linguistics and Language Study.* Monograph Series on Language and Linguistics 9:167–173. Washington, D.C.: Georgetown University Press.

Green, Edward. 1992. Sexually transmitted illness, ethnomedicine and health policy in Africa. *Social Science & Medicine* 35(2):121–130.

Green, Edward, Allison Herling Ruark and Norman Hearst. 2011. Where is the support for low-cost, highly effective solutions? *National Review,* June 9. Accessed January 2013. http://www.nationalreview.com/corner/269213/where-support-low-cost-highly-effective-solutions-edward-green.

Green, Edward, Melissa Farley, and Allison Herling Ruark. 2009. The wisdom of whores: Bureaucracies, brothels, and the business of AIDS: A review. *JAMA* 301(23):2502–2504.

Guido-O'Grady, Deborah, ed. 1995. Nepal. *Background Notes.* Washington D.C.: United States Department of State.

The Guardian. 2012. AIDS conference forces Washington's epidemic into global spotlight, July 9, 2012. Accessed January 2013. http://www.guardian.co.uk/society/2012/jul/09/aids-conference-washington-dc-epidemic.

Gurubacharya, V.L. 1998. Prevalence of HIV amongst commercial sex workers in Kathmandu. Paper presented at the Second National Conference on AIDS, Kathmandu, Nepal, August 1–4, 1998.

Hannum, Jill. 1997. *AIDS in Nepal: Communities confronting an emerging epidemic.* New York: AmfAR/Seven Stories Press.

Hausler, Sabine. 1993. Community forestry: A critical assessment—the case of Nepal. *The Ecologist* 23(3):84–90.

Herdt, Gilbert and Shirley Lindenbaum, eds. 1992. *The time of AIDS: Social analysis, theory, and method.* London: Sage Publications.

Herrell, Richard K. 1991. Research and the social sciences. *Current Anthropology* 32(2):201.

Herzlich, Claudine. 1989. The construction of a social phenomenon: AIDS in the French press. *Social Science & Medicine* 29(11):1235–1242.

Hirshfield, Lawrence A., and Susan Gelman. 1994. *Mapping the mind: Domain specificity in cognition and culture.* Cambridge, England: Cambridge University Press.

Hissaria, S. N., ed. 1999. Souvenir program and collection of papers of the 19th All Nepal Medical Conference of the Nepal Medical Association, Birganj, Nepal, January 6–9, 1999.

Holland, Dorothy. 1992a. How cultural systems become desire: A case study of American romance. In Roy D'Andrade and Claudia Strauss (eds), *Human motives and cultural models*, 61–89. New York: Cambridge University Press.

Holland, Dorothy. 1992b. The woman who climbed up a house: Some limitations of schema theory. In Theodore Schwartz, Geoffrey White, and Catherine A. Lutz (eds.), *New directions in psychological anthropology*, 68–79. New York: Cambridge University Press.

Holland, Dorothy and Naomi Quinn, eds. 1987. *Cultural models in language and thought.* Cambridge, England: Cambridge University Press.

Holmberg, David. 1989. *Order in paradox: Myth, ritual, and exchange among Nepal's Tamang.* Ithaca, N.Y.: Cornell University Press.

Howe, Ann C. 1996. Development of science concepts within a Vygotskian framework. *Science Education* 80(1):35–51.

Ibriz Interactive. 1999. Map of Nepal. Nepal Home Page. Accessed October 30, 1999. http://www.nepalhomepage.com/general/nepalmap.gif.

Institute of Medicine (IOM). 2013. Evaluation of PEPFAR. Washington, D.C.: National Academy of Sciences. Accessed January 2013. http://www.nap.edu/openbook.php?record_id=18256&page=723.

Iriyama, Higenmi, Shinji Nakahara, Masamine Jimba, Masao Ichikawa, and Susumu Wakai. 2007. AIDS health beliefs and intention for sexual abstinence among male adolescent students in Kathmandu, Nepal: A test of perceived severity and susceptibility. *Public Health* 121(1):64–72. Accessed January 2013. http://www.publichealthjrnl.com/article/S0033-3506(06)00278-2/abstract.

Jacobson-Widding, Anita. 1979. *Red-white-black as a mode of thought: A study of triadic classification by colours in the ritual symbolism and cognitive thought of the peoples of the lower Congo.* Uppsala: University of Stockholm.

Jha, Chandra Kant, David Plummer, and Randolph Bowers. 2011. Coping with HIV and dealing with the threat of impending death in Nepal. *Mortality: Promoting the Interdisciplinary Study of Death and Dying* 16(1):20–34. doi: 10.1080/13576275.2011.535999.

Jha, Chandra Kant, and Jean Madison. 2009. Disparity in health care: HIV, stigma, and marginalization in Nepal. *Journal of the International AIDS Society* 12:16. http://dx.doi.org/10.1186/1758-2652-12-16.

Johnson, Basil L. C. 1983. *Development in South Asia.* New York: Penguin Books.

Kant, Immanuel. 1929. *Critique of pure reason.* Translated by Norman Kemp Smith [from 1781 edition]. London: Macmillan.

Karan, Pradyumna P., and Hiroshi Ishii. 1994. *Nepal: Development and change in a landlocked Himalayan kingdom.* Tokyo: Institute for the Study of Languages and Cultures of Asia and Africa, Tokyo University of Foreign Studies.

Karkee R., and D. B. Shrestha. 2006. HIV and conflict in Nepal: relation and strategy for response. *Kathmandu University Medical Journal* 4(3):363–76.

Karki, B., T. Geurma, and Bal K. Suvedi. 1995. *Lynn.* Kathmandu, Nepal: National Center for AIDS and STD Control.

Karki, B.B. 1998. HIV/AIDS: A problem on a global and national level. Abstract of the Second National Conference on AIDS, Kathmandu, Nepal, August 1–4, 1998.

Karmic Society, K. C. Ambu, Mani Ram Thapaliya, and Bal K. Suvedi. 1998. Knowledge, attitude, and practice on HIV/AIDS and STDs among youth in Dang, Kailali and Surkhel. Abstract of paper presented at the Second National Conference on AIDS (Abstract no. 71), Kathmandu, Nepal, August 1–4, 1998.

Karuna, Onta. 1998. Media intervention and behavior change. Abstract of paper presented at the Second National Conference on AIDS (Abstract no. 77), Kathmandu, Nepal, August 1–4, 1998 .

Kathmandu Post, The. 1998a. Children, innocent victim of Africa's AIDS Epidemic. *The Kathmandu Post,* October 17.

Kathmandu Post, The. 1998b. Drug abuse on rise in Hetauda. *The Kathmandu Post,* October 27.

Keesing, Roger M. 1987. Models, "folk" and "cultural." In Dorothy Holland and Naomi Quinn (eds.), *Cultural models in language and thought,* 369–393. London: Cambridge University Press.

Keyser, Chris. 1993. Special report: A grass-roots effort against HIV in Nepal. *AIDS Policy & Law* February 19:6–7.

Kleinman, Arthur M. 1980. *Patients and healers in the context of culture.* Berkeley: University of California Press.

Kleinman, Arthur M. 1988. *The illness narratives.* New York: Basic Books.

Knight, Lindsay. 2008. UNAIDS: The first ten years, 1996–2006. Joint United Nations Programme on HIV/AIDS (UNAIDS). Accessed January 2013. http://data.unaids.org/pub/Report/2008/JC1579_First_10_years_en.pdf.

Kuipers, Benjamin 1978. Modeling spatial knowledge. *Cognitive Science* 2:129–153.

Labov, William. 1972. The transformation of experience in narrative syntax. In William Labov (ed.), *Language in the inner-city: Studies in the black vernacular,* 354–396. Philadelphia: University of Pennsylvania Press.

Lakoff, George. 1987. *Women, fire, and dangerous things: What categories tell us about the mind.* Chicago: University of Chicago Press.

Langaker, Ronald. 1987. *Foundations of cognitive grammar.* Stanford: Stanford University Press.

Lewis, Stephen. 2006. Statement: Stephen Lewis on World AIDS Day. Humanities and Social Sciences Online. December 1. Accessed January 2013. http://h-net.msu.edu/cgi-bin/logbrowse.pl?trx=vx&list=H-West-Africa&month=0612&week=a&msg=YZEfZRI/vIJEH0a4TbnbNQ&user=&pw=.

Lohani, Prakash C. 1984. Nepal's economy in retrospect and its prospects for the 1980s. In Pradip K. Ghosh (ed.), *Developing South Asia: A modernization perspective,* 179–238. International Development Resource Books. Westport, Conn: Greenwood Press.

Lyttleton, C. 1996. Messages of distinction: The AIDS media campaign in Thailand. *Medical Anthropology* 16(4):363–89.

Maharjan, Shiba H., Manisha Singh, Aaron Peak, and Nick Crofts. 1994. *A survey of KAPB in relation to risk of HIV and HIV prevalence among injecting drug users in Kathmandu, Nepal.* Kathmandu: Lifegiving and Lifesaving Society (LALS).

Mahat, Ganga, and Lucille Eller. 2009. HIV and universal precautions: Knowledge and attitudes of Nepalese nursing students. *Journal of Advanced Nursing* 65(9):1907–1915

Mandler, Jean M. 1984. *Stories, scripts, and scenes: Aspects of schema theory.* Hillsdale, N.J.: Lawrence Erlbaum Associates.

Mangla, B. 1993. Health worker says Nepal can't escape AIDS. *Lancet* 341(8846).

Mann, Jonathan M., ed. 1992. *AIDS in the World.* Cambridge, Mass: Harvard University Press.

Maskey, S. S. 1998. HIV Sentinel Surveillance Situation in Nepal. Paper presented at the Second National Conference on AIDS, Kathmandu, Nepal, August 1–4.

Matingly, Cheryl, and Linda G. Garro. 1994. Introduction. *Social Science & Medicine* 38(6):771–774.

Meadows J., J. Catalan, and B. Gazzard. 1993. "I plan to have the HIV test": Predictors of testing intention in women attending a London antenatal clinic. *AIDS Care* 5(2):141–148.

Mishler, Elliot G. 1986. The analysis of interview-narratives. In Theodore R. Sarbin (ed.), *Narrative psychology: The storied nature of human conduct,* 233–255. New York: Praeger.

Moss, Kelly. 2008. *International HIV and AIDS, tuberculosis, and malaria: Key changes to U.S. programs and funding.* CRS Report for Congress. Congressional Research Service. Accessed January 2013. http://fpc.state.gov/documents/organization/110385.pdf. Currently available at http://fpc.state.gov/documents/organization/107214.pdf.

Muir, Marie A. 1991. *The environmental context of AIDS.* New York: Praeger.

Nepal-Asia Center for Strategic Studies (NACSS). 2009. Press release, May 28, 2009. Inter-Asia Civil Society Archive. Accessed January 2013.

http://interlocal.skhu.ac.kr/home/bbs/board.php?bo_table=issue&wr_id=764&sfl=&stx=&sst=wr_hit&sod=desc&sop=and&page=18.

National Center for AIDS and STD Control (NCASC). 2012a. Fact sheet 1: HIV epidemic update of Nepal as of July 2012. Accessed January 2013. http://www.ncasc.gov.np/uploaded/facts_n_figure/FactSheet_2012/Factsheet%201_HIV_epidemic_update_Nov_25_2012.pdf

National Center for AIDS and STD Control (NCASC). 2012b. Factsheet 2: Cumulative HIV and AIDS Situation of Nepal, as of Asad 2069 (15 July 2012). Accessed January 2013. http://www.ncasc.gov.np/uploaded/facts_n_figure/FactSheet_2012/Factsheet_2_HIV_and_AIDS_Cases_Nov_25_Final.pdf.

National Public Radio (NPR). 1999. HIV and starting a family. *All Things Considered,* September 7. National Public Radio KPBX.

National Public Radio (NPR). 2011. Doctor spends career waging war on AIDS, June 3. Accessed January 2013. http://www.npr.org/2011/06/03/136930343/doctor-spends-career-waging-war-on-aids

National Public Radio (NPR). 2012. How AIDS care became the way it is. *Weekend Edition*, July 22. Accessed January 2013. http://www.npr.org/2012/07/22/157185934/how-aids-care-became-the-way-it-is.

Nepal, Binod. 2007. Population mobility and spread of HIV across the Indo-Nepal border. *Journal of Health, Population and Nutrition* 25(3):267–277.

Nepal, Vishnu P. and Michael W. Ross. 2010. Issues related to HIV stigma in Nepal. *International Journal of Sexual Health Volume* 22:20–31.

Newton, David E. 1992. *AIDS Issues: A handbook.* Hillside, N.J.: Enslow Publishers, Inc.

Nicholson-Lord, David. 1994. Hitting—and obliterating—the trail. *World Press Review* 41(1):48.

Nichter, Mark. 1989. Anthropology and international health: South Asian case studies. *Culture, Illness and Healing* 15. Boston Mass.: Kluwer Academic Publishers.

Nichter, Mark. 1994. Anthropological approaches to the study of ethnomedicine. Yverdon, Switzerland: Gordon and Breach Science Publishers.

Nigam, Nikhil. 1994. India: Trafficking in Nepalese women widespread. WIN (Women's International Network) News 20(4):40.

Ozgood, Charles E. 1952. The nature and measurement of meaning. *Psychological Bulletin* 49:197–232.

PACN. 2011. Peoples awarness campaign Nepal: Education. Accessed January 2013. http://pacnepal.org.np/programs/education/.

Pandy, Shanta. 1992. Community development programs in Nepal: A test of diffusion of innovation theory. *Social Science Review* 66(4):582–97.

Parish, Steven. 1991. The sacred mind: Newar cultural representations of mental life and the production of moral consciousness. *Ethos* 19(3):313–351.

Paudel, B. N., A. Khanal, P. Paudel, S. Sharma, and G.B. Singh. 2008a. A study of gastrointestinal manifestations in HIV and AIDS patients. Accessed January 2013. *Post Graduate Medical Journal of Nepal Academy of Medical Sciences* 8(1). http://www.pmjn.org.np/index.php/pmjn/article/viewFile/38/34.

Paudel, B. N., A. Khanal, P. Paudel, S. Sharma, and G. B. Singh. 2008b. retrospective study of HIV infection among migrants and house wives in ART center Dhangadi of far western Nepal. Accessed January 2013. *Post Graduate Medical Journal of Nepal Academy of Medical Sciences* 8(1). http://www.pmjn.org.np/index.php/pmjn/article/viewFile/32/28.

Paudel, B. N., S. Sharma, G. B. Singh, G. B. Dhungana, and P. Paudel. 2008c. Socio-demographic profile of HIV patients at Seti Zonal Hospital. *Journal of the Nepal Health Research Council* 6(2):107–110

Pelto, Pertti, and Gretel H. Pelto. 1996. Research designs in medical anthropology. In Carolyn F. Sargent and Thomas M. Johnson (eds.), *Medical anthropology: Contemporary theory and method*, 293–324. Revised edition. Westport, Connecticut: Praeger.

Pfaff-Czarnecka, Joana. 1997. Vestiges and visions: Cultural change in the process of nation-building in Nepal. In David N. Gellner, Joanna Pfaff-Czarnecka, and John Whelpton (eds.), *Nationalism and ethnicity in a Hindu kingdom: The politics of culture in contemporary Nepal*, 419–470. United Kingdom: Harwood Academic Publishers.

Piaget, Jean. 1932. *The moral judgement of the child*. Translated by Marjorie Gabain. New York: Free Press.

Piaget, Jean and Barbel Inhelder. 1969. *The psychology of the child*. London: Routledge & K. Paul.

Pigg, Stacy Leigh. 1992. Inventing social categories through place: Social representations and development in Nepal. *Comparative Studies in Society and History* 34(3):491–513.

Pigg, Stacy Leigh. 1993. Unintended consequences: The ideological impact of development in Nepal. *South Asia Bulletin* 13(172):45–66.

Pigg, Stacy Leigh. 1995a. The social symbolism of healing in Nepal. *Ethnology* 34(1):17–36.

Pigg, Stacy Leigh. 1995b. Acronyms and effacement: Traditional medical practitioners in international health development. *Social Science & Medicine* 41(1):47–68.

Pigg, Stacy Leigh. 1996. The credible and the credulous: The question of villagers' beliefs in Nepal. *Cultural Anthropology* 11(2):160–201.

Pigg, Stacy Leigh. 1999. Beyond behavior change: A review of *AIDS in Nepal* by Jill Hannum. *Himal* 11(10):57–61.

Pike, Kenneth. 1956. Towards a theory of the structure of human behavior. In Universidad Nacional Autónoma de México (ed.), *Estudios antropológicos en homenaje al Doctor Manuel Gamio* [Anthropological studies in honor of Dr. Manuel Gamio], 659-671. Mexico City: Universidad Nacional Autonoma de Mexico.

Pokhrel, Pallav, Shekhar Regmi, and Erica Piedade. 2008. HIV and AIDS prevention in the Nepalese context. *Evaluations & The Health Professions* 31(2):198–210.

Pollack, Andrew, and Donald McNeil. 2013a. In medical first, a baby with H.I.V. is deemed cured. *The New York Times,* March 3. Accessed January 2013. http://www.nytimes.com/2013/03/04/health/for-first-time-baby-cured-of-hiv-doctors-say.html?pagewanted=all&_r=0.

Pollack, Andrew, and Donald McNeil. 2013b. French study indicates some patients can control H.I.V. after stopping treatment. *The New York Times,* March 15. Accessed January 2013. http://www.nytimes.com/2013/03/16/world/europe/french-study-indicates-some-patients-can-control-hiv-after-stopping-treatment.html.

Poudel, Meena. 1994. Poverty, prostitution and women. *World Health* 47(6):10–11.

Poudel, Krishna, Masamine Jimba, Anand Joshi, et al. 2005. Retention and effectiveness of HIV and AIDS training of traditional healers in far western Nepal. *Tropical Medicine and International Health* 10(7):640–646.

Poudel, Pratima, and Jenny Carryer. 2000. Girl-trafficking, HIV and AIDS, and the position of women in Nepal. *Gender and Development* 8(2):74–79.

Price, Laurie. 1987. Ecuadorian illness stories: Cultural knowledge in natural discourse. In Dorothy Holland and Naomi Quinn (eds.), *Cultural models in language and thought,* 313–342. London: Cambridge University Press.

Puri Mahesh. 1998. Sexual risk behavior and risk perceptions of STDs/AIDS among non-resident men in Nepal. Paper presented at the Second National Conference on AIDS, Kathmandu, Nepal, August 1–4, 1998.

Puri Mahesh, and J. Cleland. 2006. Sexual behaviour and perceived risk of HIV/AIDS among young migrant factory workers in Nepal. *Journal of Adolescent Health* 38:237–246. Accessed January 2013. http://www.ncbi.nlm.nih.gov/pubmed/16488821.

Quinn, Naomi. 1987. Convergent evidence for a cultural model of American marriage. In Dorothy Holland and Naomi Quinn (eds.), *Cultural models in language and thought,* 173–194. London: Cambridge University Press.

Ramesh, A. 1993. He deceived me: The responsibility of life (Women's Songs). Audiocassette. Advisory Group on Nepali Women/ United Mission to Nepal.

Regmi, Pramod R., Simkhada P. Padam, and Edwin van Teijlingen. 2010. "Boys remain prestigious, girls become prostitutes": Socio-cultural context of relationships and sex among young people in Nepal. *Global Journal of Health Science* 2(1):60–72. Accessed January 2013. http://www.google.com/url?sa=t&rct=j&q=&esrc=s&source=we

b&cd=2&ved=0CDQQFjAB&url=http%3A%2F%2Fwww.ccsenet.
org%2Fjournal%2Findex.php%2Fgjhs%2Farticle%2Fdownload%2F395
1%2F4542&ei=n8qHUuisM4KOyAHi94DIBQ&usg=AFQjCNGHBYWx1
4U2tw9FogUCGRARYP9mNw&sig2=mKI8SUtYw4j5t3OihRa8mQ&bv
m=bv.56643336,d.aWc.

Riessman, Cathrine Kohler. 1993. *Narrative analysis.* Newbury Park: Sage
    Publications.

Rodrigo, Chaturaka and Senaka Rajapakse. 2010. HIV, poverty and women.
    International Health Volume 2(1):9–16.

Roy, J.K. 1998. KAB: Crisis among people under the poverty line. Paper
    presented at the Second National Conference on AIDS, Kathmandu,
    Nepal, August 1–4, 1998.

Rumelhart, D. 1980. Schemata: The building blocks of cognition. In Rand
    J. Spiro, Bertram C. Bruce, and William F. Brewer (eds.), *Theoretical
    issues in reading comprehension: Perspectives from cognitive psychology,
    linguistics, artificial intelligence and education.* Psychology of Reading
    and Reading Instruction Series, 33–58. Hillsdale, N.J.: Lawrence
    Erlbaum Associates.

Sabatier, Renée. 1988. *Blaming others: Prejudice, race and worldwide AIDS.*
    London: The Panos Institute.

Sabatier, Renée. 1989. *AIDS and the Third World.* Washington: Panos Institute.

Salter, Jim. 2013. Timothy Ray Brown, "Berlin patient," and his doctor are
    convinced HIV cure is real. Huffpost, September 12, 2012. Accessed
    January 2013. http://www.huffingtonpost.com/2012/09/13/timothy-
    ray-brown-hiv-cure-berlin-patient_n_1881004.html.

Sarkar, Kamalesh, Baishali Bal, Rita Mukherjee, Sekhar Chakraborty, Suman
    Saha, Arundhuti Ghosh, and Scott Parsons. 2008. Sex-trafficking,
    violence, negotiating skill, and HIV infection in brothel-based sex
    workers of eastern India, adjoining Nepal, Bhutan, and Bangladesh.
    Journal of Health Population Nutrition 26(2):223–231.

Sarkar, Sudeshna. 2010. Housewives now AIDS' worst victims in Nepal.
    Thaindian News, December 1, 2010. Accessed January 2013. http://
    www.thaindian.com/newsportal/health1/housewives-now-aids-worst-
    victims-in-nepal_100467858.html.

Sattar, Naila. 1996. The poverty virus coming soon to a family near you.
    Himal Southasian 9(3):34–37.

Sattaur, Omar. 1993. *Child labour in Nepal.* Child Labor Series 13.
    Kathmandu, Nepal: Anti-slavery International.

Savada, Andrea Matles, ed. 1991. *Nepal and Bhutan: Country studies.*
    Washington D.C.: Department of the Army.

Schloss, Aran. 1983. *The politics of development: Transportation policy in Nepal.*
    Monograph Series 22: Center for South and Southeast Asia Studies, University
    of California, Berkeley. Lanham, Md.: University Press of America.

Schoepf, Brooke Gunderfest. 1990. *Understanding AIDS in Africa: Political economy and culture in Zaire.* Cambridge, Mass: MIT.

Schoepf, Brooke Gunderfest. 1992 . Women at risk: Case studies from Zaire. In Gilbert Herdt and Shirley Lindenbaum (eds.), *The time of AIDS,* 259–285. Newbury Park: Sage Publications.

Schwartz, Theodore, Geoffrey M. White, and Catherine A. Lutz, eds. 1992. *New directions in psychological anthropology.* New York: Cambridge University Press.

Sebus, J. H. and A. K. Oderwald. 1991. Metaphors and medicine. *Curare* 14:119–126.

Seddon, David. 1995. AIDS in Nepal: Issues for consideration. *Himalayan Research Bulletin* 15(2):2–11. Accessed January 2013. http://digitalcommons.macalester.edu/cgi/viewcontent.cgi?article=1486&context=himalaya.

Shah, Igbal. 1991. Knowledge and perceptions about AIDS among married women in Bangkok. *Social Science & Medicine* 33(11):1287–1293.

Shannon, Gary W. Gearald F. Pyle, and Rashid Bashshur. 1991. *The geography of AIDS: Origins and course of an epidemic.* New York: The Guilford Press.

Sharma, Bhuwan. 2010. Nepal: Multiple problems mar fight against HIV and AIDS. *The Global Realm.* June 21, 2010. Accessed January 2013. http://theglobalrealm.com/2010/06/21/nepal-multiple-problems-mar-fight-against-hivaids/.

Sharma, Muna. 2008. Impact of educational intervention on knowledge regarding HIV and AIDS among adults. *Journal of Nepal Health Research Council* 6(13):102–106.

Shore, Bradd. 1996. *Culture in mind: Cognition, culture and the past of meaning.* New York: Oxford.

Shrestha, I.L. 1998. Seroprevalence of HIV among injecting drug users in Nepal. Paper presented at the Second National Conference on AIDS, Kathmandu, Nepal, August 1–4, 1998.

Shrestha, J., and V. L. Gurubacharya. 1998. Prevalence and control of STD/HIV among commercial sex workers (CSW). Paper presented at the Second National Conference on AIDS, Kathmandu, Nepal, August 1–4, 1998.

Shrestha, Nanda R. 1993. Enchanted by the mantra of Bikas: A self-reflective perspective on Nepalese elite and development. *South Asia Bulletin* 13(1–2):5–22.

Shrestha, Nirakar M. 1992. Alcohol and drug abuse in Nepal. *British Journal of Addiction* 87(9):1241–1248.

Sidibé, Michel. 2009. Message on the occasion of World AIDS Day: "Universal Access and Human Rights," December 1. Accessed January 2013. http://www.unaids.org/en/media/unaids/contentassets/dataimport/pub/speechexd/2009/20091201_exd_wad_message_en.pdf.

Sill, Mike. 1991. On the development trail. *Geographical* 63(9):4–7.

Silverman, Jay, Michele R. Decker, Jhumka Gupta, Ayonija Maheshwari, Brian M. Willis, and Anita Raj. 2007. HIV prevalence and predictors of infection in sex-trafficked Nepalese girls and women. *JAMA* 298(5).

Silwal, Pradeep. 1998. Big dilemma for Nepal as AIDS cases increase. *The Kathmandu Post,* 8 May.

Singer, Merrill. 1999. Anthropology and the politics of AIDS fatigue. *Anthropology Newsletter* 40(3):58.

Singh, Sonal, Eward Mills, Steven Honeyman, Bal Krishna Suvedi, and Nur Prasad Pant. 2005. HIV in Nepal: Is the violent conflict fuelling the epidemic? *PLoS Medicine* 2(8):e216. Accessed January 2013. doi:10.1371/journal.pmed.0020216.

Singh, Shilendra Kumar, N. Manandhar, M. Prasia, S. Patoary, and G. Krishna. 2005. An awareness study of HIV and AIDS among adolescent students of Chitwan District, Nepal. *Journal of the Institute of Medicine* 27(3):17–20.

Singh, Kedar Man. 1993. Counting the cost. *Far Eastern Economic Review* 156(38):95.

Smith, J.H., and A. Whiteside. 2010. The history of AIDS exceptionalism. *Journal of the International AIDS Society* 13:47 doi: 10.1186/1758-2652-13-47.

Smith, Sally L. 1996. A participatory action research study of health education, knowledge, attitudes and practices regarding sexual information in Nepal. M.A. Thesis. Leeds Metropolitan University, UK.

Sontag, Susan. 1988. *AIDS and its metaphors.* Toronto: Collins Publishers.

Spaeth, Anthony. 1996. A silent scourge. *Time Magazine* (International Edition), July 29.

Spradley, James, ed. 1972. *Culture and cognition: Rules, maps, and plans.* San Francisco: Chandler Publishing Co.

Steiner, Claude. 1974. *Scripts people live: Transactional analsysis of life scripts.* New York: Bantam Books.

Stone, Linda. 1976. Concepts of illness and curing in a Central Nepal village. *Contributions to Nepalese Studies* 3:55–80.

Stone, Linda. 1983. Hierarchy and food in Nepalese healing rituals. *Social Science & Medicine* 20(11): 1151–1159.

Stone, Linda. 1986. Primary health care for whom?: Village perspectives from Nepal. *Social Science & Medicine* 22(3):293–302.

Stone, Linda. 1988. *Illness beliefs and feeding the dead in Hindu Nepal: An ethnographic analysis.* Lewiston, New York: The Edwin Mellen Press.

Stone, Linda. 1992. Cultural influences in community participation in health. *Social Science & Medicine.* 35(4):409–417.

Stone, Linda. 1997. *Kinship and gender: An introduction.* Boulder, Colo.: Westview Press.

Stone, Linda, and Gabriel Campbell. 1984. The use and misuse of surveys in international development: An experiment from Nepal. *Human Organization* 43(1):27–37.

Strauss, Claudia. 1992. Introduction. In Roy D'Andrade and Claudia Strauss (eds.), *Human motives and cultural models*, 1–22. London: Cambridge University Press.

Streefland, Peter 1985. The frontier of modern western medicine in Nepal. *Social Science & Medicine* 20(11):1151–1159.

Suvedi, Bal K. 1998. Presentation of AIDS in Nepal. *Journal of the Institute of Medicine* 20(1):53–57.

Suvedi, Bal K. 1999. AIDS and STD prevention models used in Nepal. In S.N. Hissaria (ed.), *Souvenir program and collection of papers presented at the 19th All Nepal Medical Conference of the Nepal Medical Association*, Birganj, Nepal, January 6–9, 1999, 27–36. Kathmandu: Nepal Medical Association.

Suvedi, Bal K., Jean Baker, and Shyam Thapa. 1994. HIV/AIDS in Nepal: An update. *Journal of the Nepal Medical Association* (JNMA) 32:204–213.

Tannen, Deborah. 1993. *Framing in discourse*. New York: Oxford University Press.

Taylor, Christopher. 1990. Condoms and cosmology: The fractal person and sexual risk in Rwanda. *Social Science & Medicine* 31(9):1023–1028.

The Register-Guard. 1997. AIDS fatalities declining. *The Register-Guard*, July 15, 1997.

Time. 1998. Good news on AIDS. *Time*, November 9.

Tones, Keith. 1994. *Health education: Effectiveness, efficiency and equity*. Second edition. London: Chapman and Hall.

Treichler, Paul A. 1992. AIDS, HIV, and the cultural construction of reality. In Gilbert Herdt and Shirley Lindenbaum (eds.), *The time of AIDS*, 65–98. Newbury Park: Sage Publications.

Tyler, Stephen A. 1969. *Cognitive anthropology*. New York: Holt, Reinhart and Winston, Inc.

UN (United Nations). 1993. *Policy analysis through macro-models: Issues, techniques and applications in selected developing Asian countries*. Development Papers 14,14. Bangkok, Thailand: United Nations Economic and Social Commission for Asia and the Pacific.

UNAIDS. 1999. Fact sheet: The global AIDS epidemic. Accessed January 2003. http://www.unaids.org/documents/20101123_FS_Global_em_en.pdf.

UNAIDS. 2010. UNAIDS report on the global epidemic. *Global Report*. Accessed January 2013. http://www.unaids.org/globalreport/Global_report.htm.

UNAIDS. 2010. Methodology: Understanding the latest estimates. *Global Report*. Accessed January, 2013. http://www.unaids.org/documents/20101115_GR2010_methodology.pdf.

UNAIDS. 2011. UNAIDS World AIDS Day report. Accessed January 2013. http://www.unaids.org/en/media/unaids/contentassets/documents/unaidspublication/2011/jc2216_worldaidsday_report_2011_en.pdf.

UNAIDS. 2012. Global factsheet: World AIDS Day 2012. Accessed January 2013. http://www.unaids.org/en/media/unaids/contentassets/documents/epidemiology/2012/gr2012/20121120_FactSheet_Global_en.pdf.

UNAIDS and WHO. 2009. AIDS epidemic update. Accessed January, 2013. http://data.unaids.org/pub/report/2009/jc1700_epi_update_2009_en.pdf.

UNDP. 2013. National human development report for Nepal. Accessed January 2013. http://hdrstats.undp.org/en/countries/profiles/NPL.html

UNICEF. 1992. *Children and women of Nepal: A situation analysis.* Kathmandu: National Planning Commision, HMG: UNICEF.

UNICEF. 2008. Children and HIV and AIDS. Accessed January 2012. http://www.unicef.org/aids/index_epidemic.html.

Uppal, Jogindar. 1977. *Economic development in South Asia.* New York: St. Martin's Press.

Uprety, Aruna. 2012. Voices: World AIDS Day: The price of ignorance. The *Kathmandu Post,* November 30.

USAID. 2004. *Assessment of youth reproductive health/HIV programs in Nepal.* Kathmandu, Nepal: USAID.

USAID. 2008. HIV/AIDS health profile. USAID: Nepal. Accessed August 25, 2008. http://www.apachanet.org/facts/nepal_profile.pdf.

USAID. 2012. HIV and AIDS. Accessed January 2012. http://www.usaid.gov/what-we-do/global-health/hiv-and-aids.

USAID. 2013a. HIV/AIDS. Accessed January 2013. http://www.usaid.gov/nepal/hivaids.USAID. 2013b. USAID forward. Accessed January 2013. http://www.usaid.gov/usaidforward.

Van Gelder, Paul. 1996. Talkability, sexual behavior, and AIDS: Interviewing male Moroccan immigrants. *Human Organization* 55(2):133–140.

Viney, Linda L. 1988. Which data collection methods are appropriate for a constructivist psychology? *International Journal of Personal Construct Psychology* 1:191–203.

Viney, Linda L., and Lynne Bousfield. 1991. Narrative analysis: A method of psychosocial research for AIDS-affected people. *Social Science & Medicine* 32(7):757–765.

Vygotsky, Lev. 1962. *Thought and language.* New York: Wiley.

Wasti, Sharada. P., Padam Simkhada, Julian Randall, and Edwin VanTeijlingen. 2009. Issues and challenges of HIV and AIDS prevention and treatment programme in Nepal. *Global Journal of Health Science* 1(2):62–72.

Watters, David. 1975. Siberian shamanistic traditions among the Kham Magar of Nepal. *Contributions to Nepalese Studies* 2(1):123–168.

Watters, David. 2011. *At the foot of the snows.* Poulsbo, Wash.: Engage Faith Press.

Watters, Daniel P., and Narendra B. Rajbhandary. 2000. *Nepali in context: A topical approach to learning Nepali.* Kathmandu: Ekta Books.

Weller, Susan C. and A. Kimball Romney. 1988. *Structured interviewing.* Newbury Park, Calif.: Sage.

WHO (World Health Organization). 2000. European Commission, WHO and UNAIDS take a united stand against killer diseases. *Press Release,* September 28, 2000. WHO/61. Accessed May 2013. Available now at http://europa.eu/rapid/press-release_IP-00-1072_en.htm?locale=FR.

WHO (World Health Organization). 2008. HIV/AIDS (HIV). Accessed May 2013. http://www.nep.searo.who.int/en/section4/section28.htm. No longer available at this URL.

WHO (World Health Organization). 2010. 2010/2011 Tuberculosis global facts. World Health Organization. Accessed May 2013. http://www.who.int/tb/publications/2010/factsheet_tb_2010.pdf.

WHO (World Health Organization). 2010. World malaria report. World Health Organization. Accessed May 2013. http://www.who.int/malaria/world_malaria_report_2010/malaria2010_summary_keypoints_en.pdf.

Wikipedia. 2012. AIDS fatigue. *Wikipedia.* Wikimedia Foundation. Accessed May 2013. http://en.wikipedia.org/wiki/AIDS_fatigue .

World Bank. 2008. HIV/AIDS in Nepal. The World Bank. Accessed January 2013. http://siteresources.worldbank.org/INTSAREGTOPHIVAIDS/Resources/496350-1217345766462/HIV-AIDS-brief-Aug08-NP.pdf.

World Food Program. 2012. Breaking the cycle of HIV, hunger and poverty. World Food Program. Accessed May 2013. http://www.wfp.org/stories/breaking-cycle-hiv-hunger-and-poverty.

Worobey, M., M. Gemmel, D. E. Teuwen, T. Haselkorn, K. Kunstman, M. Bunce, J. J. Muyembe, J. M. Kabongo, R. M. Kalengayi, E. Van Marck, M. T. Gilbert, and S. M. Wolinsky. 2008. Direct evidence of extensive diversity of HIV-1 in Kinshasha by 1960. Nature, 455(7213). doi:10.1038/nature07390.

Young, James. 1981. *Medical choice in a Mexican village.* New Brunswick, N.J.: Rutgers University Press.

Zhongwei Jia, Ruan Yuhua, Qianqian Li, Peiyan Xie, Ping Li, Xia Wang, Ray Y Chen, and Yiming Shao. 2012. Antiretroviral therapy to prevent HIV transmission in serodiscordant couples in China (2003–11): A national observational cohort study. *Lancet,* Dec 1. doi:10.1016/S0140-6736(12)61898-4.

Zurick, David N. 1993.The road to Shangri La is paved: Spatial development and rural transformation in Nepal. *South Asia Bulletin* 13(1–2):35–43.

Zvosec, Deborah L. 1996. Perceptions and experiences of tuberculosis in rural eastern Nepal: A biobehavioral perspective. Ph.D. dissertation. University of Hawaii.

Subject and Author Index

SIL International Publications
Additional Releases in the
Publications in Ethnology Series

41. **The Norsk Høstfest: A celebration of ethnic food and ethnic identity,** by Paul Thomas Emch, 2011, 121 pp., ISBN 978-1-55671-265-4.
40. **Our company increases apace: History, language, and social identity in early colonial Andover, Massachucetts,** by Elinor Abbot, 2007, 279 pp., ISBN 978-1-55671-169-5.
39. **What place for hunters-gatherers in millenium three?** by Thomas N. Headland and Doris E. Blood, eds. 2002, 130 pp., ISBN 978-1-55671-132-9.
38. **A tale of Pudicho's people,** by Richard Montag. 2002, 181 pp., ISBN 978-1-55671-131-2.
37. **African friends and money matters,** by David E. Maranz, 2001, 237 pp., ISBN 1-55671-117-4.
36. **The value of the person in the Guahibo culture,** by Marcelino Sosa, translated by Walter del Aguila, 1999, 158 pp., ISBN 978-1-55671-085-8.
35. **People of the drum of God—Come!,** by Paul Neeley, 1999, 310 pp., ISBN 978-1-55671-013-1.
34. **Cashibo folklore and culture: Prose, poetry, and historical background,** by Lila Wistrand-Robinson, 1998, 196 pp., ISBN 978-1-55671-048-3.

SIL International Publications
7500 W. Camp Wisdom Road
Dallas, TX 75236-5629 USA

Voice: + 1-972-708-7404
Fax: + 1-972-708-7363
publications_intl@sil.org
www.ethnologue.com/bookstore.asp

www.ingramcontent.com/pod-product-compliance
Lightning Source LLC
Chambersburg PA
CBHW072047020426
42334CB00017B/1420